Fundamentals of
Traditional Chinese Medicine

World Century Compendium to TCM

Volume 1   Fundamentals of Traditional Chinese Medicine
by Hong-zhou Wu, Zhao-qin Fang and Pan-ji Cheng
(translated by Ye-bo He)
(Shanghai University of Traditional Chinese Medicine, China)
ISBN: 978-1-938134-28-9 (pbk)

Volume 2   Introduction to Diagnosis in Traditional Chinese Medicine
by Hong-zhou Wu, Zhao-qin Fang and Pan-ji Cheng
(translated by Chou-ping Han)
(Shanghai University of Traditional Chinese Medicine, China)
ISBN: 978-1938134-13-5 (pbk)

Volume 3   Introduction to Chinese Materia Medica
by Jin Yang, Huang Huang and Li-jiang Zhu
(translated by Yunhui Chen)
(Nanjing University of Chinese Medicine, China)
ISBN: 978-1-938134-16-6 (pbk)

Volume 4   Introduction to Chinese Internal Medicine
by Xiang Xia, Xiao-heng Chen, Min Chen and Yan-qian Xiao
(translated by Ye-bo He)
(Shanghai Jiaotong University, China)
ISBN: 978-1-938134-19-7 (pbk)

Volume 5   Introduction to Formulae of Traditional Chinese Medicine
by Jin Yang, Huang Huang and Li-jiang Zhu
(translated by Xiao Ye and Hong Li)
(Nanjing University of Chinese Medicine, China)
ISBN: 978-1-938134-10-4 (pbk)

Volume 6   Introduction to Acupuncture and Moxibustion
by Ren Zhang (translated by Xue-min Wang)
(Shanghai Literature Institute of Traditional Chinese Medicine, China)
ISBN: 978-1-938134-25-8 (pbk)

Volume 7   Introduction to Tui Na
by Lan-qing Liu and Jiang Xiao (translated by Azure Duan)
(Shanghai University of Traditional Chinese Medicine, China)
ISBN: 978-1-938134-22-7 (pbk)

World Century Compendium to TCM – Vol. 1

Fundamentals of Traditional Chinese Medicine

Hong-zhou Wu
Zhao-qin Fang
Pan-ji Cheng
Shanghai University of Traditional Chinese Medicine, China

translated by

Ye-bo He

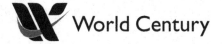 World Century

Published by

World Century Publishing Corporation
27 Warren Street
Suite 401-402
Hackensack, NJ 07601

Distributed by

World Scientific Publishing Co. Pte. Ltd.
5 Toh Tuck Link, Singapore 596224
USA office: 27 Warren Street, Suite 401-402, Hackensack, NJ 07601
UK office: 57 Shelton Street, Covent Garden, London WC2H 9HE

Library of Congress Control Number: 2013931122

British Library Cataloguing-in-Publication Data
A catalogue record for this book is available from the British Library.

World Century Compendium to TCM
A 7-Volume Set

FUNDAMENTALS OF TRADITIONAL CHINESE MEDICINE
Volume 1

Copyright © 2013 by World Century Publishing Corporation

Published by arrangement with Shanghai Scientific & Technical Publishers.

Originally published in Chinese
Copyright © Shanghai Scientific & Technical Publishers, 2007
All Rights Reserved.

ISBN 978-1-938134-34-0 (Set)
ISBN 978-1-938134-28-9 (pbk)

Typeset by Stallion Press
Email: enquiries@stallionpress.com

Printed in Singapore

Contents

THE FIRST WEEK

CHAPTER 1

Introduction

Traditional Chinese medicine (TCM), with a history of thousands of years, is the crystallization of the ancient Chinese people's experience in their struggle against diseases. It is also an integral part of the splendid Chinese culture. Under the influence and direction of classical Chinese philosophies, it has undergone long-term medical practice and infiltrated into, as well as absorbed from, other subjects at that time, thus gradually evolving into a unique medical theoretical system that contributed significantly to the health care of the Chinese people and the prosperity of the Chinese nation.

The basic theories of TCM are the theoretical foundations for guiding traditional Chinese preventive medicine and clinical medicine, and encompass such aspects as the philosophical foundation for TCM, the understandings of TCM on the physiology and pathology of the human body, and the principles in TCM for life-cultivation, rehabilitation, diagnostics, and therapeutics. In this sense, these basic theories are regarded not only as an important part of TCM, but also as a compulsory course fundamental to the studying and researching on TCM.

SECTION 1   A SUMMARY OF THE DEVELOPMENT OF BASIC THEORIES OF TCM

The Warring States Period — The Eastern Han Dynasty

The end of the Warring Sates Period has witnessed a dramatic change in society with remarkable advancement of politics, economics and culture, thus providing a considerable impetus to the development of academic thoughts that became increasingly dynamic and brisk. It is exactly during this period that the earliest medical classic in China, The *Yellow Emperor's Canon of Medicine* (*Huang Di Nei Jing*, 黄帝内经), or Nei Jing for short, came into existence. It covered the achievements before the Warring States Period from various subjects, such as philosophy, astronomy, calendar, meteorology, mathematics, biology and geography. Particularly, under the far-reaching influence of yin-yang and wuxing (five elements) theories, it summarized the medical achievements and experience before the period of Warring States and established the unique theoretical system of TCM, thereby laying a solid foundation for the development of traditional Chinese medicine.

Nei Jing is composed of two parts: *Ling Shu* (*Miraculous Pivot*, 灵枢) and *Shu Wen* (*Plain Conversation*, 素问), 18 volumes and 162 chapters in total. Through the conversation between Huangdi and Qibo, it adopts a question and answer approach to discuss systematically the relationship between man and nature, the physiology and pathology of the human body, and the diagnosis, treatment and prevention of diseases, thus laying a theoretical foundation for TCM. It covers aspects such as visceral manifestation, meridians and collaterals, etiology, pathogenesis, diagnostics, therapeutics, life cultivation, yunqi (five successive evolutive phases corresponding to five elements), acupuncture and moxibustion, etc. While addressing the medical theories, it also probes into some philosophical thoughts being the focus of attention at that time, such as yin-yang, five elements, qi, correspondence between man and nature, and the relationship between body and spirit. In such a way, it not only promoted the development of TCM by assimilating the advanced philosophical theories during that period, but also enriched and improved, in turn, the philosophical theories on the basis of medical progress. Many viewpoints in this book were really advanced at that time. For example, in *Ling Shu-Jingshui* (*Miraculous Pivot-Meridians and Vessels*, 灵枢·经水), it was clearly pointed out that, "After death, he or she can be examined by anatomy." And in the same book, it was also recorded that the ratio of the esophagus to the intestine is 1: 35, which is very close to the modern finding of 1:37. In *Su Wen-Wei Lun* (*Plain Conversation-Discussion on Paralysi*, 素问·痿论), it was put forth that, "The heart governs the blood and vessels of the body." And in *Su Wen·Ju Tong Lun* (*Plain Conversation-Discussion on Pain*), it was emphasized that the blood "circulates around the body in an endless circle." These statements have survived the lapse of time and, till today, they are still considered to be correct. For this reason, *Nei Jing* has been revered as an essential textbook for medical learners since its advent.

Nan Jing (*Canon of Difficult Issue*, 难经), written in the Eastern Han Dynasty, addresses 81 difficult issues in a question and answer approach. The book aims to elucidate the theories in *Nei Jing* and covers many different fields such as physiology, pathology, diagnostics and therapeutics. For pulse diagnosis, "exclusive examination on cunkou (a specific location on the radial artery at the wrist)" is particularly emphasized. And it further developed the theories of mingmen (gate of life) and sanjiao (triple energizer) in *Nei Jing*. For this reason, it was thought of as another important medical classic after *Nei Jing*.

Shang Han Za Bing Lun (*Treatise on Damage Cold and Miscellaneous Disease*, 伤寒杂病论), written by Zhang Zhongjing, a great physician at the end of the Eastern Han Dynasty, summarized the clinical experience of many doctors before the Eastern Han Dynasty, as well as the author himself under the guidance of theories in *Nei Jing*. It discussed cold-induced diseases in terms of six-meridian theory and miscellaneous diseases in terms of zang-fu theories, and put forth the principle of treatment according to syndrome differentiation encompassing principle, method, prescription and medicine, thus serving as a significant and indelible milestone in the rapid development of Chinese clinical medicine. The original *Shang Han Za Bing Lun* (*Treatise on Damage Cold and Miscellaneous Disease*, 伤寒杂病论) was once lost, and during the Song dynasty, it was divided into two books: *Shang Han Lun* (*Treatise on Exogenous Febrile Diseases*, 伤寒论) and *Jin Gui Yao Lue* (*Synopsis of Prescriptions in the Golden Chamber*, 金匮要略). The former formulated the outline and specific methods for treatment of six-meridian disorders based on syndrome differentiation, expounded the characteristics of the syndromes of the six meridians (taiyang, yangming, shaoyang, taiyin, shaoyin and jueyin), and established the principles and methods for the mechanisms of transmission from one meridian to another as well as their treatment according to syndrome differentiation. In this sense, it has laid a theoretical foundation for the diagnosis and treatment of exogenous febrile diseases. The second book, *Jin Gui Yao Lue* (*Synopsis of Prescriptions in the Golden Chamber*,

金匮要略), took the viscera and meridians as the outline, and put forth more than 40 therapeutic methods based on syndrome differentiation and 262 meticulously-formulated prescriptions perfect in principles, methods and herbs, thereby providing effective methods and approaches for the diagnosis and treatment of miscellaneous diseases due to internal damage.

Shen Nong Ben Cao Jing (*Shen Nong's Classic of the Materia Medica*, 神农本草经), complied in the Eastern Dynasty, is the earliest monograph on materia medica extant in China. In this book, 365 kinds of medicinal substances are recorded and, according to their properties and actions, divided into tree grades: the superior, the mediocre, and the inferior. It also deals with the medicinal theories or concepts, e.g., the classification of herbs in a prescription into four types: monarch, minister, assistant and guide, the four properties, and the five flavors, etc. It has laid a theoretical foundation for the development of Chinese Materia Medica. All of these clearly pointed to the fact that this was a critical phase when experiential knowledge was chanelled into systematic theories.

The Wei Dynasty, Jin Dynasty, and Southern-Northern Dynasties

During this period, medical theories were systematically summarized by Wang Shu. He rearranged Shang Han Lun, and wrote *Mai Jing* (*The Pulse Classic*, 脉经), the earliest most elaborate monograph on pulse-taking. This book elaborate the theories, methods and clinical significances of sphygmology in addition to the standardization of the titles for different pulses. Huang Fumi in the Jin Dynasty complied *Zhen Jiu Jia Yi Jing* (*A-B Classics of Acupuncture and Moxibustion*, 针灸甲乙经), the earliest comprehension monograph on acupuncture and moxibustion. This book, which rich in content, complete in theories and practical in application, covers areas such as viscera, meridians, acupoints, pathogenesis, diagnostics, therapeutics and medication taboos, etc. In *Ben Cao Jing Ji Zhu* (*Collective Commentaries on the Classic of Materia Medica*, 本草经集注), Tao Hongjing proposed the classification of medicinal substances according to their natural sources and the application of an universally-applicable medicine for all diseases, which had a significant influence on the later generations. *Lei Gong Pao Zhi Lun* (*Master Lei's Discourse on Medicinal*

Processing, 雷公炮炙论) complied by Lei Xiao, dealt exclusively with the theories about the properties and flavors of medicinal substances and the methods for their preparation and decoction.

The Sui and Dang Dynasties

During this period, the theoretical system of TCM continued to evolve owing to its rich medical practice. *Huang Di Nei Jing Tai Su (Grand Simplicity of Yellow Emperor' Canon of Medicine,* 黄帝内经太素) complied by Yang Shangshan is the earliest thickest? annotation edition. In *Bu Zhu Huang Di Nei Jing Su Wen (Supplementary Commentaries on Plain Conversation of Yellow Emperor' Canon of Medicine,* 补注黄帝内经素问), Wang Bing expounded and developed some theories in *Nei Jing,* and advocated that "restraining predominant yang by strengthening yin and restraining predominant yin by reinforcing yang," which was highly regared by the later generations. He also supplemented seven chapters about five movements and six climates, in which the theory of Yun Qi was rooted. *Zhu Bing Yuan Hou Lun (Treatise on Causes and Manifestations of Various Diseases,* 诸病源候论), the earliest monograph on etiology and symptomatology, was compiled by Chao Yuanfang. In this book, he made penetrating elucidations on the causes and symptoms of various diseases due to internal damage. Moreover, Sun Simiao devoted all his life to the writing of two great books: *Qian Jin Yao Fang (Valuable Prescriptions,*千金要方) and *Qian Jin Yi Fang (Supplement to Valuable Prescription,* 千金翼方). The two books highly regarded in the medical history of China because they cover a relatively comprehensive discussion on various medical fields from basic theories to clinical subjects.

The Song, Jin and Yuan Dynasties

This period witnessed the tremendous development in the theoretical system of TCM. In the Song Dynasty, and Chen Wuze wrote *San Yin Ji Yi Bing Zheng Fang Lun (Treatise on Diseases, Patterns and Formulas Related to the Unification of the Three Etiologies,* 三因极一病证方论). In this book, he put forth the well-known "theory of triple factors in causing diseases," which further improved the theory of etiology in TCM.

Cha Bing Zhi Nan (*Guide to Diagnosis*, 察病指南) written by Shi Fa is a book recording 33 pictures, each depicting the characteristics of a certain pulse. In *Ao Shi Shang Han Jin Jing Lu* (*Ao's Golden Mirror Records for Cold Damage*, 敖氏伤寒金镜录) written by Du Ben, there are 36 pictures depicting the morbid conditions of the tongue. It is the earliest extant book dealing exclusively with tongue examination. Zhang Yuansu summed up the essentials of many previous physicians and came-up with a comparatively systematic theory on visceral syndrome differentiation. He also proposed the theories of medicinal tropism and medicinal guide. Besides, Qian Yi is the first one to apply syndrome differentiation of the five zang-organs to treat infantile diseases, gradually developing a systematic set of fundamental principles or methods for infantile syndrome differentiation and treatment. In the Jin and Yuan Dynasties, there came forth four great medical schools represented by Liu Wansu, Zhang Congzheng, Li Gao and Zhu Zhenheng. Their achievements provided significant impetus to the development of basic theories in TCM. For example, Liu Wansu believed that "fire-heat" is the main cause of a variety of diseases, including the hyperactivity of six climatic factors and five emotions. He often treated these diseases with herbs cool or cold in nature; so his theory, known as the "School of Cold and Cool," had a far-reaching impact on the later generations and, in particular, contributed significantly to the formation of warm-disease theory. Zhang Congzheng believed that all diseases are caused by exogenous pathogenic factors and such factors should be driven out of the body by means of sweating, vomiting, and purging. For this reason his theory is known as the "School of Purgation." Li Gao put forward that internal impairment of the spleen and the stomach would bring about various diseases and therefore emphasized that the spleen and stomach are the foundation for the primordial qi. Improper diet, overstrain or emotional stimulation may all impair the spleen and stomach, giving rise to a variety of diseases. So he suggested that the most important thing in clinical treatment should be warming and invigorating the spleen and the stomach. That is why he was regarded as the founder of the "School of Reinforcing the Earth (spleen and stomach)." Zhu Zhenheng advocated forcefully that yang is usually redundant while yin is frequently deficient, which is based on the theory of ministerial fire (kidney fire). Clinically he often used the prescriptions for nourishing yin and reducing fire to treat patients. So his theory was known as the "School of Nourishing Yin." Besides, he was also a master at treating miscellaneous diseases, and came up with many ingenious ideas such as "almost all diseases are caused by phlegm" and "stagnation is responsible for a myriad of diseases."

The Ming and Qing Dynasties

In the Ming Dynasty, Zhao Xianke put forth the theory of mingmen (gate life) and emphasized that the gate of life is the pivot for regulating the yin and yang and the visceral activities of the whole body, which further enriched the theory of visceral manifestation in TCM. Li Zhongzi also stated that the kidney is the prenatal foundation while the spleen is the postnatal foundation. Even today, this remark is still widely used to guide clinical practice. It is noteworthy that, during this period, the theory of warm disease, emerged. Although it is a clinical subject focusing on the occurrence and development patterns of seasonal warm disease, as well as its treatment based on syndrome differentiation, the theory is of great significance to the improvement of the theoretical foundation of TCM. In the late Ming Dynasty, Wu Youxing first put forward the idea in *Wen Yi Lun* (*Treatise on Warm-Heat Pestilence*, 温疫论) that the cause of pestilence was different from the six abnormal climatic factors comprising of wind, cold, summer-heat, dampness, and so on. He believed that it is a special pathogenic factor in the natural world and that the channel of infection by pestilence is through the mouth and nose. All of these great contributions have revealed, from theory to practice, the causes of pestilence and warm disease, as well as their routes of transmission. In the Qing Dynasty, Ye Tianshi and Wu Jutong established the theories and methods for the treatment of warm disease based on syndrome differentiation and centered on "wei, qi, ying and blood" and the "triple energizer." In such a way, the theory of warm disease was further developed and became self-consistent in etiology, pathogenesis or treatment based on syndrome differentiation. Moreover, Wang Qingren wrote *Yi Li Gai Cuo* (*Corrections on Medical Errors*, 医林改错). In this book, he rectified some errors in a number of medical classics with regard to the human anatomy and, more noticeably, developed the theory of pathogenic blood stasis, thereby making certain contributions to the development of the basic theories of TCM.

Daily Exercises

1. Why it is said that *Huang Di Nei Jing* has laid the theoretical foundation for TCM?
2. What are the main viewpoints of the four great medical schools in the Jin and Yuan Dynasty?
3. In which book were the remarks made by Wu Youxing on the etiology of pestilence originated?

SECTION 2   THE MAIN CHARACTERISTICS OF BASIC THEORIES OF TCM

The theoretical system of TCM has evolved in the long course of clinical practice under the guidance of ancient Chinese philosophies. It originates from practice and, in turn, guides the practice. This unique theoretical system is essentially characterized by the concept of holism and the treatment based on syndrome differentiation.

Concept of Holism

Concept of holism views everything as holistic and integral objects, and deems the connection among them as inseparable. In light of this concept, the human body is regarded in TCM as an organic whole of which the constituent parts are inseparable in structure, interdependent in physiology, and inter-affected in pathology. The unity between the body and its external environment is also emphasized in TCM. It is just through the process of actively adapting to and remolding the natural environment that human beings maintain their normal life activities. For this reason, the concept of holism is highly valued in TCM, and is widely used in various branches of TCM such as physiology, pathology, diagnostics, syndrome differentiation and therapeutics.

The Human Body is an Organic Whole

The human body is composed of five zang-organs (the heart, liver, spleen, lung and kidney), six fu-organs (the stomach, small intestine, large intestine, triple energizers, urinary bladder, and gallbladder), five body constituents (the skin, vessels, muscles, tendons and bones) and seven orifices (the eyes, nose, ears, mouth, tongue, external genitalia and anus). Though different in physiological functions, they are interconnected rather than isolated. The unity of the body, according to the theory of TCM, is realized through the dominance of the five zang-organs, the assistance of the six fu-organs, and the communication of the meridians. The meridians, pertaining to the viscera in the interior and connecting with the limbs and joints in the exterior, can circulate essence, qi, blood and body fluid so as to nourish and coordinate various organs and tissues. In this sense, it is considered that TCM approaches the human body from a holistic perspective, e.g., digestion, absorption and excretion of food must rely on the coordinated action of the stomach in decomposition, the spleen in transformation and the large intestine in transportation; besides, the metabolism of water and fluid is also a concerted effort of the spleen in transformation and transportation, the lung in dredging and regulating waterways, and the kidney in distribution and excretion.

Such activities in a coordinated fashion are the prerequisite for the soundness of the body. If a pathological change takes place in a local area, there will be functional disorders not only in this specific region, but also in its related organs or even in the organs and tissues of the whole body. Take the spleen and stomach for example. The spleen and stomach are the postnatal foundation of the body, and if they fail to ascend and descend properly, there will be disordered reception and transformation and, consequently, the malnutrition of the organs of the whole body, or general weakness. Besides, the heart controls blood, while the lung governs qi. Blood is promoted by qi, whereas qi is carried by blood. If the lung qi is stagnated, the heart blood will fail to circulate smoothly; in contrast, if the heart blood is obstructed, the lung qi will fail to disperse properly. Moreover, if the essence qi of the five zang-organs are in deficiency, the organs or tissues related to them will be in disorder accordingly, e.g., insufficiency of liver blood leading to dizziness and dry eyes, or even contraction of the tendons and vessels; and insufficiency of kidney yin resulting in dizziness and tinnitus, or even soreness and weakness of the waist and knees.

Since the various organs and tissues of the body are physiologically interdependent and pathologically affected, external manifestations, such as the changes in the five sensory organs, body constituents, complexion and pulse, can be used to identify and diagnose the disorders of the internal organs, so as to make a correct diagnosis and treatment. What's more, the treatment of regional disease has to take the whole body into consideration. There are a number of therapeutic principles in TCM developed under the guidance of this holistic concept, such as treating the ear from the perspective of the kidney, treating the nose from the lung, and treating the eye from the liver, in addition to "drawing yin from yang and drawing yang from yin; treating the right for curing diseases on the left and treating the left for curing diseases on the right" and "needling the acupoints on the lower part of the body for diseases in the upper part and needling the acupoints on the upper part of the body for diseases in the lower part."

The Close Connection Between Man and Nature

Man lives in the natural world, and the changes in nature will inevitably affect the human body in a direct or indirect fashion, causing different reactions of the body. This is called "correspondence between man and nature." Take seasonal changes for example. Usually spring is marked by warmth, summer by hotness, autumn by coolness and winter by coldness. Under the influence of such changes, the living things on the earth will also change in order to adapt to environmental changes. In spring and summer when yang qi is predominant, the body's qi and blood tends to flow to the superficies, making the muscular interstices open and causing perspiration; in autumn and winter when yang qi begins to decline, the body's qi and blood tend to flow inward, making the muscular interstices closed and causing excessive urination. The seasonal variations are influential on the human body, so are the changes within a day. The morning is likened to spring, the noon to summer, the dusk to autumn and the midnight to winter. Although the temperature change within a day is not so dramatic as that of the four seasons, it has certain influences on the body, too. This also points to the fact that the human body can adapt its physiological activities to the natural changes of the day and night, as well as the yin and yang.

The differences in geographical environment and local climate may also affect the human body. It has been observed that in the south of the lower reaches of the Yangtze River with low-lying terrain and warm, humid climate, people are characterized by loose muscular interstices. Once these inhabitants move to other geographically distinct areas, they may encounter discomforts at the beginning, but after a period of time, they will gradually get accustomed to the new environment.

Human beings can take the initiative to adapt themselves proactively to the natural environment. For this reason, normal climatic changes will not cause adverse effects. However, if the body fails to adjust itself to such changes, or when the changes are so extreme that it exceeds the regulative capacity of the body, there will be occurrence of diseases. That is why some diseases are prominent in a certain season, e.g., spring is marked by wind diseases, summer by febrile diseases, autumn by dry diseases, and winter by cold diseases. Besides, sudden changes in the living environment may also lead to the conditions of "one's system disagreeing with a new natural environment." For these who are old, weak, or with chronic diseases, they may have physical discomfort and disease onset or aggravation whenever the seasons alternate. Some patients may experience the process of "feeling comfortable in the morning, being at ease in the daytime, worsening at dusk, and aggravating at night." In this sense, the treatment must take the natural climate and geographical environment into consideration, and always keep in accordance with the time and locality.

Social environment may also influence people psychologically and emotionally. A sound environment is good for people's health, whereas a negative environment may become the disease-inducing factor. Therefore, people should always strengthen their will and cultivate their mind so as to better adapt to the social environmental changes.

Treatment Based on Syndrome Differentiation

Treatment based on syndrome differentiation, another important feature of TCM, is a basic principle in TCM for diagnosing and treating diseases.

Syndrome is a pathological generalization of a disease at a certain stage in its course of development. It includes the location, cause and nature of the disease, as well as the relationship between pathogenic factors and healthy qi, and can reveal the overall conditions of the pathological changes at a certain stage of the disease.

Differentiation of syndrome implies that the patient's symptoms and signs collected through the four diagnostic methods (inspecting, smelling-listening, inquiring and pulse-taking) are analyzed so as to identify the etiology, nature and location of a disease, and the relationship between healthy qi and pathogenic factors, thereby generalizing them into a certain syndrome.

Treatment refers to the selection of the corresponding therapy according to the result of syndrome differentiation. Syndrome differentiation is the prerequisite and foundation for the determination of proper therapies, whereas treatment is the purpose of syndrome differentiation. The course of treatment based on syndrome differentiation is actually a process of understanding the nature of disease as well as treating the disease. In this sense, syndrome differentiation and treatment are interconnected and inseparable in the process of disease diagnosis and treatment.

The relationship between disease and syndrome is dialectically dealt with by treatment based on syndrome differentiation, which is the basic principle guiding clinical diagnosis and treatment. It is believed that one disease may include several different syndromes, while different diseases may manifest the same syndrome during the course of development. That is why TCM uses two different clinical methods to deal with the relationship between disease and syndrome: "treating the same disease with different therapies" and "treating different diseases with the same therapy."

"Treating the same disease with different therapies" means that the same disease may manifest different syndromes or pathogeneses at different stages or under different conditions in terms of time, locality and individuality. As a result, the therapies will also be different. For example, common cold is differentiated into several syndromes: wind-cold, wind-heat and summer-damp, so it can be treated by the following methods: dispelling wind and dissipating cold, dispersing wind and clearing away heat, relieving summer-heat and resolving dampness. "Treating different diseases with the same therapy" means that different diseases may manifest similar syndrome or the same pathogenesis in the process of development, which can be treated with the same therapy. For example, proctoptosis due to prolonged dysentery, gastroptosis and uterine prolapse are different diseases. However, if they show the same syndrome of sinking of middle qi (gastrosplenic qi), all of them can be treated with the therapeutic method of lifting middle qi. This demonstrates that the treatment of diseases in TCM does not concentrate on the difference or similarity of diseases, but on the difference of pathogenesis. In other words, diseases with similar pathogenesis can be treated with therapeutic methods that are basically the same, while diseases with different pathogeneses have to be treated with different therapeutic methods. For this reason, "treating the same disease with different therapies" and "treating different diseases with the same therapy" are regarded as the specific manifestations of differentiating syndrome to decide treatment.

Daily Exercises

1. What are the main characteristics of the theoretical foundation of TCM?
2. Why it is said that the human body is an organic whole?
3. How can we understand the "correspondence between man and nature"?

SECTION 3   THE ESSENTIALS OF BASIC THEORIES IN TCM

The basic theories of TCM cover many aspects, primarily the essence, qi and spirit, the yin-yang and five elements, the visceral manifestation, the meridians and collaterals, the qi, blood and body fluid, as well as the etiology, pathogenesis, and the preventive and curative principles, etc.

The theory of essence, qi and spirit, and the theories of yin-yang and five elements are ancient philosophical thoughts in China. The theory of essence, qi and spirit holds that all the things in the universe are composed of qi, which is in constant motion and variation. The world is made up of qi, and the motion of all the things on earth is, as a matter of fact, a reflection of the movement of qi. If qi varies, everything will change accordingly. Hence, the theory of essence, qi and spirit is actually a doctrine of monish about the origin and essence of the world. The theory of yin-yang believes that anything in the world can be divided into either yin or yang. Yin and yang are mutually opposed and inter-rooted, which means that neither of the two can exist in isolation. Besides, yin and yang are constantly waxing and waning within a certain entity which, when yin prevails, is essentially yin in nature; otherwise, it is yang in nature. So yin and yang are interchangeable. Since all the things on earth can be divided into two aspects, the theory of yin-yang is deemed as a dualism about the origin and essence of the world. The theory of five element looks upon the world as a combination of wood, fire, earth, metal and water, which are inter-generated and inter-restricted. Such a relationship among them maintains the dynamic balance of all things in the universe. So the theory of five elements is a doctrine of pluralism about the origin and essence of the world. With tremendous influence on TCM, the three philosophical thoughts have already infiltrated into every field of TCM and become its philosophical foundation.

The theories of visceral manifestation and meridians explore chiefly into the physiological function, pathological change and interrelation of the five zang-organs, six fu-organs, twelve meridians and eight extraordinary meridians, as well as the intimate association between the viscera and meridians and the external environment. Among them, the theory of visceral manifestation, in the light of ancient anatomy, divided the internal organs into three types according to the physiological function of the viscera: five zang-organs, six fu-organs and the extraordinary fu-organs. Despite their relative independence, these organs are mutually connected and coordinated during their life activities, making up an entirety in which one zang-organ is related to another zang-organ, one fu-organ to another fu-organ, different zang-organs to different fu-organs, and different zang-fu organs to the various body constituents and orifices. While located deep inside the body, the zang-fu organs can manifest their functional hyperactivity or debilitation on certain regions of the body surface through the connection of meridians. So by observing the external signs or manifestations, we can further understand the visceral functions and their interconnections. So it is believed, according to the theory of meridians, that the meridians and collaterals, ubiquitous inside the body or on the body surface in a crisscross pattern, are passages for circulating qi and blood as well as an intricate network for connecting the viscera, limbs, tendons, muscles and skin. Pathologically, the meridian system can also become the routes for pathogenic invasion and transmission. For this reason, the meridians and collaterals are of great and unusual value in the diagnostic and therapeutic practice.

The theory of qi, blood and body fluid probes into the production, distribution and physiological function of the basic substances for life. They are viewed in TCM as the basic materials for constituting the human body and the fundamental substances for maintaining the life activities. Qi is an extremely fine substance in constant motion; blood is a red fluid circulating inside the vessels; while body fluid is a collective term for all the normal fluids within the body. All of them are metabolic products of the physiological activities of the viscera on the one hand, and on the other hand, they can provide necessary substances or energy in turn so as to maintain the normal physiological function of the viscera and meridians. In this sense, they also serve as the material foundation for the functional activities of the viscera and meridians.

The theories of etiology and pathogenesis expound mainly the properties, characteristics and pathogenic manifestations of various pathogenic factors, as well as the occurrence, development, change and prognosis of diseases. In TCM, etiological factors are divided into four types: exogenous pathogenic factors, endogenous pathogenic factors, pathological products, and other pathogenic factors. Exogenous pathogenic factors, including wind, cold, summer-heat, dampness, dryness, fire and the highly epidemic qi, derive from nature and invade the body through the skin, muscles, nose and mouth. Endogenous pathogenic factors damage the internal organs directly due to abnormal emotions or behaviors, including joy, anger, worry, thinking, sorrow, terror, and fright, or overstrain, excessive rest, and improper diet. Metabolic products, such as water-damp, phlegmatic fluid and blood stasis, are produced during the process of some diseases and may also become pathogenic factors engendering other diseases. Other etiological factors include external injury and medicinal damage. Pathogenesis can be discussed in terms of basic pathogenesis and system pathogenesis. The former refers primarily to the exuberance and debilitation of pathogenic factors and healthy qi, imbalance between yin and yang, and disorders of qi, blood and body fluid. These are the most fundamental pathogeneses which may occur in any disease. The latter refers to the pathological mechanisms of the viscera, meridians, body constituents, orifices and exogenous febrile diseases. These are the specific manifestations of the basic pathogenesis in different regions of the body or in different diseases.

Preventive and therapeutic principles are basic laws for preventing and treating diseases. Prevention before the occurrence of diseases is highly valued in TCM, which is of great significance to the controlling of the occurrence and development of diseases. The basic therapeutic principles mainly incorporate treating diseases from the perspective of the root, strengthening the healthy qi and expelling pathogenic factors, balancing yin and yang as well as suiting measures to individual, seasonal and geographical conditions, etc.

The above-mentioned are important constituent parts of the theoretical system of TCM, coming from practice and, in turn, directing practice. They also serve as the foundation for studying other branches of TCM, especially the clinical subjects.

Daily Exercises

1. What are the main contents of the basic theories of TCM?
2. Summarize the main contents of the theory of etiology in TCM.

CHAPTER 2

The Theory of Essence, Qi and Spirit

The theory of essence, qi and spirit is an ancient philosophical thought. Qi is an intangible substance in constant motion. Essence, or jing in Chinese, is the most important part of qi. Spirit, or shen, refers to motion and variation of substances in nature and their intrinsic regularities. All of them have a tremendous influence on TCM.

The Essentials of the Theory of Essence, Qi and Spirit

The ancient philosophers in China believed that everything in the world is made up of qi. For example, Liu An described in *Huai Nan Zi* (*The Book of the Prince of Huai Nan*) the process of the heaven, earth, water, fire, sun and moon coming into being out of qi. It was considered that the universe is in a chaotic state before its formation. This phase is called the taishi period in Chinese, which means the primordial origin. After the formation of the universe, qi came into being. The light and lucid part of qi ascends and disperses, forming the sky; while the heavy and turbid part of qi descends and congeals, constituting the earth. Besides, water and fire, as well as the sun and moon, are also made up of qi. As for the mechanism of qi producing everything, most ancient philosophers explained it with the theory of "interaction between the heavenly qi and earthly qi" and regarded the movements of qi as qi dynamic, which is highly generalized into four motive types: ascending, descending, exiting and entering. Ascending means moving from down to up, descending from up to down, exiting from inside to outside, and entering from outside to inside. These movements never cease, and under normal circumstances, the ascending and descending, as well as the entering and exiting, maintain a relative balance. Such actions of qi will inevitably engender various changes, called qi transformation. The manifestations of qi transformation are very complicated, e.g., from intangible qi to tangible substances, or from tangible substances to intangible qi. Since everything is composed of qi, the variation of all things is, in essence, a kind of qi transformation, such as the birth, growth, maturity, aging and death of animals or sprouting, growing, transforming, reaping, and storing of the plants. This indicates that qi transformation is eternal. Qi motion and qi transformation are closely related, and only through the movements of qi can such transformations be carried out. Once the ascending, descending, entering and exiting of qi stop, the transformation of qi also ends. So the motion of qi is prerequisite to qi transformation. Without qi movement there will be no qi transformation and every variation in the world. According to the ancient philosophers, qi is in constant motion and variation, which bring forth the movements and changes of everything in the world. And every movement or change in the world is the specific manifestation of qi in constant motion and variation.

A famous ancient philosopher, Guan Zi has said that essence is the quintessence of qi, which indicates that essence is the most import part of qi and the origin of life. So Guan Zi also said, "The human being is borne by the heaven proving essence and the earth giving form." In *Huai Nan Zi* (*The Book of the Prince of Huai Nan*), it is also said, "the non-essential qi produces the insects whereas the essential qi gives birth to the human beings." It is evident that the human beings are produced by combining the essence qi from the heaven and earth, which is the most basic substance making up the body.

Moreover, many ancient philosophers have clearly pointed out that spirit, or shen, refers to the various motion and variation as well as their intrinsic regularities in mysterious nature, as well as the comprehensive external manifestations of vitality in all living organisms.

Daily Exercises

1. List the types of qi movements.
2. What is qi transformation, and what are the specific forms of qi transformation as far as animals and plants are concerned?

3. What is essence, and is it the basic substance for constituting the human body?
4. What is spirit?

The Application of the Theory of Essence, Qi and Spirit in TCM

Essence

The theory of essence, qi and spirit is widely applied in various areas of TCM. Among them, essence is the basic substance constituting the human body and maintaining its life activities. Essence in a broad sense includes cereal nutrients, visceral essence, and kidney essence. The cereal nutrients are transformed from water and food, and when they are distributed to the viscera, they will become the visceral essence. Kidney essence originates from parents and is nourished by water and food. The essence in a narrow sense refers to a substance with reproductive capability within the kidney, so it is also called reproductive essence.

Essence is divided into prenatal essence and postnatal essence in terms of origin. The former, a primitive substance for embryonic development, refers to the reproductive essence acquired from parents and endowed since birth. The postnatal essence is transformed from water and food, and then distributed to the zang-fu organs and finally to the kidney. Despite their different origins, the prenatal essence and postnatal essence are both related to the kidney and are mutually promoted. The prenatal essence depends on the constant nourishment and replenishment of the postnatal essence, whereas the production of the postnatal essence, in turn, relies on the activation of the prenatal essence. The two are mutually complemented, so as to maintain the abundance of essence within the kidney.

The functions of essence are multi-faceted.

a. For reproduction

The reproductive essence is the primitive substance for life with the capability of giving birth to offspring. This is reflected not only in the combination of parental essence which creates new life, but also in the development and maturity of a new life which leads to the abundance of kidney essence and the production of Tai Gui, a substance signifying the ability to reproduce. So essence is the material foundation for reproduction. If the kidney essence is abundant, the reproductive capacity will be strong; otherwise, the reproductive capacity will be abnormal.

b. For promotion of growth and development

From the formation of the embryo to the growth and development of fetus, essence is the main material foundation for constituting various tissues and organs of the body and also the substance for promoting the growth and development of the fetus. After birth, essence continues to promote the growth and development of the body from infancy to adolescence. If the kidney essence is insufficient, the body will develop slowly and abnormally.

c. For nourishment

The cereal nutrients are distributed to the viscera and other organs for nourishment so as to maintain the physiological activities of the human body. Water and food are received, digested and absorbed by the stomach and spleen, and then transformed into essence, a part of which is for the nourishment of the body, and the rest of which is stored in the kidney for reservation. The kidney essence is stored on the one hand and discharged on the other. In this way, life activities go on ceaselessly. In this sense, it is safe to say that essence is the basic substance for maintaining the life activities of the human body. If the essence is abundant, the body will be full of vitality and can adapt to the external environment and resist the invasion of the pathogenic factors; on the contrary, if the essence is deficient, the body will lack vitality have poor adaptability and resistance.

Qi

Qi is not only the basic substance for the constitution of the human body, but also the main substance for the maintenance of life activities. The life activities of the body rely on the nutrients from the heavenly qi and earthly qi, which nourish the visceral qi and maintain the physiological activities of the body. So we can say that qi is also the motive force of human life.

The five zang-organs, six fu-organs, body constituents, orifices, blood and body fluid are all tangible parts and can exert their actions only through the promotion of qi. For example, the heart controls blood circulation, the lung manages respiration, the spleen governs transformation of water and food, the kidney takes charge of storing prenatal essence, the liver promotes free flow of qi and the stomach receives water and food. All these functions, however, are carried out under the promotion of qi. Hence, the sufficiency of qi is a sign of normal life activities. In TCM, it is believed that before birth, the human body has already acquired the postnatal essence which, after birth, combines the lucid qi inhaled by the lung from nature and cereal nutrients transformed by the spleen and stomach from water and food. The three substances thus combine and transform into the essence qi of the human body. Such a kind of qi can promote the physiological functions of the viscera, meridians, body constituents and orifices of the body. If it is sufficient, the life activities will be normal; and otherwise, the force promoting the local or general physiological functions will be weak, leading to deficiency manifestations of the whole body or in some specific regions.

The movements of qi inside the body have four forms: ascending, descending, entering and exiting. Under normal circumstances, ascending and descending, as well as entering and exiting, should maintain a relative balance. Such a balance, if disturbed, may lead to morbid conditions such as qi adverseness marked by excessive ascending and inadequate descending, or qi sinking marked by inadequate ascending and excessive descending, etc. All of these are collectively called disorders of qi movement. Qi adverseness manifested as cough, wheezing, belching and vomiting can be treated by lowering down qi. Qi sinking manifested as anal prolapse or visceroptosis can be treated by lifting up qi. The purpose is to restore the balance of qi movements. If the flow of qi is smooth, the circulation of blood and fluid will be unobstructed, and the body will remain healthy. Otherwise, if the flow of qi is not smooth, which is called qi stagnancy, there will be sensations of stuffiness, distension and pain in the affected region. This can be treated by promoting the flow of qi. If the stagnancy of qi persists, there will be accumulation of blood and body fluid, which should be treated by promoting qi to activate blood and resolve stasis, as well as promoting qi to resolve phlegm and drain dampness.

Spirit

Spirit reflects and dominates the mind, consciousness, perception, cognition, and motion of the human body. The material foundation for spirit is essence. Spirit has already existed since the beginning of life when the embryo takes shape. Every activity of the spirit relies on postnatal nourishment. Only when cereal nutrients are sufficient, and the five zang-organs are harmonized, can the vitality of spirit be exuberant.

The spirit inside the body is most closely connected with the five zang-organs. In Su Wen, it is said, "the heart stores spirit, the lung stores ethereal soul, and liver stores corporeal soul, the spleen stores ideation, and the kidney stores will." Although different in names, the ethereal soul, corporeal soul, ideation and will all pertain to spirit. In addition, the heart governs other zang-organs, so spirit can generalize and represent the ethereal soul, corporeal soul, ideation and will. TCM holds that the body and spirit are inseparable, and with or without spirit is the decisive factor for life and death. The co-existence of spirit and body is a major sign of life. The reason why eyes can see, ears can listen, mouth can talk, and limbs can move are all attributed to spirit; all the mental activities and body movements are the functional manifestations of spirit. Hence, a healthy person must have exuberant vitality, whereas an unhealthy one is usually impaired in spirit, manifested as lusterless eyes, depression, speech disorder, involuntary movements, and even coma. All these symptoms point to an extremely severe case. In this sense, clinically the examination of spirit can give a hint about the severity and prognosis of a disease.

The Relationship Between Essence, Qi and Spirit

Essence, qi and spirit are called the "triple treasures" in TCM which, although being independent entities, are closely associated. Essence may transform into qi, and qi may transform into essence, so they are inter-transformed. Essence and qi can generate and nourish spirit which, in turn, can control essence and qi. Therefore, people with abundant essence and qi must have a vigorous spirit. Contrarily, those with insufficient spirit are mostly due to the inadequacy of essence and qi.

Because they are interconnected, over-consumption of essence may affect the generation of qi whereas the over-depletion of qi may also impede the transformation of essence; both will lead to insufficiency of spirit. Besides, although spirit originated from essence and qi, it may impair them, in turn, if abnormal emotional activities damage the spirit, leading to weakness of the body, too.

In TCM, it is believed that spirit is the most important one among the three factors because it is the dominator of essence, qi, and all the life activities.

Daily Exercises

1. What are the functions that essence possesses?
2. Why is it said that qi is the motive force of human life?
3. Why is it said that spirit is most closely associated with the five zang-organs?
4. Why is it said that essence, qi and spirit, although being independent entities, are closely associated?

Weekly Review

As a TCM learner, one should be familiar with the history of TCM in the development of basic theories. During the period from the Warring Sates to the Eastern Han Dynasty, The *Yellow Emperor's Canon of Medicine* (*Huang Di Nei Jing*, 黄帝内经） and *Nan Jing* (*Canon of Difficult Issue*, 难经) came into existence. These two books indicate that TCM has developed from the phase of pristine experiential accumulation to the phase of systematic theoretical summarization, thus providing theoretical guidance and foundation for the development of TCM. *Shang Han Za Bing Lun* (*Treatise on Damage Cold and Miscellaneous Disease*, 伤寒杂病论), written by Zhang Zhongjing, put forth the principle of treatment according to syndrome differentiation encompassing principle, method, prescription and medicine. It also discussed the diagnostics and therapeutics of cold-induced diseases and miscellaneous diseases. For these reasons, the book is considered an indelible milestone in the development of Chinese clinical medicine. *Shen Nong Ben Cao Jing (Shen Nong's Classic of the Materia Medica*, 神农本草经) is a systematic monograph on materia medica, thus laying a theoretical foundation for the development of Chinese Materia Medica.

During the Wei Dynasty, Jin Dynasty, and Southern-Northern Dynasties, the medical theories were systematically compiled. Wang Shu He wrote *Mai Jing* (*The Pulse Classic*, 脉经), the earliest comprehensive monograph on pulse-taking. Huang Fumi in the Jin Dynasty complied *Zhen Jiu Jia Yi Jing* (*A-B Classics of Acupuncture and Moxibustion*, 针灸甲乙经), the earliest monograph on acupuncture and moxibustion. In *Ben Cao Jing Ji Zhu* (*Collective Commentaries on the Classic of Materia Medica*, 本草经集注), Tao Hongjing further elucidated the theories on Chinese materia medica. *Lei Gong Pao Zhi Lun* (*Master Lei's Discourse on Medicinal Processing*, 雷公炮炙论) complied by Lei Xiao, dealt exclusively with the theories and methods of preparation and decoction of Chinese medicinals.

During the Sui Dynasty, Dang Dynasty, and the Five Dynasties, the theoretical system of TCM continued to evolve owing to the rich medical practice. *Huang Di Nei Jing Tai Su* (*Grand Simplicity of Yellow Emperor' Canon of Medicine*, 黄帝内经太素) complied by Yang Shangshan is the earliest annotation edition. And in *Bu Zhu Huang Di Nei Jing Su Wen* (*Supplementary Commentaries on Plain Conversation of Yellow Emperor' Canon of Medicine*, 补注黄帝内经素问), Wang Bing expounded and developed some theories in *Nei Jing*. He also supplemented seven chapters about five movements and six climates, in which the theory of Yun Qi was rooted. *Zhu Bing Yuan Hou Lun* (*Treatise on Causes and Manifestations of Various Diseases*, 诸病源候论), the earliest monograph on etiology and symptomatology, was compiled by Chao Yuanfang. Moreover, Sun Simaio devoted all his life to the writing of two great books: *Qian Jin Yao Fang* (*Valuable Prescriptions*, 千金要方) and *Qian Jin Yi Fang* (*Supplement to Valuable Prescription*, 千金翼方). The two books played an important role in the medical history of China in that they cover a relatively comprehensive discussion on various medical fields from basic theories to clinical subjects.

The Song, Jin and Yuan Dynasties witnessed tremendous development in the theoretical system of TCM. In the Song Dynasty, Chen Wuze wrote *San Yin Ji Yi Bing Zheng Fang Lun* (*Treatise on Diseases, Patterns and*

Formulas Related to the Unification of the Three Etiologies, 三因极一病证方论), which further improved the theory of etiology in TCM. Zhang Yuansu summed up the essentials of many previous physicians and came-up with a comparatively systematic theory on visceral syndrome differentiation. He also proposed the theories of medicinal tropism and medicinal guide. In the Jin and Yuan Dynasties, there came forth four great medical schools represented by Liu Wansu, Zhang Congzheng, Li Gao and Zhu Zhenheng. Their achievements provided significant impetus to the development of basic theories in TCM. For example, Liu Wansu advocated the theory of "fire-heat." Zhang Congzheng proposed the method of "purging the pathogenic factors." Li Gao suggested "warming and invigorating the spleen and the stomach." Zhu Zhenheng believed that "yang is usually redundant while yin is frequently deficient," which is based on the theory of "ministerial fire (kidney fire)."

In the Ming Dynasty, Zhao Xianke put forth the theory of mingmen (gate life), which further enriched the theory of visceral manifestation in TCM. Besides, Li Zhongzi held that the kidney is the prenatal foundation while the spleen is the postnatal foundation. Even today, this remark is still widely used to guide clinical practice. In the late Ming Dynasty, Wu Youxing revealed the causes of pestilence and warm disease as well as their routes of transmission, which is a major theoretical breakthrough. In the Qing Dynasty, Ye Tianshi and Wu Jutong established the theories and methods for treatment of warm disease based on syndrome differentiation and centered on "wei, qi, ying and blood" and the "triple energizer," generalizing the knowledge on warm-diseases into a systematic theory. Moreover, Wang Qingren wrote *Yi Li Gai Cuo* (*Corrections no Medical Errors*, 医林改错). In this book, he developed the theory of pathogenic blood stasis, which is of great clinical significance.

The theoretical system of TCM is essentially characterized by the concept of holism and treatment based on syndrome differentiation. Concept of holism views everything as holistic and integral objects, and deems the connection among them as inseparable. In light of this concept, the human body is regarded in TCM as an organic whole of which the constituent parts are inseparable in structure, interdependent in physiology, and inter-affected in pathology. The human body is composed of five zang-organs, six fu-organs, five body constituents (the skin, vessels, muscles, tendons and bones) and seven orifices (the eyes, nose, ears, mouth, tongue, external genitalia and anus). Though different in physiological functions, they are interconnected through the meridians rather than isolated. The unity between the body and its external environment is also emphasized in TCM. It is just through the process of actively adapting to and remolding the natural environment that human beings maintain their normal life activities. For this reason, the concept of holism is highly valued in TCM, and is widely used in various branches of TCM such as physiology, pathology, diagnostics, syndrome differentiation and therapeutics.

Treatment based on syndrome differentiation is a basic principle in TCM for diagnosing and treating diseases. Differentiation of syndrome implies that the patient's symptoms and signs collected through the four diagnostic methods (inspecting, smelling-listening, inquiring and pulse-taking) are analyzed so as to identify the etiology, nature and location of a disease, and the relation between healthy qi and pathogenic factors, thereby generalizing them into a certain syndrome. Treatment refers to the selection of the corresponding therapy according to the result of syndrome differentiation. The course of treatment based on syndrome differentiation is actually a process of understanding the nature of disease, as well as treating the disease. It is one of the basic characteristics of TCM.

The theory of essence, qi and spirit, an ancient philosophical thought, has tremendous influence on TCM and is widely applied in various areas of TCM. In TCM, it is believed that essence is the basic substance constituting the human body and maintaining its life activities. Essence in a broad sense and essence in a narrow sense refer to deferent substances. According to its origin, essence can also be divided into prenatal essence and postnatal essence. The functions of essence are to reproduce, to nourish, and to promote growth and development. Qi is not only the basic substance for the constitution of the human body, but also the main substance for the maintenance of life activities. The movements of qi inside the body have four forms: ascending, descending, entering and exiting. Under normal circumstances, ascending and descending, as well as entering and exiting, should maintain a relative balance. Such a balance, if destroyed, may lead to morbid conditions. Spirit is the concentrated reflection and dominator of the mind, consciousness, perception and motion of the human body. The spirit inside the body is most closely connected with the five zang-organs. Although they are different in names, ethereal soul, corporeal soul, ideation and will, as a matter of fact, all pertain to spirit. TCM holds that the body and spirit are inseparable, and with or without spirit is the decisive factor for life and death. The co-existence of spirit and body is a major sign of life.

In TCM, essence, qi and spirit are called the "triple treasures" which, although being separate entities, are closely associated. Essence may transform into qi, and qi may transform into essence, so they are inter-transformed. Essence and qi can generate and nourish spirit which, in turn, can control essence and qi. In TCM, it is considered that spirit is the most important one among the three factors because it is the dominator of essence, qi, and all the life activities.

Daily Exercises

1. Understand the general information on the development of the basic theories of TCM.
2. Master the basic characteristics of the basic theories of TCM.
3. Master the application of the theory of essence, qi and spirit in TCM.

THE SECOND WEEK

CHAPTER 3

The Theory of Yin and Yang

The theory of yin and yang, an ancient philosophical thought in China, is a world outlook and methodology for recognizing and interpreting the world by Chinese ancestors. The initial connotations of yin and yang are quite simple, the side facing the sun being yang and the reverse side being yin. But later on, ancient Chinese came to understand that all things or phenomena in the natural world could be viewed as having a dual aspect of either yin or yang, i.e. all those being bright, warm, ascending, or motive pertain to yang, while all those being dark, cold, descending or quiet pertain to yin. Besides, the ancient philosophers gradually recognized that the generation, development and variation of the natural world are actually the result of the interaction between yin and yang. They even explained the phenomenon of earthquake in the light of yin-yang theory. In *Yi Jing* (*Book of Change*), it is regarded that yin and yang are the natural law of the universe. The occurrence, development and motion of all things in nature are deemed as a result of the interaction between yin and yang, which are both opposite and unified.

Yin and yang represent the attributes of things that are both interrelated and contradictory. Generally speaking, those being motive, outward, upward, warm or bright pertain to yang whereas those being still, inward, downward, cold or dark pertain to yin. Take heaven and earth as an example, the heavenly qi, being light and clear, pertains to yang, while the earthly qi, being heavy and turbid, pertains to yin. For water and fire, the former is cold, cool and moistening downward, so it pertains to yin; the latter is warm, hot and flaming upward, so it pertains to yang. In terms of motion and stillness, the former pertains to yang for the reason that yang-heat controls motion, and the latter pertains to yin because yin-cold governs stillness. When it comes to the motion and variation of substances, those pertaining to yang are steaming and transforming into qi, while those pertaining to yin are congealing and forming into shape. As for the cold and heat in temperature, day and night in time, up and down in direction, or sunny and rainy in weather, they are all manifestations of yin and yang in opposition. With regard to the life activities of the human body, those being propelling, warming, exciting, and stimulating pertain to yang; those being congealing, moistening, suppressing, and calming pertain to yin. In this sense, it is considered that yin and yang can represent a pair of things in both opposition and unity, or signify two opposite aspects within the same entity.

The Essentials of Yin-Yang Theory

Interaction Between Yin and Yang

The theory of yin and yang holds that all things stem from the interaction between yin and yang, which is the root for the emergence and variation of myriad things. In nature, the generation and transformation of all things are caused by the communication between the heavenly yang qi and earthly yin qi; the descent of heavenly yang qi and the ascent of earthly yin qi provide the prerequisite for such a change. In other words, the interaction of the physical and chemical factors between the heaven and earth gives rise to all things in nature, and without such an interaction, there would be no generation and transformation of myriad things on earth. As far as the human beings are concerned, the intercourse between man and woman give birth to new lives, and the sustaining of life also relies on the inter-communication between his or her own yin and yang. If yin and yang are separated or insolated, life will be terminated, too.

The interaction between yin and yang is the precondition for the generation and transformation of all things. For this reason, TCM stressed that different components of the body interact constantly, and so do the physiological functions. This ensures the normal proceeding of life activities. For instance, the mutual interaction of yin, qi and yang qi leads to normal physiological functions whereas disorders of such an interaction may give rise to a series of pathological manifestations.

Interaction between yin and yang is carried out incessantly. It may be manifested as mutual restriction, interdependence, mutual waning and waxing, inter-transformation and inter-preponderance, etc. That is to say, all these manifestations take place in the process of yin-yang interaction.

Mutual Restriction Between Yin and Yang

The theory of yin and yang holds that all things in nature have two aspects: yin and yang. They are mutually contradictory in nature and mutually restricted in relation. Such a relationship, called yin and yang in opposition ancient philosophers, can be exemplified by the opposite aspects of up and down, left and right, motion and stillness, exiting and entering, ascent and descent, darkness and brightness, day and night, cold and heat, or water and fire, etc. Take the seasonal variation as an example. In spring and summer it is warm and hot because the yang-heat qi becomes gradually predominant, suppressing the cool and cold qi of the autumn and winter; In autumn and winter it is cool and cold because the yin-cold qi becomes gradually predominant, suppressing the warm and hot qi of the spring and summer. From the Winter Solstice to the Beginning of Spring, yang qi waxes gradually while yin qi wanes accordingly. Yang qi reaches its prime in summer when yin qi hides inside. From the Summer Solstice to the Beginning of Autumn, yin qi waxes gradually while yang qi wanes accordingly. Yin qi reaches it prime in winter when yang qi hides inside. In such a cycle yang qi and yin qi wax and wane year in and year out. This is how the seasonal cycle of warm spring, hot summer, cool autumn and cold winter is explained by the relationship of mutual opposition and restriction between yin and yang.

The two opposite aspects of yin and yang are inter-restricted, so excessive exuberance of one side will inevitably lead to relative insufficiency of the other side. On the contrary, excessive debilitation of one side may also result in the relative hyperactivity of the opposite side. Such a change must be controlled within certain limits so as to maintain its relative dynamic equilibrium. If it gets out of control, the balance between yin and yang will be broken, causing relative exuberance or debilitation of yin and yang which points to the occurrence of diseases.

Daily Exercises

1. What are the initial connotations of yin and yang?
2. What are the attributes of yin and yang?
3. Why yin and yang are mutually opposite in nature?
4. Why yin and yang are mutually restricted in relationship?

The Essentials of Yin-Yang Theory

The interdependence and inter-promotion of yin and yang

Yin and yang are a unity of opposites. They are opposed to and, at the same time, depend on each other. Neither can exist in isolation. In other words, without yin there would be no yang, without the upper there would be no lower, and without cold there would be no heat, and vice versa. All of these indicate that yin and yang are inter-rooted, and the survival of one side relies on the existence of the other. Such a relation of interdependence is called inter-promotion between yin and yang by the ancient philosophers. On the basis of yin-yang interdependence, they are also inter-promoted and mutually reinforced. For instance, the ascent of earth-qi pertains to yang while the descent of heaven-rain to yin; water vapor rises with earth-qi and forms could, which is prerequisite to the descent of rain and this, in turn, may provide the preconditions for the re-ascent of earth-qi by replenishing the water-vapor on the ground. Substance pertains to yin whereas function to yang. They are inter-depended and inter-promoted for the reason that functional activities are the result of material movements while the composition of substance relies on the functional activities. Neither of them can exist in isolation.

Yin and yang depends on each other. Without yin, there would be no yang, and vice versa. If this relation is disrupted, it will lead to such a morbid condition described by the ancients as "solitary yin cannot generate and solitary yang cannot grow." When it comes to the human body, diseases may be induced or even life activities will be terminated as a result.

Waning-Waxing of Yin and Yang in a Balance

The inter-restriction, inter-dependence and inter-promotion between yin and yang are not invariable but in constant motion and change. This is called waxing-waning or balance of yin and yang. Such a balance is neither static nor absolute, but a relative equilibrium in which one waxes while the other wanes. This is completely consistent with the laws of motion which hold that movement is absolute while quiescence is relative, and waxing-waning is absolute while balance is relative. In other words, the absolute movement and relative quiescence do not preclude each other, nor do the absolute waxing-waning and relative balance contradict each other. In such a process, a myriad of things germinate, grow, and thrive constantly on earth. For example, seasonal variation from winter to spring and then to summer is a process of yin waning and yang waxing, with the weather turning from cold to warm and then to hot, whereas from summer to autumn and then to winter is a process of yang waning and yin waxing, with the weather turning from hot to cool and then to cold. The seasonal variations and weather changes, marked by either yin waning and yang waxing or yin waxing or yang waning, are in a relative and dynamic balance when viewed from the perspective of the climatic changes of the whole year.

Despite that waxing-waning is absolute and balance is relative, the importance and necessity of relative balance can never be neglected. Only through the synthetic action of both can things develop normally and may the human body maintain its proper life activities. If this relationship goes to extremes or beyond certain limits, the relative balance of yin and yang will be broken, leading to the relative exuberance or debilitation of yin and yang or the morbid waxing and waning of yin and yang.

Inter-Transformation Between Yin and Yang

This refers to the transformation of yin or yang into its opposite side under certain circumstances, namely yin transforming into yang or yang transforming into yin. It is an alternation of the overall attribute of yin or yang of things. Each thing is either yin or yang in nature, which is determined by whether yin or yang is in predominance. However, such a relation is not invariable, but in constant change which, beyond certain limits, may cause the change of things in nature from yin to yang or yang to yin. Hence, the alternation often occurs when it goes to extremes, which is known as "things always reverse their nature after reaching an extreme."

Take the seasonal variation again, when the climate changes from warm spring to hot summer, the trend will be reversed, as is signified by the appearance of cool autumn; and when cool autumn turns to cold winter, the weather may become warm again with the appearance of spring. Such a fundamental change will not occur if it does not go to extremes. So it is said in *Su Wen* (*Plain Conversation*, 素问) that "extreme cold produces heat, and extreme heat produces cold" and "extreme yin turns to yang, extreme yang turns to yin." Only when the development goes to extremes can fundamental change occur. This is also true for the alternation of day and night and the changes of weather in nature. In *Su Wen*, the ascent or descent of the heavenly qi and earthly qi is also indicative of the inter-transformation between yin and yang.

Many ancient philosophers have penetrating remarks on this point. For instance, Lao Zi said in *Dao De Jing* (*Classic of the Virtue of the Tao*) that fortune and misfortune go hand in hand, which clearly points out the fact that fortune and misfortune are mutually transformed. In *Su Wen*, it is indicated that life and death are inter-connected, and negative factors are contained in fresh things while positive factors are conceived in perishing things. All these transformations are realized through the process of constant motion, or incessant waning and waxing of yin and yang. In this sense, it is safe to say that interdependence between yin and yang is the intrinsic cause responsible for such a transformation while waxing and waning of yin and yang provides the essential conditions.

In conclusion, yin or yang is the relative attribute of things and can be subdivided infinitely. The inter-restriction, inter-dependence, inter-promotion, and inter-transformation of yin and yang are an illustration of the interaction between yin and yang which is not solitary and static, but inter-connected, inter-restricted and inter-produced. A good understanding of these basic points is helpful for the application of yin-yang theory in the practice of TCM.

Daily Exercises

1. What are inter-dependence and inter-promotion of yin and yang?
2. What are waxing-waning balance between yin and yang?
3. What is inter-transformation between yin and yang?

The Application of Yin-Yang Theory in TCM

The theory of yin-yang runs through the entire theoretical system of TCM, and is widely used to generalize the structure, physiology and pathology of the body as well as to direct clinical diagnosis and treatment.

For Generalization of the Organic Structure of the Body

Despite the fact that the human body is an organic whole, it can be divided into two aspects in opposition: yin and yang. This is based on the different attributes of the body constituents. In terms of position, the upper pertains to yang while the lower to yin; the exterior to yang while the interior to yin; the back to yang while the abdomen to yin; the lateral side of the four limbs to yang while the medial side to yin. In terms of the viscera, the five zang-organs pertain to yin for the reason that they store essence without discharging, while the six fu-organs to yang because they transport foodstuff without storing; among the five zang-organs, the heart and lung, located in the upper part (thoracic cavity), pertain to yang (yang within yin), and the spleen, liver and kidney, located in the lower part (abdominal cavity), pertain to yin (yin within yin). So each zang-organ can be subdivided into two aspects of yin and yang. All those with the functions of activating, warming and propelling pertain to yang, such as the heart yang, liver yang and kidney yang; all those with the functions of inhibiting, moistening and tranquilizing pertain to yin, such as the heart yin, liver yin and kidney yin. In terms of the basic substances constituting the human body, qi is intangible and pertains to yang, whereas blood and body fluid are tangible and pertain to yin. In a nutshell, the opposition and unity of yin and yang exist in all parts of the body, e.g., the upper and lower, interior and exterior, anterior and posterior, and the zang-organs and fu-organs.

For Generalization of the Physiological Functions of the Body

TCM holds that normal life activities of the human body are a result of the coordination between yin and yang in a unity of opposites. As far as the function and substance are concerned, the former pertains to yang and the latter to yin. And the functional activities can be subdivided into either yin or yang, e.g., ascending pertains to yang and descending to yin; exiting to yang and entering to yin; exiting to yang and inhibiting to yin; warming and propelling to yang while moistening and nourishing to yin; transforming of tangible substances into intangible qi pertains to yang while transforming of intangible qi to tangible substances pertains to yin. When it comes to the physiological activities of the human body, yang qi is predominant in the daytime which is marked by excitement; whereas yin qi is exuberant at night which is marked by inhibition. From midnight to midday, yang qi grows slowly and, at the same time, the physiological functions of the body change from inhibition to excitement, which is a process of yang waxing while yin waning; From midday to dusk, yang qi declines slowly while yin qi grows gradually and, at the same time, the physiological functions of the body change from excitement to inhibition, which is a process of yin waxing while yang waning. Others such as function and substance, as well as decomposition and composition, are constantly undergoing the process of either yang waxing while yin waning or yin waxing while yang waning. Such a dynamic balance is indispensable to normal life activities. The waxing-waning of yin and yang stems from the inter-restriction between yin and yang.

The inter-dependence and inter-promotion of yin and yang is prevalent in the physiological activities of the human body. For example, both qi and blood are basic substances for the composition of the body, and the former pertains to yang while the latter to yin. Qi can produce blood and promote blood circulation, whereas blood can house qi and nourish qi. Such a relationship is a typical illustration of the inter-dependence and inter-promotion of yin and yang. As for activation and inhibition, the basic functions indispensable for the life activities of the body, the former pertains to yang while the latter to yin. They are inter-dependent and inter-promoted. Without activation, there would be no inhibition. A well-functioned activation relies on adequate inhibition, and when activation is predominant, certain inhibitive factors still exist. Otherwise, it will lead to either depression or mania. Likewise, without inhibition, there would be no activation. Normal inhibition relies on sufficient activation, and when inhibition is predominant, certain active factors still exist.

Otherwise, it will lead to either insomnia and dreaminess or lethargy and coma. Another case in point is the relation between function and substance. The former pertains to yang and the latter to yin. Function is a result of the movements of substance, while substance relies on the functional activities for its composition. They are also interdependent and inter-promoted. *Huang Di Nei Jing* (*The Yellow Emperor's Canon of Medicine*, 黄帝内经) says, "yin dwells in the interior as the substantial base of yang; while yang is sent outside as the functional manifestation of yin." This remark highly generalized the interdependence and inter-promotion between substance and substance, function and function, or substance and function in the light of interdependence and inter-promotion of yin and yang.

For Generalization of the Pathological Changes of the Body

The theory of yin-yang holds that although the pathological manifestations of a disease are complicated and various, they can be generalized by imbalance of yin and yang in waxing-waning or inter-restriction, i.e., the relative exuberance or debilitation of yin and yang. Relative exuberance refers to that the predominance of either yin or yang leads to over-restriction or even impairment of the opposite side. For instance, when pathogenic yang-heat invades the body, it may cause relative excess of yang qi and damage of yin fluid. This is because yang is marked by heat while yin by cold, and if yang is in excess while yin is insufficient, there will be heat manifestations. By contrast, pathogenic yin-cold tends to damage yang qi and may lead to cold manifestations. This is called in *Nei Jing* that predominance of yin may lead to yang disorders and cold manifestations, whereas exuberance of yang can result in yin disorders and yang manifestations; Relative debilitation refers to that the weakness of either yin or yang leads to inadequate restriction or even relative hyperactivity of the opposite side. This is called in *Nei Jing* that deficiency of yin may lead to yang hyperactivity and heat manifestations, whereas deficiency of yang can result in yin exuberance and cold manifestations;

Since yin and yang are interdependent and inter-promoted, when the deficiency of yin or yang exceeds certain limits, the opposite side will inevitably be involved. For example, excessive deficiency of yin may fail to transform yang, leading to the insufficiency of yang at the same time. This is called "deficiency of yin involving yang." Similarly, excessive deficiency of yang may fail to produce yin, leading to the insufficiency of yin at the same time. This is called "deficiency of yang involving yin." The former can be exemplified by blood deficiency failing to nourish qi and leading to qi deficiency, while the latter is illustrated by qi deficiency failing to produce blood and leading to blood deficiency. Ultimately there will be simultaneous deficiency of yin and yang. If extreme deficiency of yin leads to collapse of yang, or extreme deficiency of yang lead to depletion of yin, the inter-dependence and inter-promotion of yin and yang will be seriously damaged, and the life activities of the human body will also be terminated. This is called in *Nei Jing* that disassociation of yin and yang will result in exhaustion of essence qi.

The pathological manifestations due to imbalance between yin and yang, under certain circumstances, may transform into their opposite aspects. For instance, in acute febrile diseases marked by high fever or severe toxicity, there may be such symptoms as shock, collapse, paleness or cyanotic complexion, cold limbs, profuse sweating and sudden dropping of body temperature, etc. This is a case in which yang or heat syndrome transforms into yin or cold syndrome. Conversely, cold syndrome can transform into heat syndrome. For example, under certain conditions, exterior-cold syndrome may transform into interior-heat one. Another point to consider is that in patients with mental disorders, the alternation of mania (yang syndrome) and depression (yin syndrome) often occurs. This is actually a pathological manifestation of inter-transformation between yin and yang. Such a transformation, however, necessitates certain conditions. Whether the healthy qi or pathogenic factors are strong or not, and whether the treatment is proper or not, can be the main factors responsible for the inter-transformation between yin and yang.

Daily Exercises

1. How to generalize the organic structure of the human body with the theory of yin-yang?

2. How to generalize the physiological functions of the human body with the theory of yin-yang?
3. How to generalize the pathological changes of the human body with the theory of yin-yang?

The Application of Yin-Yang Theory in TCM

An Overview of Exogenous Pathogenic Factors

In TCM, pathogenic wind, cold, summer-heat, dampness, dryness and fire are collectively called "six excesses." Due to their different natures and pathogenic characteristics, the six excess can be divided into either yin or yang, i.e., pathogenic wind, summer-heat, dryness and fire (heat) pertain to yang whereas pathogenic cold and dampness pertain to yin. Pathogenic yang tends to impair yin fluid, while pathogenic yin is apt to damage yang qi.

For Diagnosis of Diseases

Because the underlying factor responsible for the occurrence and development of diseases is imbalance between yin and yang, all the diseases, though complicated and changeable in clinical symptoms, can be generalized into either yin or yang, e.g., those with fever, agitation, dry stool, reddish and scanty urine, bright and lustrous complexion, loud and clear voice, and a floating, surging, slipping, rapid or excessive pulse pertain to yang; in contrast, those with intolerance of cold, depression, loose stool, clear and profuse urine, dark and lusterless complexion, low and faint voice, and a sinking, thin, rough, retard, and deficient pulse pertain to yin. In other words, those marked by fever, dark color, thick or sticky excreta or secreta, dry manifestations with yin damage, and agitation pertain to yang; these marked by cold manifestations, white or pale color, thin or loose excreta and secreta, moistening manifestations with internal retention of water-damp, and quiescence pertain to yin. Hence, it is self-evident that the differentiation of yin and yang is fundamental to the application of the four major diagnostic methods (inspecting, smelling and listening, inquiring, and pulse-taking). The correct differentiation of yin and yang, however, necessitates a good understanding of their attributes.

For Treatment of Diseases

Imbalance between yin and yang is the root for the occurrence and development of diseases. Therefore, restoring the relative balance between yin and yang by regulating yin and yang or supplementing the insufficiency and reducing the excess becomes the basic principle in the treatment of diseases. The theory of yin and yang is used in disease treatment by generalizing the nature of herbs and determining the principles of treatment.

1. *Generalization of the herbal nature*

The nature of a herb is determined by its property, flavor and functional tendencies of ascending, descending, floating and sinking. They can be generalized into either yin or yang. As for the four properties (cold, hot, warm and cool), cool and cold (cool is second to cold only in degree) pertain to yin while warm and hot (warm is second to hot only in degree) pertain to yang. Generally speaking, herbs with the function of alleviating or eliminating heat syndromes, such as Huangqi (Baical Skullcap Root) and Zhizi (Fructus Gardeniae), are cold or cool in nature. By contrast, herbs with the function of alleviating or eliminating cold syndromes, such as Fuzi (Prepared Common Monkshood Daughter) and Ganjiang (Dried Ginger), are warm or hot in nature. As for the five flavors, there are mainly pungency, sweetness, sourness, bitterness, and saltiness. Besides, there are bland taste and astringent taste, and the latter pertains to sourness. Different flavors have different actions marked by either yin or yang. Yin herbs are used for yang disorders while yang herbs for yin disorders. As for the functional tendencies of herbs, ascending and floating pertain to yang while sinking and descending to yin. In other words, those with the functions of ascending yang, dispersing, vomiting, and orifice-opening pertain to yang and are marked by upward and outward moving, as well as ascending and floating; and those with the function of clearing away heat, purging, subduing with heaviness, suppressing hyperactive yang, descending adverseness, and astringing pertain to yin and are marked by downward and inward moving, as well as sinking and descending.

2. Determination of therapeutic principles

Relative exuberance or excess of yin or yang can be treated by reducing the redundant, or purging the excess. For instance, cold due to predominance of yin can be treated with warm or hot herbs, which is called treating cold syndromes by warming; while heat due to predominance of yang can be treated by cool or cold herbs, which is also called treating heat syndromes by cooling. Relative debilitation or deficiency of yin or yang can be treated by supplementing or nourishing the insufficiency. For instance, heat due to deficiency of yin cannot be directly treated by cold herbs; rather, it should be treated by strengthening water and nourishing yin so as to suppress the hyperactive internal heat. This is called in *Nei Jing* that treating yang disorders from the perspective of yin, or by Wang Bing in the Tang dynasty that strengthening water-source to restrain yang-heat. Cold due to deficiency of yang cannot be directly treated by warm, hot or dispersing herbs; instead, it should be treated by strengthening fire and invigorating yang so as to suppress the hyperactive internal cold. This is called in *Nei Jing* that treating yin disorders from the perspective of yang, or by Wang Bing that strengthening the fire-source to dissipate yin-cold.

For treatment of relative debilitation of yin or yang, "seeking yin from yang" or "seeking yang from yin" proposed by Zhang Jingyue can be used, which is established on the basis of interdependence and inter-promotion between yin and yang. For example, patients with yang deficiency can be treated by adding proper amount of yin-nourishing herbs to yang-warming ones. This is called "seeking yang from yin," as is exemplified by You Gui Pill, a representative formula for warming and nourishing the kidney yang. In this formula, Shudi (prepared rhizome of rehmannia) is used in large quantity to obtain yang from yin. By contrast, patients with yin deficiency can be treated by adding proper amount of yang-warming herbs to yin-nourishing herbs. This is called "seeking yin from yang," as is exemplified by Zuo Gui Pill, a representative formula for nourishing the kidney yin. In this formula, Lujiaojiao (Deerhorn Glue), with the function of warming kidney yang, is used among the large quantity of yin-nourishing herbs to obtain yin from yang. Moreover, nourishing qi to produce blood and nourishing blood to invigorate qi are both methods established on the basis of interdependence and inter-promotion between yin and yang.

Daily Exercises

1. How to apply yin-yang theory in disease diagnosis?
2. How to apply yin-yang theory in generalizing exogenous pathogenic factors?
3. How to apply yin-yang theory in determining therapeutic principles?

CHAPTER 4

The Theory of Five Elements

The theory of five elements, an ancient Chinese philosophy, refers to a universe outlook and methodology for recognizing, interpreting and exploring the world and the natural laws by analogy with the characteristics and the inter-promotion or inter-restriction of the five substances in nature, namely wood, fire, earth, metal and water. This theory is evolved from "the theory of five directions" and "the theory of five materials." As early as the Yin Shang period, our ancestors have used the five directions, namely east, west, north, south and middle, to determine the spatial orientations. The five materials refer to water, fire, metal, wood and earth, which are daily necessities for life and work of the ancestors. By contrast, the five elements refer not only to the five substances of water, fire, metal, wood and earth, but also to the motion, change and interrelationship between them. Each of the five elements stands for a functional attribute, e.g., water is characterized by moistening and downward flowing, fire by flaming up, wood by growing freely and peripherally, metal by change, and earth by cultivation and reaping. The inter-promotion and inter-restriction of the five elements maintain their overall dynamic balance, and thus ensure the survival and development of things.

The theory of five elements holds that the world is in essence material and made-up of five basic substances, namely wood, fire, earth, metal and water. All the things in this world are produced and transformed through the "inter-mingling" and "inter-harmonizing" of these five basic elements. Hence, everything on earth or beyond can be reasoned out, deduced and classified in the light of five-element theory, and the inter-promotion and inter-restriction of the five elements are general laws for the motion, change and interrelation of various things in the universe.

This theory has a far-reaching influence on the theoretical systems of TCM, and as early as the period of *Nei Jing*, it has been frequently discussed and used in the medial field. It can be employed to recognize the correlation among the different parts of the body, or between parts and entirety, superficies and internal organs, as well as human body and external environment. The theory is also used to interpret the physiology and pathology of the body, and to direct clinical diagnosis and treatment. In this sense, it is undeniable that this theory has become an integral part of the theoretical systems of TCM.

The Essentials of Five-Element Theory

The Characteristics of Five Elements

In the long-term practice in life and work, the ancient people gradually accumulated a simple and plain recognition about the five basic materials of wood, fire, earth, metal and water, and abstracted them into concepts of reason. On such a basis, the characteristics of the five elements are generalized and used to classify different things and study the connections between them. Therefore, the characteristics of the five elements, though deprived from the five materials per se, have exceeded far beyond the original meanings and possessed a more extensive and abstract connotation.

1. *Wood is characterized by growing freely and peripherally*

This refers originally to the morphological characteristics of trees with luxuriant foliage and outreaching branches, and it was later used to describe traits such as growth, ascending, dispersing and smoothing. So anything with such characteristics or functions pertains to the category of wood.

2. *Fire is characterized by flaming-up*

This refers originally to the warmth of burning and ascending nature of fire, and was later used to generalize the things marked by warmth, hotness, and ascent, all of which pertain to fire.

3. *Earth is characterized by cultivation and reaping*

This refers originally to the growth and harvest of crops, and was later used to generalize the things marked by generating, transforming, supporting and receiving, all of which pertain to earth. The ancients deemed earth as the most important one among the five elements. As the saying goes, "earth supports water, air, fire and earth," "all things grow from earth," "all things may perish and be buried in earth" or "earth is the mother of all things."

4. *Metal is characterized by change and compliance*

It refers originally to the compliance of metal with man's will of casting it into weapons, or the change of metal from mineral. And later it was used to describe the things marked by purifying, eliminating, sinking and astringing, all of which pertain to metal.

5. *Water is characterized by moistening and flowing downward*

It was later used to describe the things marked by moistening, descending, cooling, and storing, all of which pertain to water.

The Classification of Things According to the Attributes of Five Elements by Analogy and Deduction

The theory of five elements is used to classify different things according to the attributes of the five elements, so the five-element attributes of things are not exactly identical with the characteristics of the wood, fire, earth, metal and water per se. They are, as a matter of fact, an analogy or deduction of the basic traits of these five materials. There are two specific methods for this process: one is by analogy, the other is by deduction. The former is conducted by first finding the specific features of things (form, function and nature) which can reflect their essence, and then make a comparison between these features and the five-element attributes so as to determine their classification. For instance, the sun rises in the east, which is similar to wood marked by ascending and dispersing, so the east pertains to wood; the south is characterized by hotness, which is similar to fire with the tendency of flaming up, so the south pertains to fire; the sun sets in the west, which is similar to metal marked by sinking and descending, so the west pertains to metal; the north is characterized by cold, which is similar to water with the feature of cold and storage, so the north pertains to water; and in the middle plain area, the soil is fertile and all things flourish, which is similar to earth marked by supporting and generating, so the middle pertains to earth. The latter refers to the determination of the five-element attributes of some things by deducing from other things of which the five-element attributes are already known. For instance, if we have already known that long summer (June in lunar calendar, or the interval between summer and autumn) pertains to earth, then it can be deduced that dampness also pertains to earth because it is predominant in the long summer; likewise, autumn pertains to metal, so dryness also pertains to metal given the fact that it is predominant in the autumn; the liver pertains to wood, so the gallbladder, tendons, eyes, tear, and anger also pertain to metal given that the liver is internally and externally connected with the gallbladder, governs tendons, has its outward luster on the nails, opens into the eyes, is associated with tears in fluids and anger in emotions; the heart pertains to fire, so it can be deduced that the small intestine, vessels, complexion, tongue, sweat and joy also pertain to fire for the same reason; the spleen pertains to earth, so it can be deduced that the stomach, muscles, lips, mouth, slobber, and thinking also pertain to earth; the lung pertains to metal, so it can be deduced that the large intestine, skin, hair, nose, snivel, and worry also pertain to metal; the kidney pertains to water, so it can be deduced that the urinary bladder, bones, hair, ears, two lower orifices, saliva and terror also pertain to water. Now the five-element attributes of things or phenomena related to nature and the human body are listed as follows.

Daily Exercises

1. According to the theory of five elements, which are the five basic substances that constitute the world?
2. What are the characteristics of the five elements?
3. How many methods are there in classifying the various things according to the attributes of the five elements?

Weekly Review

The theory of yin and yang, an ancient philosophical thought in China, is a world outlook and methodology for the ancients to recognize and explain the world. It holds that all things in the universe can be generalized into either yin or yang, and each thing or object can be divided into yin or yang, which can also be subdivided into to yin or yang. Yin and yang are inter-restricted, interdependent, inter-transformed and constantly waxing and waning in a delicate balance. Interaction between yin and yang is carried out incessantly. It may be manifested as mutual restriction, interdependence, mutual waning and waxing, inter-transformation and inter-preponderance, etc. Yin and yang are both inter-opposite and inter-restricted, such as the upper and down, left and right, motion and stillness, or cold and heat, etc. All of them are manifestations of inter-opposition and inter-restriction of yin and yang. However, relative exuberance or debilitation of one side will inevitably lead to the relative insufficiency or hyperactivity of the other, so the waxing-waning due to inter-restriction of yin and yang should be kept within certain limits and otherwise, there may be imbalanced situations such as relative exuberance or debilitation of yin and yang.

The interdependence and inter-promotion of yin and yang means that neither yin nor yang can exist in isolation. If this relationship is disrupted, it will lead to a morbid condition described by the ancients as "solitary yin cannot generate and solitary yang cannot grow." The waning-waxing of yin and yang in a balance indicates that movement is absolute while quiescence is relative, and waxing-waning is absolute while balance is relative. If this relationship goes to extremes and beyond certain limits, the relative balance of yin and yang will be broken, leading to the relative exuberance or debilitation of yin and yang and the morbid waxing and waning of yin and yang. The inter-transformation between yin and yang refers to the transformation of yin or yang into its opposite side under certain circumstances. Interdependence between yin and yang is the intrinsic cause responsible for such a transformation while waxing and waning of yin and yang provides the essential conditions. A good understanding of these basic points is helpful for the application of yin-yang theory in the practice of TCM.

The theory of yin-yang runs through the entire theoretical system of TCM, and is widely used to generalize the structure, physiology and pathology of the body as well as to direct clinical diagnosis and treatment. Despite the fact that the human body is an organic whole, it can be divided into two aspects in opposition: yin and yang. This is based on the different attributes of the body constituents. TCM holds that the normal life activities of the human body are a result of the coordination between yin and yang in a unity of opposites. As far as the function and substance are concerned, the former pertains to yang and the latter to yin. And the functional activities can be subdivided into either yin or yang, e.g., exciting pertains to yang and inhibiting to yin. Waxing-waning of yin and yang, stems from the inter-restriction between yin and yang. The inter-dependence and inter-promotion of yin and yang is prevalent in the physiological activities of the human body. For example, both qi and blood are basic substances for the composition of the body, and the former pertains to yang while the latter to yin. Qi can produce blood and promote blood circulation, whereas blood can house qi and nourish qi. Such a relationship is a typical illustration of the inter-dependence and inter-promotion of yin and yang. As for activation and inhibition, the basic functions indispensable for the life activities of the body, the former pertains to yang while the latter to yin. They are inter-dependent and inter-promoted. *Nei Jing* says, "yin dwells in the interior as the substantial base of yang; while yang is sent outside as the functional manifestation of yin." This remark highly generalized the inter-dependence and inter-promotion between substance and substance, between function and function, or between substance and function in the light of yin-yang inter-dependence and inter-promotion.

The theory of yin-yang holds that although the pathological manifestations of a disease are complicated and various, they can be generalized by the relative exuberance or debilitation of yin and yang. Relative exuberance refers to that the predominance of either yin or yang leads to over-restriction or even impairment of the opposite side. Relative debilitation refers to that the weakness of either yin or yang leads to inadequate-restriction or even relative hyperactivity of the opposite side. When the deficiency of yin or yang exceeds certain limits, its opposite will inevitably be involved, leading to "deficiency of yin involving yang" or "deficiency of yang involving yin" and ultimately simultaneous deficiency of yin and yang. The pathological manifestations due to imbalance between yin and yang, under certain circumstances, may transform into their opposite aspects.

All the diseases, although complicated and various in clinical symptoms, can be generalized into either yin or yang, e.g., those with fever and dry stool pertain to yang; by contrast, those with intolerance of cold and loose stool pertain to yin. So the differentiation of yin and yang is fundamental in carrying out the four major diagnostic methods (inspecting, smelling and listening, inquiring, and pulse-taking). The correct differentiation of yin and yang, however, necessitates a good understanding of their attributes. Imbalance between yin and yang is the fundamental cause for the occurrence and development of diseases. Therefore, restoring the relative balance between yin and yang by regulating yin and yang or supplementing the insufficiency and reducing the excess becomes the basic principle in the treatment of diseases. The theory of yin and yang is used in disease treatment by generalizing the nature of herbs and determining the therapeutic principles. The nature of an herb is determined by its property, flavor and functional tendencies of ascending, descending, floating and sinking; all of them can be generalized into either yin or yang. Cool and cold pertain to yin while warm and hot pertain to yang. As for the functional tendencies, ascending and floating pertain to yang while sinking and descending to yin, etc. There are many therapeutic methods established based on the theory of yin and yang, such as reducing the redundant, purging the excess, cooling the hot, warming the cold, strengthening water-source to restrain yang-heat, strengthening the fire-source to dissipate yin-cold, seeking yin from yang and seeking yang from yin, etc.

The theory of five elements, an ancient Chinese philosophy, refers to a universe outlook and methodology for recognizing, interpreting and exploring the world and the natural laws by analogy with the characteristics and the inter-promotion or inter-restriction of the five substances in nature, namely wood, fire, earth, metal and water. The theory of five elements holds that the world is in essence material and made-up of five basic substances, namely wood, fire, earth, metal and water. In the long-term life and work of the ancient people, they gradually accumulated a plain recognition about the five basic materials of wood, fire, earth, metal and water, and abstracted them into concepts of reason. On such a basis, the characteristics of the five elements are generalized and used to classify different things and study the connection between them. Therefore, the characteristics of the five elements, though deprived from the five materials per se, have gone far beyond their original meanings and possessed a more extensive and abstract connotation. For instance, wood is characterized by growing freely and peripherally, and it is often used to describe traits such as growth, ascending, dispersing and smoothing. So anything with such characteristics or functions pertains to the category of wood. Fire is characterized by flaming-up, and it is often used to generalize the things marked by warmth, hotness, and ascent, all of which pertain to fire. Earth is characterized by cultivation and reaping, and it is often used to generalize the things marked by generating, transforming, supporting and receiving, all of which pertain to earth. Metal is characterized by change and compliance, and it is often used to describe the things marked by purifying, sinking and astringing, all of which pertain to metal. Water is characterized by moistening and flowing downward, and it is often used to describe the things marked by moistening, descending, cooling, and storing, all of which pertain to water. The theory of five elements is used to classify different things according to the attributes of the five elements, and there are two specific methods: one is by analogy, the other is by deduction.

Daily Exercises

1. To master the basic content of yin-yang theory
2. To mater the application of yin-yang theory in TCM.
3. How many specific methods of classifying things by deduction or analogy according to the theory of five elements?

THE THIRD WEEK

The Essentials of Five-Element Theory

Inter-Generation, Inter-Restriction, Over-Restriction and Counter-Restriction of the Five Elements

The correlation between things and the five elements are not static and isolated. The inter-generation and inter-restriction of the five elements are used to explore and explain the association, coordination and unification of things. Besides, the over-restriction and counter-restriction of the five elements are also used to explore and explain the interaction among things after the disruption of balance. These are the main functions of the inter-generation, inter-restriction, over-restriction and counter-restriction of the five elements.

1. *Inter-generation*

Inter-generation, or mutual promotion, refers to that one kind of object generates, reinforces and brings forth another in a fixed sequence, i.e., wood generates fire, fire generates earth, earth generates metal, metal generates water, and water, in turn, generates wood. So inter-generation cannot be simply viewed as a disordered two-way interaction, but an orderly and endless cycle. Each of the five elements is marked by such relations as "being generated" and "generating." This relationship of the five elements is called the "mother-child" relationship. For example, wood generates fire, so it is the element generating; fire generates earth, so earth is the element being generated. It can concluded that wood is the mother of fire and earth is the child of fire. Wood and fire form a relationship of mother-child, so do fire and earth.

2. *Inter-restriction*

Inter-restriction, or mutual restraint, implies suppression or inhibition. Inter-restriction of the five elements refers to the alternate restricting activity among wood, fire, earth, metal and water in a circular order: wood restricting earth, earth restricting water, water restricting fire, fire restricting metal, metal restricting wood, and wood, in turn, restricting earth. So inter-restriction cannot be simply viewed as a disordered two-way interaction, but an orderly and endless cycle. That is to say, wood, fire, earth, metal and water restrict one another alternately. In this circular order, each of the five elements is marked by "being restricted" and "restricting." The former refers to the element that is not restraining, and the latter refers to the element that is restraining. For example, wood restricts earth, so the element restricting is wood, and earth is the element that is restrained by wood. And metal restricts wood, so wood is the element being restricted, and metal is the element that is not retrained by wood.

The theory of five elements believes that the inter-generation and inter-restriction are two aspects indispensable to the maintenance of normal relationship among different things. Without inter-generation there would be no birth and development, and without inter-restriction there would be disasters due to excessive growth. Both are opposite and complementary to each other, thus maintaining coordination and balance among things. As far as the relation of the five elements are concerned, generation is contained in restriction, and restriction is conceived in generation, e.g., wood generates fire, fire generates earth, and earth generates metal, whereas wood restricts earth, metal restricts wood, wood restricts earth, earth restricts water and, moreover, water generates wood, and fire generates earth. Wood, fire, earth, metal and water generate one another one by one, but restrict one another alternately. So generation and restriction are intermingled and interacted in an endless cycle.

3. *Over-restriction*

Over-restriction, or subjugation, refers to the launching of an attack on a counterpart when it is weak. In five elements, it means the excessive restriction of one element on another in the same circular order as inter-restriction: wood over-restricting earth, earth over-restricting water, water over-restricting fire, fire over-restricting metal, and metal over-restricting wood. This is due to either "over-action" or "under-action." The former means that one element is hyperactive, and thus may restrict another element excessively, leading to the deficiency of this element as well as abnormal interaction of the five elements. For example, under normal circumstances, wood restricts earth in a proper manner; however, if wood is hyperactive and restricts earth excessively, earth will be subjugated and debilitated under the over-restriction of wood. This is called "wood over-restricting earth due to hyperactivity of wood." The latter means that one element is too weak to resist the normal restriction by its restraining element, and thereby becomes more debilitated. Take wood restricting earth again, under normal circumstances, wood restricts earth in a proper manner. However, if earth is too weak to withstand the normal restriction by wood, the restraining force will become relatively stronger and the restricted earth will become relatively deficient. This is called "wood over-restricting earth due to deficiency of earth." Although restriction and over-restriction are identical in sequence, they vary in that the former functions in a proper manner whereas the latter takes place under abnormal conditions. So it is called "over-restriction" or "subjugation" instead of "restriction."

4. *Counter-restriction*

Counter-restriction, or reverse-restriction, literally means the strong bullies the weak. In five elements, it refers to the restriction of one element on another in an opposite order. The counter-restriction of five elements follows such an order that wood counter-restricts metal, metal counter-restricts fire, fire counter-restricts water, water counter-restricts earth, and earth, in turn, counter-restricts wood. Similar to over-restriction, there are two aspects causing counter-restriction: "over-action" and "under-action." The former means that when one element is hyperactive, it may restrict the element originally being the restricting one. For example, when wood is hyperactive, it may restrict metal which, under normal circumstances, is supposed to restrain wood; this is called "wood counter-restricting metal." The latter means that when one element is too weak, it may not only fail to restrict the next element, but also be counter-restricted by this element which, under normal conditions, is supposed to be restrained. For instance, normally metal restricts wood, and wood restricts earth; however, if wood is too weak, it may not only be over-restricted by metal, but also be counter-restricted by earth, which is called "earth counter-restricting wood."

Over-restriction and counter-restriction are both abnormal restrictions due to the damaged interaction among the five elements. Both of them can be caused by "over-action" or "under-action" of any of the five elements.

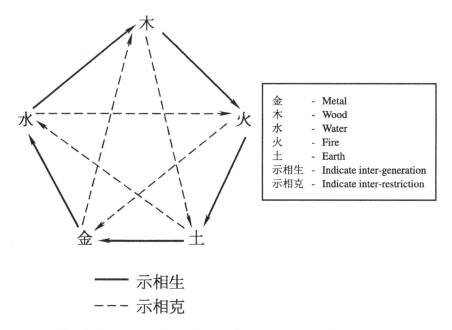

Fig. 1 Inter-generation and inter-restriction among the five elements.

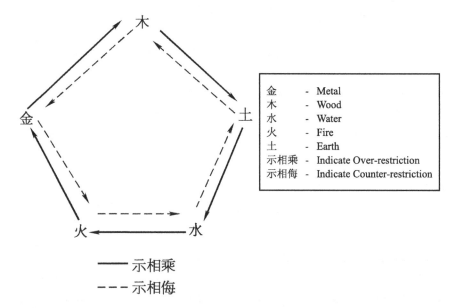

Fig. 2 Over-restriction and counter-restriction among the five elements.

Over-restriction and counter-restriction have similarities as well as differences. They differ in that the former follows the normal order of inter-restriction whereas the latter is in the opposite order. They are similar in that over-restriction and counter-restriction take place synchronically, and in essence, they are two sides to the same coin.

Daily Exercises

1. What is inter-generation of five elements?
2. What is inter-restriction of five elements?
3. What is over-restriction of five elements?
4. What is counter-restriction of five elements?

The Application of Five-Element Theory in TCM

The theory of five elements is used in TCM to classify the viscera and meridians into five categories and explain their characteristics according to the properties of the five elements, to analyze the relationships among the viscera, meridians and various physiological functions according to the inter-generation and inter-restriction of five elements, and to explain their interactions under pathological conditions according to the over-restriction and counter-restriction of five elements.

To Explain the Physiological Function of the Five Zang-Organs

Each of the internal organs, according to the theory of five elements, pertains to one of the five elements. So their physiological functions are illustrated by the characteristics of the five elements. For example, the liver prefers to grow freely and dislikes depression, and can regulate qi and blood as well as emotions, so it pertains to wood marked by growing, ascending, dispersing and free-reaching; the heart yang has the function of warming, so it pertains to fire marked by warming, heating and ascending. The spleen, as the source of qi and blood, can transport and transform water and food into nutrients for the nourishment of the viscera, limbs and bones, so it pertains to earth marked by generating and supporting a myriad of things. The lung, characterized by purifying and descending, takes the downward action as the normal tendency, so it pertains to metal marked by clarifying, descending, and astringing. The kidney stores essence and controls water, so it pertains to water marked by moistening, descending and storing.

In addition to explaining the physiological functions of the five zang-organs, the theory of five elements is also used for analyzing the various structures, tissues and functions of the entire body by analogy and deduction. At the same time, it is further extended to correlate the five orientations, five seasons, five properties, five flavors and five colors in nature with the five zang-organs, six fu-organs, five sensory organs and five body constituents of the human body. In such a manner the internal environment and external environment of the body are connected into an entirety. Take the liver as an example, it says in *Su Wen*, "the east engenders wind, wind generates wood, wood produces sourness, sourness forms liver, liver controls eyes and gives birth to tendon, and tendon promotes heart." That is how the east, spring, wind and sourness in nature are correlated with wood in five elements and liver, tendons and eyes in the human body, indicating the holistic concept of correspondence between man and nature.

To Explain the Inter-Connection Among the Five Zang-Organs

The functional activities of the five zang-organs are not isolated, but interconnected. The attribution of the five zang-organs to the five elements is helpful for the discussion of the functional characteristics of the five zang-organs, as well as the intrinsic connection among the physiological functions of the viscera. The five elements are inter-generated and inter-restricted, so are the five zang-organs.

1. *The Inter-Generation of the Five Zang-Organs*

Liver promoting heart, or wood generating fire, means that the liver stores blood to nourish the heart. Heart promoting spleen, or fire generating earth, means that the heart yang warms the spleen earth so as to facilitate its transportation and transformation. Spleen promoting lung, or earth generating metal, means spleen qi disperses nutrients over the lung. Lung promoting kidney, or metal generating water, means the lung qi flows downward to regulate waterways and facilitate the kidney water. Kidney promoting liver, or water generating wood, means the kidney stores essence to nourish liver blood.

2. *The inter-restriction of the five elements*

Liver restraining spleen, or wood restricting earth, means the free flow of liver qi helps to unblock the stagnation of the spleen earth. Spleen retraining kidney, or earth restricting water, means the spleen transforms water and dampness to prevent kidney water from overflowing. Kidney restraining heart, or water restricting fire, means the upward flow of kidney water for curbing heart fire. Heart restraining lung, or fire restricting metal, means that the warmth of heart fire is helpful for the dispersion of lung qi and may prevent it from excessive descent. Lung restraining liver, or metal restricting wood, means lung qi moves downward to prevent over-ascent of the liver qi.

It should be pointed out that the physiological functions of the five zang-organs and their inter-generation and inter-restriction are illustrated through the characteristics of the five elements and their interactions. Despite all of these, the functions of the five zang-organs, and their relations, are very complicated. So the characteristics of the five elements cannot cover all the functions of the five zang-organs, nor can the interactions among the five elements explain all the intricate physiological relations among the five zang-organs. Therefore, when studying the intrinsic connection and regulatory mechanism of the physiological functions of the viscera, we cannot confine our attention only to the inter-generation and inter-restriction of the five elements.

To Illustrate the Pathological Interaction Among the Five Zang-Organs

The theory of five elements is not only used to indicate the inter-connection among the viscera under physiological conditions, but also used to explain the interaction among the viscera under pathological circumstances. The disorder of one organ may be transmitted to another. This pathological interaction is called transmission, which is divided into two types: inter-generation transmission and inter-restriction transmission.

1. *Inter-generation transmission*

This refers to the disorder of one organ that may be transmitted to another organ in the order of inter-generation of the five elements: from liver to heart, spleen, and lung, then to kidney, and finally to liver, again. In a specific disease, there are often such an inter-generation relationship between two organs, i.e., mutual transmission between the mother organ and the child organ, including "mother organ involving child organ" and "child organ involving mother organ." Mother organ involving child organ refers to the transmission of disease from the mother organ to the child organ. For example, the kidney pertains to water and the liver to wood, so the kidney is the mother organ and the liver is the child organ; if the kidney disease involves the liver, this is regarded as mother organ involving child organ. A case in point is "water failing to nourish wood," which is very common clinically. This is due to deficient kidney water that fails to nourish the liver yin, leading to yin deficiency of both the liver and the kidney as well as hyperactivity of liver yang, which is called "water failing to nourish wood." Child organ involving mother organ refers to the transmission of disease from the child organ to the mother organ. For example, the liver pertains to wood and the heart to fire, so the kidney is the mother organ and the liver is the child organ because wood produces fire; if the heart disease involves the liver, this is regarded as child organ involving mother organ. Blood deficiency of heart and liver or fire hyperactivity of heart and liver, which are very common clinically, are both classified into this category. This is due to that deficient heart blood fails to nourish the liver yin, leading to blood deficiency of the liver and heart, or due to that hyperactive heart fire involves the liver, leading to fire hyperactivity of both heart and liver.

2. *Inter-restriction transmission*

This refers to the disorder of one organ that may be transmitted to another organ in the order of inter-restriction of the five elements: from liver to spleen, from spleen to kidney, from kidney to heart, from heart to lung, and finally, from lung to liver. This usually takes place between two organs that are mutually restricted. Such a transmission is divided into two types: "over-restriction" transmission in the normal order of inter-restriction of the five elements and "counter-restriction" transmission in the reverse order of inter-restriction of the five elements.

Over-restriction means the excessive restraint of one element one another. There are mainly two reasons for over-restriction among the five zang-organs: one is due to that the restricting organ is so hyperactive that it restricts another organ excessively; the other is due to that the restricted organ is too weak to withstand the excessive inhibition of the restricting organs. For example, as far as the relation between the liver wood and spleen earth are concerned, there are mainly two types: "hyperactive wood over-restricts earth" (hyperactive liver over-restricts spleen) and "deficiency of earth incurs over-restriction of wood" (deficiency of spleen incurs over-restriction of liver). It is generally called "hyperactive wood over-restricting earth" when the stagnation of liver qi impairs the transportation and trans-formation of the spleen and stomach, leading to fullness and distension in the chest and hypochondria, distending pain in the gastric and abdominal region, bitterness sensation in the mouth, acid regurgitation, belching, nausea, and loose stool, etc. By contrast, if the spleen and stomach are too weak to bear the restriction of the liver, leading to dizziness, lassitude, indigestion, belching, fullness and distension in the chest and hypochondria, distending pain in the gastric and abdominal region, rugitus and diarrhea, this is called "deficiency of earth incurring over-restriction of wood."

Counter-restriction means the reverse restraint of one element on another. There are mainly two reasons for counter-restriction among the five zang-organs: over-action and under-action. For instance, the lung-metal is supposed to restrict the liver-wood, but when the liver qi rises adversely and liver fire burns hyperactively, the lung metal will be counter-restricted by liver wood instead of restricting it. This is called "hyperactive wood counter-restricting metal" or "hyperactive wood fire scorching metal." Clinically there will be adverse rising of liver qi and hyperactive of liver fire due to sudden, intense anger, marked by irascibility, reddened complexion and eyes, fullness and distension in the chest and hypochondria, or even cough with dyspnea, sputum with blood and hemoptysis, etc. Counter-restriction due to under-action refers to the reverse inhibition on the organ that is supposed to be the restricting one by the organ that is supposed to be the restricted one due to the weakness of the former. For instance, if the spleen-earth cannot inhibit the kidney-water, there will be such symptoms as general edema. This is called "deficiency of earth incurring counter-restriction by water."

In a nutshell, the pathological interaction among the five zang-organs can be illustrated by the over-restriction, counter-restriction and mother-child relation of the five elements. If the disease transmits in the order of inter-generation, it is a relatively mild one when the mother organ involves the child organ; however, when the child organ involves the mother organ, it will be a relatively severe one. Contrarily, if the disease transmits in the order of inter-restriction, it is a relatively severe one when there is over-restriction and a milder one when there is counter-restriction. Nevertheless, the inter-generation and inter-restriction of the five elements cannot be used to explain all the complicated physiological relations among the five zang-organs, and similarly, the over-restriction, counter-restriction and mother-child relation of the five elements cannot be used to illustrate all the pathological interactions among the five zang-organs. So clinically we should proceed from practice so as to truly command the transmission patterns of disease.

Daily Exercises

1. How to describe the inter-generation and inter-restriction of the five elements?
2. What is transmission in the order of inter-generation?
3. What is transmission in the order of inter-restriction?

The Application of Five-Element Theory in TCM

For Diagnosis of Diseases

The human body is an organic entirety, the internal disorders of which must be manifested externally. The manifestations may be various. The abnormal changes of the functional activities of the viscera and their interrelations can be reflected on the corresponding tissues and organs of the superficies, marked by morbid changes in color, luster, voice, shape, and pulse. The five zang-organs have specific connections with the five colors, five sounds, and five flavors. Such a hierarchic classification of the five-zang system provides the theoretical foundation for the clinical diagnosis of diseases. Hence, during the clinical diagnosis, the information collected through the synthetic application of inspecting, listening and smelling, inquiring and pulse-taking can be used to deduce the disease conditions in the light of five-element attribution and the inter-generation, inter-restriction, over-restriction and counter-restriction of the five elements.

1. *For inspection of the complexion*

Each of the five zang-organs are associated with a certain type of color, i.e., the liver is associated with blue, heart with red, spleen with yellow, lung with white, and kidney with black. This is determined by the five-element attribution. So clinically the changes of facial color may indicate the disorder of a certain organ, e.g., facial colors such as blue, red, yellow, white and black are indicative of disorders in the liver, heart, spleen, lung and kidney, respectively. Besides, the changes in color can also be used to infer the transmission of diseases among the zang-organs. For example, if blue color is shown in spleen diseases, it is mostly due to "hyperactive wood over-restricting earth" or "over-restriction of wood due to deficiency of earth:" if black complexion is shown in heart diseases, it is mostly due to "water over-restricting fire." The prognosis of diseases may be deduced from the inter-generation and inter-restriction among the five colors. When the facial color is inconsistent with the disease, this is called color-disease contradiction in which colors in an inter-generation relationship indicate a favorable prognosis while colors in a inter-restriction relationship signify an unfavorable turn. For instance, liver disease with blue complexion, called correspondence between color and disease, is a common manifestation. However, if the complexion turns black (water generating wood) or red (wood generating fire), the prognosis is favorable although the color contradicts the disease because there are inter-generation between the color and the disease. If the complexion turns yellow (wood restricting earth) or white (metal restricting wood), the prognosis is unfavorable because there are inter-restriction between the two. In favorable cases, color generating disease indicates the positive of fortune; whereas disease generating color signifies the negative of fortune.

In unfavorable diseases, color restricting disease indicates the negative of misfortune, whereas disease restricting color signifies the positive of misfortune. This is also applicable to other viscera. The diagnostic signifi-cance of five colors and their application in predicting disease prognosis according to the inter-generation and inter-restriction of the five elements bear certain theoretical and practical value. It is very common clinically that kidney deficiency leads to a black complexion and spleen deficiency results in a yellow one. Nevertheless, some deductions from this theory are not congruent with practical manifestations, so clinically this method should be used flexibly and be combined with the four major diagnostic methods so as to achieve a satisfactory therapeutic effect.

2. *For inquiry of flavors*

The abnormal changes of flavors are also pathological manifestations of the five zang-organs, so the organs in disorder can be deduced from the five-element attribution: sourness pertains to liver, bitterness to heart, sweetness to spleen, pungency to lung and saltiness to kidney. Therefore, sourness in the mouth indicates hyperactivity of liver fire (hyperactive liver fire invading stomach); bitterness in the mouth indicates relative exuberance of heart fire; sweetness in the mouth indicates obstruction of dampness in the spleen (or Pi Dan); pungency in the mouth indicates dis-order of the lung metal (unusual in the clinic); and saltiness in the mouth indicates deficiency of the kidney. The diagnostic significance of five flavors is much valued clinically. For example, if pathogenic dampness accumulates in the spleen and stomach and turbid qi flows upward to the mouth, there will be sweet and greasy flavor in the mouth; if heat accu-mulates in the liver and stomach and goes upward to the mouth, there will be sourness sensation in the mouth; if kidney yang is deficient with upward flowing of cold water, there will salty flavor in the mouth. There are also conditions in which the same abnormal flavor indicates more than one disease, e.g., bitterness in the mouth can be seen in up-flaming of heart fire, or up-flowing of gallbladder qi (because bile is bitter in flavor), or even all the fire-heat syndromes.

3. *For combined diagnosis of color and pulse*

Combined diagnosis of color and pulse refers to the judgment of progno-sis of diseases through the generation and inter-restriction between color and pulse. Generally speaking, liver disease with blue color and taut pulse is marked by correspondence between color and pulse; if there is floating pulse instead of the taut one, the prognosis will be unfavorable because the pulse restricts the color (metal restricts wood); if there is sinking pulse, the prognosis will be favorable because the pulse promotes the color (water generates wood). This is also applicable to other zang-organs. Despite its diagnostic significance, this method cannot replace the synthetic application of the four major diagnostic methods in the clinical judgment of prognosis for the reason that it is not invariably correct.

Daily Exercises

1. Explain why disordered viscera can be identified by examining the changes of facial color and luster?
2. What are the viscera pathological states of which can be indicated by the unusual changes of oral flavors?
3. What is combined diagnosis of color and pulse?

The Application of Five-Element Theory in TCM

For Treatment of Diseases

The application of the five-element theory in TCM is mainly reflected in directing visceral medication, controlling disease transmission, and determining therapeutic principles and methods, etc.

1. Directing visceral medication

Different herbs have different colors and flavors. Colors include blue, red, yellow, white and black, while flavors include sourness, bitterness, sweetness, pungency and saltiness. The correlation of the five colors and five flavors with the five zang-organs are based on the natural property, function and attribution of the herbs according to characteristics of the five elements. To be specific, the five colors of blue, red, yellow, white and black and the five flavors of sourness, bitterness, sweetness, pungency and saltiness pertain to the liver, heart, spleen, lung and kidney, respectively.

Baishao (White peony Alba) is white in color, sour in flavor and attributed to the liver meridian, so it can nourish the liver; Zhusha (Cinnabar) is red in color and attributed to the heart meridian, so it can tranquilize the heart; Shigao (Gypsum) is white in color, pungent in flavor and attributed to the lung meridian, so it can clear away lung-heat; Huanglian (Golden Thread) is bitter in flavor, so it is used for clearing away lung-heat; Baizhu (Largehead Atractylodes Rhizome) is yellow in color and sweet in flavor, so it is used for nourishing spleen qi; Xuanshen (Figwort Root) is black in color and salty in flavor, so it is used for nourishing the kidney yin, etc. Clinically the medication for visceral diseases should be conducted in the light of the four properties (cold, hot, warm and cool) and functional tendencies (ascending, descending, floating and sinking) of the herbs in addition to their five colors and five flavors.

2. *Controlling disease transmission*

Disorder of one zang-organ may be transmitted to other zang-organs following the order of inter-generation or inter-restriction of the five elements. During the treatment, not only the organ in disorder is regulated but also other related organs are coordinated according to the inter-generation, inter-restriction, over-restriction, and counter-restriction of the five elements. Reducing the excess and nourishing the insufficient are often used to control the transmission and recover their normal activities. For example, hyperactivity of liver wood may over-restrict spleen earth, so according to the sequence of inter-restriction, the spleen earth can be nourished beforehand to prevent it from being over-restricted by liver wood. In this way the disease will discontinue the transmission and be cured eventually. Apparently it is actually a preventive measure with great therapeutic significance. It is clear that nourishing the spleen to treat the liver, a therapeutic principle for controlling disease transmission, is established on the basis of over-restriction of the five elements. The factors responsible for disease transmission are multi-faceted, and the principal one is the functional conditions of the viscera, i.e., if the zang-organs are in deficiency, the transmission will proceed, and if in excess, the transmission will stop.

3. *Determining therapeutic principles and methods*

The therapeutic principles and methods can be established according to the inter-generation or inter-restriction of the five elements.

(1) The therapeutic principles established according to the inter-generation of the five elements are nourishing the mother in the case of deficiency and reducing the child in the case of excess. The former means that a deficiency syndrome is treated by nourishing not only the organ in deficiency, but also its mother organ (the generating zang-organ), thus facilitating its recovery through the action of inter-promotion. For instance, in the case of deficiency of liver yin-blood, not only the liver is nourished, but also the kidney is supplemented, thus the liver disease can be cured thought the mechanism of water generating wood. The latter means that an excess syndrome is treated by purging not only the organ in excess, but also its child organ (the generated zang-organ), thus reducing the excess through the mechanism that qi of one organ is housed in its child-organ. For instance, in the case of hyperactivity of liver fire, not only the liver fire is purged, but also the heart fire is subdued because "the heart receives qi from the liver" and "the liver qi is housed in the heart."

(2) Commonly the therapeutic methods established according to the inter-generation of the five elements are as follows:

Replenishing water to nourish wood: It refers to the method of replenishing kidney yin to nourish liver yin, applicable to the syndrome of liver-yin deficiency or liver-yang hyperactivity due to insufficiency of kidney yin.

Invigorating fire to reinforce earth: It refers to the method of warming kidney yang to supplement spleen yang, applicable to the syndrome of spleen-yang inactivation due to insufficiency of kidney yang. What must be mentioned here is that the heart pertains to fire and spleen to earth, so originally fire failing to generate earth means that heart-fire fails to promote spleen-earth. However, since the emergence of life-gate theory, it gradually refers to that the life-gate fire, or kidney yang, fails to warm the spleen-earth.

Reinforcing earth to generate metal: It refers to the method of invigorating spleen qi to nourish lung qi, applicable to the syndrome of lung-qi deficiency, with or without malfunction of the spleen in transformation.

Mutual generation of metal and water: it refers to a method of mutual nourishment of the kidney yin and the lung yin. The lung pertains to metal and kidney to water, so the kidney yin can be nourished by supplementing the lung yin because metal can generate water. It is a method of simultaneous treatment of the kidney and the lung.

(3) The therapeutic principles established according to the inter-restriction of the five elements suppress the strong and support the weak. Clinically the abnormal restrictions among the five elements, such as over-restriction or counter-restriction, are caused by either over-action or under-action. The former is strong and characterized by hyperfunction while the latter is weak and characterized by hypofunction. So the principle of suppressing the strong and supporting the weak at the same time should be adopted to treat such cases. Suppressing the strong should be given particular emphasis so as to recover the weak. If one element is too powerful, and the other element is not excessively restricted yet, the weak one should be reinforced in advance so as to prevent the disease from further developing.

Suppressing the strong is mainly used to treat disorders due to over-restriction and counter-restriction when a certain element is extremely powerful. For example, transverse invasion of liver qi into the spleen and stomach may lead to imbalance between the liver and spleen, or between the liver and stomach. This is called hyperactive wood over-restricting earth, and should be treated by soothing and calming the liver. Wood is supposed to restrict earth, but when earth qi is excessive, it will restrict wood reversely, which is called earth counter-restricting wood. Clinically this is marked mainly by damp-heat in the spleen and stomach or accumulation of cold-damp, which impedes the free flow of liver qi. It should be treated by activating the spleen and expelling pathogenic factors. Therefore, by suppressing the strong, the weak will naturally be recovered. Supporting the weak is mainly used to treat disorders due to over-restriction and counter-restriction when a certain element is too weak. When the spleen and stomach are weak, the liver qi will find its way to invade, leading to imbalance between liver and spleen, called over-restriction of wood due to deficiency of earth. It should be treated by invigorating the spleen and nourishing qi. Earth is supposed to restrict water, but if the spleen qi is too weak, it will not restrict water. Instead, it may be restricted by water reversely, leading to overflow of water due to spleen deficiency. This is called counter-restriction of water due to deficiency of earth, and should be treated mainly by warming the kidney and invigorating the spleen. Therefore, by supporting the weak, the normal visceral functions can be recovered.

(4) Commonly the therapeutic methods established according to the inter-restriction of the five elements are as follows:

Subduing wood to reinforce earth. This is a method of treating hyperactivity of liver and deficiency of spleen by soothing the liver and invigorating the spleen, or calming the liver and harmonizing the stomach. It is applicable to the syndrome of hyperactive wood over-restricting earth, or deficient earth incurring over-restriction of wood. Besides, during the practice, the wood-suppressing method and earth-reinforcing method should be used with different emphasis. For example, in the syndrome of hyperactive wood over-restricting earth, the wood-suppressing method should be given priority and the earth-reinforcing method should be used as an auxiliary approach; whereas in the syndrome of deficient earth incurring over-restriction of wood, the earth-reinforcing method should be given priority and the wood-suppressing method should be used as an auxiliary approach.

Consolidating earth to control water. This is a method of treating accumulation of water-damp by invigorating the spleen and relieving edema. It is also called building-up earth to promote flow of water or warming the kidney and invigorating the spleen. It is applicable to the treatment of edema, distension and fullness due to spleen deficiency with overflowing of water-damp.

Supporting lung to suppress liver. This is a method of descending lung qi and clearing liver fire at the same time, also called purging liver and clearing lung. It is applicable to the syndrome of wood-fire scorching metal due to excessive ascending of live qi and insufficient descending of lung qi.

Purging the south and nourishing the north. This is a method of combined application of purging heart fire and nourishing kidney yin, also called purging fire to replenish water or nourishing yin to descend fire. It is applicable to the syndrome of disharmony between the heart and kidney due to relative exuberance of heart fire and insufficiency of kidney water.

In a word, the five-element theory is widely used clinically. It is not only applicable to herbal medication, but also to acupuncture and moxibustion, or even mental therapeutics.

Daily Exercises

1. How to use the theory of five elements to guide visceral medication?
2. What is the therapeutic principle for treating hyperactivity of liver-wood?
3. What is nourishing the mother-organ in the case of deficiency?
4. What is reducing the child-organ in the case of excess?

CHAPTER 5

The Theory of Visceral Manifestation

The phrase of visceral manifestation, or Zang Xiang in Chinese, first appeared in the *Chapter of Six Sections of Discussion on Visceral Manifestation* in *Su Wen*. According to the explanation in some Chinese medical classics, "zang" refers to the interior organs which are stored inside the body, and "xiang" refers to the exterior manifestations of the physiological functions and pathological changes of the internal organs. In *Lei Jing* (*Canon of Classification*) compiled by Zhang Jingyue, it was recorded, "Xiang means image; the viscera are stored inside the body and the image is manifested outwardly. For this reason, it is called "visceral manifestation." Apparently, Zang Xiang refers to the external reflection of the physiological activities and pathological changes of the internal organs. Such a reflection can help to deduce and determine the functional changes of the viscera because they are indicative of the visceral variation in an objective manner.

Visceral manifestation is a theory focusing on the study of the physiological functions and pathological changes of the internal organs or tissues of the body as well as their inter-relations. On the basis of their long-term life and work activities and the preliminary recognition on the human anatomy, the ancient doctors developed this theory after comprehensive analysis, comparison, deduction and generalization. It aims to study the functional activities of the internal organs through the external manifestations so as to effectively direct the prevention and treatment of diseases. It plays an important role in building up the theoretical system of TCM.

The theory of visceral manifestation is based on the viscera. "Viscera" is a collective term for all the internal organs which, according to the differences in physiological function, can be divided into three categories: zang-organs, fu-organs and extraordinary fu-organs. The five zang-organs refer to the heart, lung, spleen, liver and kidney. The six fu-organs refer to the gallbladder, stomach, small intestine, large intestine, urinary bladder and triple energizer. The extraordinary fu-organs, different in shape and function from the six fu-organs, refer to the brain, marrow, bones, vessels, gallbladder and uterus. Among them, the gallbladder is unique in that it is both a fu-organ and an extraordinary fu-organ.

The five zang-organs and six fu-organs are different in physiological functions. The common physiological functions of the former are to transform and store essence qi, while these of the latter are to receive, transport and transform water and cereal. So in the *Chapter of Special Dissuasion on Five Zang-organs* in *Su Wen*, it was described, "The so called five zang-organs refers to the organs that only store essence but not excrete it; that is the reason why they can be full but not solid. The six fu-organs are in charge of transporting and transforming food, so they can be solid but not full." These remarks not only generalize the physiological characteristics of the viscera, but also points out the differences between the zang-organs and fu-organs. "Fullness with solidness" and "solidness without fullness" are descriptions for the essence qi and water-cereal, respectively. Just as what was said by Wang Bing, "Essence is characterized by fullness and food by solidness. The five zang-organs can only store essence, so they are full, but not solid; the function of the six fu-organs is to receive food rather than to store essence, so they are solid, but not full."

The extraordinary fu-organs are different from zang-organs in construction or structure, but are similar to the zang-organs in physiological function because both of them can store essence. Besides, the extraordinary fu-organs are different from the six fu-organs in morphology and physiological function and have no direct contact with water and cereal. Moreover, they are relatively hermetic. All of these account for the reason why they are named "extraordinary fu-organs." In addition, the gallbladder belongs not only to the six fu-organs but also to the extraordinary fu-organs. This is because the secretion and excretion of bile, marked by unblocked discharging, are beneficial to the digestion of food. In this way it is similar to and thus belongs to the six fu-organs marked by transportation and transformation of food without storage. On the other hand, the gallbladder stores clean, pure bile and have no direct contact with water and food. So it is not a passage for transportation and transformation of food. This is different from the six fu-organs, and that is why it is also regarded as an extraordinary fu-organ.

The theory of visceral manifestation is basically characterized by a holistic concept centering on the five zang-organs, which is reflected in the following aspects:

The zang-organs and fu-organs are interiorly and exteriorly associated: The zang-organs pertain to yin and fu-organs to yang, and they are interiorly and exteriorly associated, making up an entirety. This is due to that in the meridian and collateral system, the yin meridians pertaining to zang-organs and yang meridians pertaining to fu-organs are mutually connected. For instance, the meridian of hand taiyin pertains to the lung and connects with the large intestine, the meridian of hand yangming pertains to the large intestine and connects with the lung, the meridian of hand shaoyin pertain to the heart and connects with the small intestine, the meridian of hand taiyang pertains to the small intestine and connects with the heart. In a similar fashion, the pericardium meridian of hand jueyin connects externally and internally with the triple-energizer meridian of hand shaoyang, the spleen meridian of foot taiyin with the stomach meridian of the foot yangming, and the kidney meridian of foot shaoyin with the urinary bladder meridian of foot taiyang. The zang-organs and fu-organs in an interior-exterior relationship are coordinated in physiological functions, e.g., the dispersion-descent of the lung and the transportation of the large intestine, the ascent of the lucid by the spleen and the descent of the turbid by the stomach, the free flow of liver qi and the secretion and excretion of bile, etc. Some zang-organs are directly connected with certain fu-organs, e.g., the liver is connected with the gallbladder, the spleen with the stomach, and the kidney with the urinary bladder. Pathologically, they are also mutually affected, e.g., the downward moving of heart-fire into the small intestine, the abnormal secretion and excretion of bile due to impeded flow of liver qi, and the inconsolidation of the urinary bladder due to weakness of kidney qi. Generally speaking, in the theory of visceral manifestation, the discussion on the physiology and pathology of the zang-organs is more specific and detailed than those of the fu-organs. So the zang-organs serve as the core while the fu-organs are subordinate to the zang-organs.

The five zang-organs are connected with the body constituents and orifices in an entirety: All the five zang-organs have their external manifestations and have specific connections with the body constituents and orifices. This is another embodiment of the holistic concept of the theory of visceral manifestation. For instance, the heart is associated with the vessels in body constituents, opens into the tongue, and manifests in the skin hair; the spleen is associated with fleshes, opens into the mouth and manifests on the lips; the liver is associated with tendons, opens into the eyes and manifests on the nails; the kidney is associated with bones, opens into the ears, external genitalia and anus, and manifests in the hair. The warming and nourishing actions of qi, blood, yin and yang of the five zang-organs are indispensable to the normal physiological function and the normal color and luster of the body and its organs and orifices. Pathologically, the abnormalities of the body constituents, organs and orifices in function or color and luster are often external reflection of the disorders in the corresponding zang-organs.

The physiological functions of the five zang-organs are closely related to the emotions: The emotions, consciousness and mental activities of the human body are closely associated with the physiological functions of the five zang-organs. The theory of visceral manifestation holds that joy, anger, worry, thinking and terror are associated with the heart, liver, lung, spleen and kidney, respectively. Heart is related to joy, so excessive joy impairs the heart; liver to anger, so excessive anger impairs the liver; lung to worry, so excessive worry impairs the lung; spleen to thinking, so excessive thinking impairs the spleen; kidney to terror, so excessive terror impairs the kidney. Besides, the spirit, ethereal soul, corporeal soul, ideation and will are attributed to the heart, lung, liver, spleen and kidney, respectively. It is thus clear that the emotional and mental activities are all associated with the five zang-organs. All of these indicate that the emotional and mental activities rely closely on the physiological functions of the five zang-organs, and in turn the emotional and mental activities can also act on the five zang-organs and affect their physiological functions.

In summary, the theory of visceral manifestation attributes the fu-organs, body constituents, orifices and emotional or mental activities to the five zang-organs which serve as the core, constituting the five major physiological and pathological systems represented by the heart, lung, spleen, liver and kidney. The mutual promotion and restriction among the five systems synthetically maintain the coordination and balance of the internal environment of the body, embodying the holistic and unified nature of the body. The formation of the theory of visceral manifestation relies partly on the ancient knowledge about anatomy, but more importantly on the observatory and researching approach of "what is inside must be manifested outside" and on the theories of yin-yang and five elements. Hence the physiological functions and pathological changes of the viscera discussed in the light of visceral manifestation will inevitably go far beyond the scope of human anatomy, forming a unique theoretical system of visceral physiology and pathology.

Daily Exercises

1. What is the concept of "visceral manifestation"?
2. What are extraordinary fu-organs?
3. What are the common characteristics of the physiological function of the five zang-organs and six fu-organs?
4. What are the basic characteristics of visceral manifestation?

Weekly Review

The correlation between things and the five elements are not static and isolated. The inter-generation and inter-restriction of the five elements are used to explore and explain the association, coordination and unification of things. Besides, the over-restriction and counter-restriction of the five elements are also used to explore and explain the interaction among things after the disruption of balance. Inter-generation, or mutual promotion, refers to that one kind of object generates, strengthens and brings forth another in a fixed sequence. This relationship of the five elements is called the "mother-child" relationship. Inter-restriction of the five elements refers to the alternate restricting activity among wood, fire, earth, metal and water in a circular order. Over-restriction, or subjugation, refers to the launching of an attack on a counterpart when it is weak. For the five elements, it means the excessive restriction of one element on another in the same circular order as inter-restriction. Counter-restriction refers to the restriction of one element on another in an opposite order.

The theory of five elements is used in TCM to classify the viscera and meridians into five categories and explain their characteristics according to the properties of the five elements, e.g., the liver pertains to wood, heart to fire, spleen to earth, lung to metal, and kidney to water. The inter-generation and inter-restriction of the five elements are used to analyze the relationship among the viscera, meridians and various physiological functions, e.g., the liver stores blood to nourish the heart; the heart yang warms the spleen earth to facilitate digestion; the spleen disperses essence to the lung; the lung qi descends to regulate waterways and facilitate the kidney water; the kidney stores essence to nourish liver blood; the free flow of live qi helps to unblock the obstruction of the spleen earth; the spleen transports water-damp to control overflow of kidney water; the ascent of kidney water helps to restrain heart fire; the warmth of heart fire helps to disperse lung qi; and the descent of lung qi subdues the hyperactivity of liver qi etc. The over-restriction and counter-restriction of the five elements are used to illustrate the interaction among the viscera under pathological conditions. There are two types of transmission: inter-generation transmission and inter-restriction transmission. Inter-generation transmission refers to that the disorder of one organ may be transmitted to another organ in the order of inter-generation among the five elements. It is also called mutual transmission between mother organ and child organ, including "mother organ involving child organ" and "child organ involving mother organ." Inter-restriction transmission refers to that the disorder of one organ may be transmitted to another organ in the order of inter-restriction among the five elements. Such a transmission is divided into two types: "over-restriction" transmission in the normal order of inter-restriction and "counter-restriction" transmission in the reverse order of inter-restriction.

The five zang-organs have specific connection with the five colors, five sounds, and five flavors, and such a hierarchic classification of the five-zang system provides the theoretical foundation for the clinical diagnosis of diseases. For inspection of the complexion, the liver is associated with blue, heart with red, spleen with yellow, lung with white, and kidney with black. For inquiry of flavors, sourness pertains to liver, bitterness to heart, sweetness to spleen, pungency to lung and saltiness to kidney. The application of the five-element theory in TCM is mainly reflected in directing visceral medication, controlling disease transmission, and determining therapeutic principles and methods, etc. Disorder of one zang-organ may be transmitted to other zang-organs following the order of inter-generation or inter-restriction of the five elements. During treatment, not only the organ in disorder is regulated but also other related organs are coordinated according to the inter-generation, inter-restriction, over-restriction, and counter-restriction of the five elements so as to control the transmission. Apparently it is a preventive measure with great significance in clinical practice. The therapeutic principles established according to the inter-generation of the five elements nourish the mother in the case of deficiency and reduce the child in the case of excess. The specific methods replenish water to nourish wood, invigorating fire to reinforce earth, reinforcing earth to generate metal, and mutual generation of metal and water, etc. The therapeutic principles established according to the inter-restriction of the five elements suppress the strong and support the weak, e.g., subduing wood to reinforce earth, consolidating earth to control water, supporting the lung to suppress the liver, purging the south and nourishing the north, etc.

Zang Xiang refers to the external reflection of the physiological activities and pathological changes of the internal organs. Such a reflection can help to deduce and determine the functional changes of the viscera because they are indicative of the visceral variation in an objective manner. The theory of visceral manifestation focuses on the study of the physiological functions and pathological changes of the internal organs and tissues of the body as well as their inter-relations. The theory of visceral manifestation is based on the viscera. "Viscera" is a collective term for all the internal organs which, according to the differences in physiological function, can be divided into three categories: zang-organs, fu-organs and extraordinary fu-organs. The five zang-organs and six fu-organs are different in physiological functions. The common physiological functions of the former are to transform and store essence qi, while these of the latter are to receive, transport and transform water and cereal. The theory of visceral manifestation is basically characterized by a holistic concept centering on the five zang-organs, which is reflected in the following aspects: the zang-organs and fu-organs are interiorly and exteriorly associated, the five zang-organs are connected with the body constituents and orifices in an entirety, and the physiological functions of the five zang-organs are closely related to the emotions, etc. The five major physiological and pathological systems represented by the heart, lung, spleen, liver and kidney are mutually promoted and restricted, synthetically maintaining the coordination and balance of the internal environment of the body, and embodying the holistic and unified nature of the body.

Daily Exercises

1. To understand the patterns of inter-generation, inter-restriction, over-restriction and counter-restriction among the five elements.
2. To master the specific application scope of the theory of five elements in TCM.
3. To master the embodiment scope and specific content of the concept of entirety in the theory of visceral manifestation centering on the five zang-organs.

THE FOURTH WEEK

SECTION 1   THE FIVE ZANG-ORGANS

The five zang-organs is a collective term for the heart, lung, spleen, liver and kidney. While each of the zang-organs has its special functions, the physiological functions of the heart play a dominant role.

The Heart

The heart is situated in the thorax, above the diaphragm and enveloped by the pericardium, resembling an inverted lotus flower bud. It is the house of spirit, the governor of blood, and the converging location of vessels. Pertaining to fire in the five elements and being yang within yin, the heart plays a major role in dominating the life activities of the human body. That is why it is called "the monarch organ" in *Su Wen* (*Plain Conversation*, 素问). It has two main functions: controlling blood and vessels and dominating spirit. Besides, it opens into the tongue, manifesting on the face, associating with joy in emotions and sweat in secretion. The two major meridians, heart meridian of hand shaoyin and small intestine of hand shaoyang, connect and tangle each other between the heart and small intestine. Hence the heart and small intestine are believed to be related internally and externally.

The Main Physiological Functions of the Heart

1. *Controlling blood and vessel*

This function of the heart involves two aspects: control of blood and control of blood vessel. The blood circulates in the vessel and relies on the propelling of the heart to reach all parts of the body, so as to perform its nourishing and moistening function. The vessel is the pathway of blood circulation, the smoothness or obstruction of which directly influences the normal flow of blood. Therefore, in the relatively independent system made up of the heart, vessel and blood, the heart plays the dominant role, and the normal pulsation of which is indispensable to the physiological functions of this system.

The normal pulsation of the heart depends on the nourishing and moistening function of the heart blood and heart yin as well as the propelling and warming functions of the heart qi and heart yang. In this way the normal cardiac efficiency, cardiac rate and cardiac rhythm are guaranteed, enabling blood to circulate all over the body for nourishment. This is manifested as rosy, lustrous complexion and slow yet forceful pulsation. The normal circulation of blood also relies on the sufficiency of blood. If the blood is deficient and the vessels are empty, it will also directly affect the normal pulsation of the heart and the normal circulation of blood. In this sense, it is considered that abundance of heart qi, sufficiency of blood and smoothness of the vessels are prerequisite to the normal circulation of blood. If the heart qi is insufficient, the blood is deficient and the vessels are unsmooth, it will inevitably lead to inhibited circulation of blood and emptiness of the vessels, marked by pale and lusterless complexion as well as thin and weak pulse; if qi and blood are stagnated and the blood vessels are obstructed, there will be grayish complexion, cyanotic lips and tongue, distress or stabbing pain in the precordium region, and knotted, intermittent, hasty or unsmooth pulses.

2. *Governing spirit*

Heart governing spirit, or heart storing spirit, refers to that the heart can dominate and control the spiritual, mental and thinking activities of the body. Spirit, in a broad sense, refers to the life activities and external manifestations of the human body. The image of the body, the complexion, language, response and body movements, are all classified into the category of spirit. So there is a saying, "One thrives with spirit yet perishes without it." In everyday Chinese language, the so called "shen qi (spirit qi)," "shen zhi (spirit mind)" and "shen se (spirit complexion)," are classified into this category. While in a narrow sense, spirit refers to the spiritual, mental and thinking activities dominated by the heart. They are all important physiological functions of the body; besides, under certain circumstances, they may affect the balance or coordination among different physiological functions of the whole body. Therefore, it is said in *Su Wen (Plain Conversation, 素问)*, "The heart is the monarch organ" and in *Ling Shu-Xie Ke (Miraculous Pivot-Pathogenic invasion, 灵枢·邪客)*, "The heart, where the spirit resides, is the supreme governor of the five zang-organs and six fu-organs."

The spirit, consciousness and thinking activities are physiological functions as well as external reflections of the brain. However, in the theory of visceral manifestation, which centers on the five zang-organs, these activities are attributed to the five zang-organs, particularly the heart; that is why it is said, "The heart stores the spirit." *Ling Shu (Miraculous Pivot,* 灵枢) pointed out clearly that the heart can receive external messages and in *Lei Jing,* Zhang Jingyue further put forward that the spiritual, mental and thinking activities, though pertain to different zang-organs respectively, are mainly controlled by the heart. Therefore, if the heart controls spirit properly, one will be full in vitality, clear in mind, agile in thinking, and sensitive in reaction to the external stimulation. However, malfunction of the heart in governing the spirit may bring about such symptoms as insomnia, dreaminess, distraction and even delirium; or slow reaction, amnesia, dispiritedness, and even coma, etc.

The function of heart governing spirit is closely related to the function of heart controlling blood and vessel. Blood is the material base for mental activities; in this sense, the function of heart controlling blood and vessel is prerequisite to that of heart governing spirit. Hence, the dysfunction of heart controlling blood and vessel will inevitably lead to abnormal changes of the spirit.

The Relationship of the Heart to the Emotions, Fluids, Body Constituents and Orifices

1. The heart is associated with joy in emotions

The physiological function of the heart is closely related to joy. The theory of visceral manifestation holds that the different emotions, namely joy, anger, worry, contemplation and terror, are derived from the physiological functions of the five zang-organs. Each of them is associated with a particular zang-organ, respectively. In *Su Wen (Plain Conversation,* 素问), it is also confirmed that joy is associated with the heart. Joy, a positive reaction to the external environment, is beneficial to the heart. However, excessive joy can impair heart spirit. In a word, joy is beneficial to the heart in governing the spirit and controlling blood and vessel only when it is not excessive.

2. *The heart is associated with sweat in fluids*

It means that sweat is the fluid of the heart, indicating the close connection between sweat and the heart. Sweat, a fluid excreted from the sweat pore after the activation of yang qi, is discussed in *Su Wen* (*Plain Conversation*, 素问) that "yang acting on yin produces sweat." The secretion of sweat relies on the control of skin striae by defensive qi. If it is open, there will be sweat, and if not, there will be no sweat. Since sweat is transformed from body fluid, which shares the same origin with blood, there is a saying that "blood and sweat shares the same origin." And because blood is controlled by the heart, it is said that "sweat is the fluid of the heart."

3. *The heart is associated with the vessel in body constituents*

It refers to the connection between the heart and all the blood vessels. Its luster is reflected on the complexion. For this reason, the physiological or pathological conditions of the heart can be indicated on the face. Because the blood vessels on the head and face are very abundant, just like what is said in *Ling Shu* (*Miraculous Pivot*, 灵枢) that the face and upper orifices receive qi and blood from all the twelve meridians and three hundred and sixty-five collaterals. So abundant heart qi and blood will lead to red and lustrous complexion, whereas insufficient heart qi and blood may result in pale complexion, and stagnated blood can cause cyanosed complexion.

4. *The heart is associated with the tongue in orifices*

The heart opens into the tongue, which means the tongue is the external manifestation of the heart. The main function of the tongue is to govern sense of taste and language expression, which rely on the function of the heart to govern spirit, blood and vessel. If the heart functions abnormally, there will be change of taste and inflexibility of the tongue. If the functions of the heart are normal, the tongue will be moist and lustrous in property, normal and sensitive in taste, and free and flexible in movement. The disorders of the heart can also be reflected on the tongue. For example, if yang qi in the heart is insufficient, the tongue will be light-colored, whitish, bulgy and tender; if the blood is deficient in the heart, the tongue will be deep-red, thin and dry; if the heart fire flames up, the tongue will be reddish or even with ulcer; if the heart vessels are stagnant, the tongue will be cyanotic or even with ecchymoses; if the physiological function of the heart in controlling the spirit is abnormal, the tongue will become curled up and stiff, leading to difficulty or inability to speak, etc.

Appendix: The Pericardium

The pericardium, called xinbao, or tanzhong, is the membrane enveloping the heart to protect it. Its shape and position are recorded in many ancient classics. In the meridian theory, it is also deemed as a zang-organ because the heart meridian of hand jueyin is connected with the pericardium and is closely related to the triple energizer meridian of hand shaoyin. But, in the theory of viscera manifestation, it is regarded as the envelope of the heart for its protection so that when there is an exogenous invasion, the pericardium will be the first barrier. In the theory of warm diseases, such symptoms as coma or delirium appearing in exogenous febrile diseases are known as "heat invading the pericardium" or "heat clouding the pericardium."

Daily Exercises

1. What is heart governing blood and vessel?
2. What is heart governing spirit?
3. Why it is said that the heart is associated with sweat in fluids?
4. What is pericardium?

The Lung

The lung, including two lobes on the left and right, is situated in the thorax, and is compared to a "canopy" because of the uppermost position among all the viscera. The lung is tender, frail and finicky, and is susceptible to pathogenic invasions; hence it is called the "delicate organ." The main physiological functions of the lung are to dominate qi and control respiration, govern ascent, dispersion, purification and descent as well as regulate water passage. It also governs management and regulation because it is associated with various vessels. It communicates with the throat, opens into the nose, and is associated with the skin and hair in the exterior. In five emotions it is related to worry and in fluids to snivel. Moreover, its meridian is internally and externally related to the large intestine.

The Main Physiological Functions of the Lung

1. *The lung controls qi and governs respiration*

It controls the qi of the whole body, or general qi, and the air it inhales and exhales. The reason why it controls qi of the whole body is that all kinds of qi belong ultimately to the lung, which is mainly reflected in the process of qi production, particularly the thoracic qi. The thoracic qi is mainly composed of the fresh air inhaled by the lung and the cereal nutrients transformed by the spleen and stomach. Hence the normal respiratory function of the lung is critical for the production of thoracic qi and the general qi. The respiration is actually a dynamic process of ascending, descending, entering and exiting of qi, thus the lung is capable of regulating qi activities of the whole body.

The lung governing the inhaled and exhaled qi means that the lung is the location where the external air and the internal qi exchange. Through this process, the external fresh air is inhaled and internal turbid qi is exhaled, thus promoting the production of qi, regulating the ascending, descending, entering and exiting motions of qi, and facilitating the metabolism of the body. Both of these two functions of the lung can ultimately be traced back to the respiratory function of the lung. The normal function of respiration is prerequisite to the production and smooth movement of qi. Otherwise, the production of thoracic qi and the movement of qi will be affected, debilitating the basic function of the lung in controlling qi and may ultimately lead to the termination of life activities. Therefore, the function of the lung in controlling general qi relies mainly on the respiratory function of the lung. The shortage of qi, the abnormal movement of qi, and the abnormal distribution and circulation of blood and body fluid, however, may also be detrimental to the respiratory function of the lung.

2. The lung manages ascent and dispersion as well as descent and purification. Ascent and dispersion mean that the lung qi can move upward

and disperse outward; descent and purification means that the lung qi can move downward and clear the foreign body away from the respiratory tract. The lung managing ascent and dispersion is mainly reflected in three aspects: a. Discharging the turbid qi within the body by dispersion and qi transformation. b. Distributing the body fluid and cereal nutrients transformed by the spleen to the whole body as well as the skin and hair in the exterior. c. Diffusing defensive qi to warm and nourish the skin and muscles, to regulate the opening and closing of the skin striae, and to discharge the metabolized body fluid in the form of sweat. Hence, the dysfunction of the lung in ascent and dispersion may lead to inhibited air tube, nasal obstruction, sneezing, unconsistent respiration, chest distress and cough, etc. Besides, if the lung qi is obstructed and fails to disperse the defensive qi, there will be stagnation of defensive qi, closing of the skin striae, absence of sweat, aversion to cold and sensation of fever, etc.

The descent and purification of the lung can also be discussed in three aspects: a. inhaling the fresh air from nature; b. distributing downward the inhaled fresh air as well as the body fluid and nutrients from water and cereal transformed by the spleen; c. purifying the foreign bodies inside the respiratory tract, and keeping it clean. Thus, if the lung fails to function properly in this regard, there will be frequent coughing and wheezing aggravated on exertion, or chest oppression and breathing obstruction, etc.

The ascent-dispersion and descent-purification of the lung are inseparable. They are a unity of opposites. That is why they are mutually affected pathologically. Without normal ascent and dispersion, there will be no regular descent and purification, and *vice versa*. Only when both function properly can the air tube be smooth, respiration be rhythmic, and the exchange of qi between the interior and exterior be normal. Otherwise, there will be syndromes such as "the lung failing to disperse and ascend" and "the lung failing to purify and descend," resulting in wheezing and coughing, etc.

3. The lung is in charge of dredging and regulating waterways, which are passages within the body for circulating and discharging water and fluid. This aspect of the pulmonary function relies on the ascent-dispersion and descent-purification of the lung to regulate the distribution, circulation and excretion of water and fluid. The ascent and dispersion of the lung cover three aspects: dispersing the body fluid and the essence from water

and cereal to all parts of the body, controlling the opening and closing the skin striae, and regulating the secretion and excretion of sweat. In contrast, the descent and purification of the lung enable the inhaled lucid qi to reach the kidney and make water and fluid within the body transported downward to the urinary bladder where they transform into urine. This process is assisted by the qi transforming action of the kidney. Besides promoting the smoothness of the urination, the lung can also distribute water and fluid downwards to all parts of the body because of its supreme location above all the other viscera (The water and fluid are taken from the external environment and then transported to the lung *via* the spleen and stomach). That is why it is called "the upper source of water." If the function of the lung in regulating waterways is abnormal, there will be retention of water, fluid and phlegm, etc.

4. The lung opens into various vessels and is in charge of regulation and management. Almost all vessels are convened in the lung which means that all the blood within the body is transported to the lung through different vessels, and after exchange of qi *via* respiration, the fresh blood is sent back to the whole body. It is thus evident that the lung is closely linked to the vessels and blood circulation. The theory of visceral manifestation holds that the motive power of blood circulation lies in the dispersion and regulation of lung qi as well as the propelling action of heart qi. The circulation of visible blood relies on the propelling action of invisible qi, which is inseparable from the lung with the functions of governing respiration and qi of the whole body. The lung opening into myriad vessels, in this sense, means that the lung qi can facilitate and promote blood circulation.

The lung in charge of regulation and management refers to that the lung can regulate and manage the physiological functions of the whole body. It is largely manifested in four aspects: a. The lung controls respiration through which the fresh air is inhaled for physiological activities, and the turbid qi, produced in the process of metabolism, is exhaled out of the body; b. The respiration of the lung regulates the ascending, descending, entering and exiting of qi; c. The lung propels and regulates blood circulation for the reason that it can manage and regulate qi activities of the whole body; d. With the function of descent and purification, the lung can manage and regulate the distribution, circulation and excretion of body fluid. That is why it is likened to a prime minister in *Su Wen*.

The Relationship of the Lung to Emotions, Fluids, Body Constituents and Orifices

1. The lung is associated with worry in emotions. Worry and sorrow may vary in degree but they have similar effects on physiological activities of the body. For this reason, they both pertain to the lung. Besides, sorrow and worry are both adverse stimuli to the body and may result in persistent qi consumption. Since the lung controls qi, sorrow and worry are liable to impair the lung. Conversely, when the pulmonary function declines, the lung may be susceptible to external adverse stimulation, and produce sorrow and worry.

2. The lung is associated with snivel in fluids. Snivel, a sort of nasal discharge from the mucous membrane, can moisten the nasal cavity. Under normal conditions, the snivel will moisten the nasal cavity without flowing out. However, dysfunction of the lung may lead to various abnormalities such as lung-cold with clear nasal discharges, lung-heat with yellow, thick and turbid discharges, and lung-dryness with dry nasal cavity and absence of discharges.

3. The lung is associated with the skin and hair in body constituents. The skin and hair, including the cutaneous covering, the sweat glands and the vellus hair, constitutes the superficies of the body. Warmed, nourished and moistened by the defensive qi and body fluid, they are the first barricade for resisting exogenous pathogenic factors. The lung controls qi and pertains to the defensive qi, and can disperse defensive qi and distribute the essence to the skin and hair. Thus, it is said in *Su Wen* that: "the lung is associated with the skin and can nourish the hair." If the physiological functions of the lung are normal, the skin will be compact and smooth, the hair will be lustrous, and the resistance against pathogenic factors will be strong. On the contrary, if the lung qi is deficient, there will be weakness of the defensive qi, profuse sweating, susceptibility to common cold, or dry, brittle and withered hair. Since the lung is associated with the skin and hair, if the exogenous pathogenic factors invade the skin and hair, the lung will also be involved, marked by closure of the skin striae, stagnation of defensive qi, and obstruction of the lung qi. Likewise, when the lung qi is obstructed, there will also be closure of the striae and stagnation of defensive qi, etc.

4. The lung is associated with the nose in body constituents. The lung opens into the nose and the throat, and they are the gateway for respiration. Thus there are some sayings about them such as "the nose is the orifice of the lung" and "the throat is the doorway of the lung." The smelling function of the nose and the sounding function of the throat are both attributed to the lung qi. So when the functions of lung qi are normal, there will be smooth respiration, keen sense of smell, and clear and loud voice. Because the lung opens into the nose and connects to the throat, the nose and throat become the first station of external invasion. The dysfunction of the lung is also frequently manifested on the nose and throat, such as nasal obstruction, nasal discharge, sneezing, itching throat, and hoarseness or loss of voice.

Daily Exercises

1. What does the statement that the lung is in charge of dispersion means?
2. What does the statement that the lung is in charge of purification and descent?
3. Why it is said that the lung can dredge and regulate waterways?
4. Why it is said that the lung governs regulation and management?

THE SPLEEN

The spleen is located in the middle energizer and below the diaphragm. Its main physiological functions are to govern transportation and transformation, ascend the lucid substances, and control blood circulation. Its meridian is connected with that of the stomach. That is why the spleen and stomach is exteriorly and interiorly related. The spleen and stomach are the major organs for digestion and transformation of water and cereal into essences and nutrients, thus they are indispensable to the ongoing of life activities and the production of qi, blood, and body fluid. For this reason, they are called "the source of qi and blood" and "the postnatal foundation of the body." The spleen opens into the mouth and manifests its luster on the lips, associating with earth in the five elements, contemplation in the five emotions, slobber in fluids, and muscles and four limbs in body constituents.

The Main Physiological Functions of the Spleen

1. The spleen is in charge of transformation and transportation; in other words, the spleen can transform the water and cereal into nutrients and transport them to all over the body. Such a function can be divided into two aspects: one is transportation and transformation of water and cereal, and the other is transportation and transformation of water and fluid.

Transportation and transformation of water and cereal refers to the digestion and absorption of water and food and the distribution of nutrients. After the initial digestion of the stomach, the water and food are transported to the small intestine for further digestion. The small intestine separates the lucid substances from the turbid ones, and then transmits the nutrients to the spleen, which further disperses them to the heart and lung and, ultimately, to various parts of the body for nourishment. The nutrients transformed by the spleen are basic materials for production of qi, blood, body fluid, essence and other substances indispensable to the constitution and sustainability of the body. This function relies greatly on the conditions of spleen qi. If the spleen qi is vigorous, the transportation and transformation of water and cereal as well as the absorption of nutrients will be normal, and so will be the production of qi, blood, body fluid and kidney essence, thus ensuring the adequate nourishment of various organs and tissues of the body and the normal physiological functions of the body. Otherwise, if this function weakens, digestion and absorption will become abnormal, leading to abdominal distension, loose stool, anorexia, or lassitude and emaciation, etc. Hence it is said that the spleen is the postnatal foundation of the body and the source of qi and blood.

Transportation and transformation of water and fluid, also called transportation and transformation of water and dampness, refers to the absorption, transmission and dispersion of water and fluid so as to maintain their metabolic balance within the body. After being received and absorbed by the stomach, water and fluid are transmitted to the lung *via* the spleen, and ultimately distributed all over the body. Through the ascending and descending function of the lung, water and fluid can nourish the viscera internally, and moisten the skin, hair and striae externally. The turbid substances are partially excreted in the form of sweat, and the rest reaches the urinary bladder *via* the kidney. It is thus evident that the spleen, through transportation and dispersion, plays a significant role in the metabolic process of water and fluid. If the spleen qi is vigorous, the circulation of water and fluid will be normal, and there will be no retention of dampness, phlegm or fluid, etc. On the contrary, if the spleen qi is weak, and the spleen fails to transport properly, there will be dampness, phlegm and fluid retention, etc. This is exactly the pathological mechanism of the production of dampness, phlegm and retained fluid due to spleen deficiency.

2. The spleen governs the ascent of lucid substances; in other words, the spleen is characterized by ascending the nutrients from water and cereal to the heart, lung, head and eye so as to produce qi and blood and nourish the whole body. Ascent and descent is a pair of opposites in terms of visceral qi activities. The ascent of lucidity by the spleen is often mentioned in relation to the descent of turbidity by the stomach, and only when they are in a dynamic balance will digestion and absorption by the body be normal. Otherwise, the deficient spleen qi will fail to ascend the nutrients from water and cereal to the head and eyes, leading to dizziness, tinnitus and fatigue, etc. Moreover, the ascent of the spleen can also prevent visceroptosis. The reason why the viscera can maintain their relative position lies in the ascending function of the spleen. Only when the ascending function of the spleen is normal can the viscera maintain their original position. On the contrary, if the spleen qi is deficient, and the ascending force is weak, there will be sinking of qi marked by falling and distending sensation of the lower abdomen, frequent urination, chronic diarrhea, anal prolapse, metroptosis, nephroptosis or gastroptosis, etc.

3. The spleen controls blood, which means that the spleen can contain blood within the vessel, preventing it from flowing out. This is all due to the controlling function of qi. In *Jin Gui Yao Lue Zhu* written by Shen Mu Nan, it is said that spleen qi controls blood from the five zang-organs and six fu-organs. So the function of the spleen in controlling blood and the function of qi in controlling blood are not contradictory. The spleen controlling blood is closely related to the fact that the spleen is the source of qi and blood. If the spleen qi is vigorous, the production of qi and blood will be normal, and the function of containing blood within the vessel will also be sound. Otherwise, the function of producing qi and blood will be debilitated, so will the function of controlling blood. Since the spleen governs the ascent of lucid substances and the spleen qi

is characterized by ascending, we often attribute hematochezia, blood urine and metrorrhagia and metrostaxis to the spleen because it fails to control blood.

The Relationship of the Spleen to Emotions, Fluids, Body Constituents and Orifices

1. The spleen is associated with contemplation in emotions, which is also related to the heart. So there is a saying that contemplation stems from the heart while it dwells on the spleen. Moderate contemplation is not detrimental to the body while excessive thinking can affect the normal physiological activities, particularly the qi movement, leading to qi stagnation. In terms of the physiological functions of the viscera, the transportation and transformation of the spleen are most likely to be affected. As a result, excessive thinking often leads to anorexia, distending sensation in the gastric and abdominal region, and dizziness, etc.

2. The spleen is associated with slobber, or thin saliva derived from the mouth. It can protect the oral mucosa and moisten the oral cavity. And during the intake of food, slobber will be excreted more than usual so as to facilitate the swallowing and digesting of food. Slobber comes from the spleen and flows into the stomach. Under normal circumstances, slobber will rise upward to the mouth in moderate quantity. However, if there is disharmony between the spleen and stomach, or shortage of spleen qi, it will flow out of the mouth, which is a morbid condition.

3. The spleen is associated with muscle in body constituents. The spleen and stomach are source of qi and blood. All the muscles of the body rely on the nutrients transformed by the spleen and stomach from water and cereal. So only when the transportation and transformation of the spleen are normal can the muscles be strong and firm. Otherwise, the muscles will be thin, weak and even atrophied. In contrast to the body, the four limbs are the extremities, so they are also called "the four extremities," which need the nutrients transformed by the spleen and stomach to maintain their normal physiological activities, too. Moreover, the transportation of the nutrients to the four limbs relies on the ascending and dispersing of lucid yang. Hence if the spleen qi is vigorous, the four limbs

will be adequately nourished and forceful; otherwise, the four limbs will be malnourished due to lucid yang failing to ascend and disperse, marked by lassitude or even atrophy.

4. The spleen is associated with the mouth in orifices; in other words, the spleen opens into the mouth. So food and flavor are closely associated with the spleen. Whether the taste is normal or not depends on the transformation and transportation function of the spleen and stomach, or the ascent of lucidity by the spleen and the descent of turbidity by the stomach. If the spleen functions properly in transportation and transformation, the taste will be normal; if not, there will be abnormal tastes such as bland, sweet or greasy sensation in the mouth which may affect one's appetite. The color and luster of the lips reflect not only the conditions of qi and blood all over the blood, but also the state of the spleen in transportation and transformation. So in *Su Wen*, it is said that the spleen is associated with the muscles, and reflects its luster on the lips.

Daily Exercises

1. What does it mean to say that the spleen governs transportation and transformation?
2. What does it mean to say that the spleen controls blood?
3. Why it is said that the spleen governs ascent of the lucid?
4. Why it is said that the spleen is associated with thinking in the five mental activities?

The Liver

The liver is situated in the upper abdomen, below the diaphragm, and inside the right hypochondria. It is the house of soul, the depot of blood, and the ancestral temple of tendons. The liver pertains to wood in five elements and is characterized by ascending and moving. So it is said in *Su Wen* (*Plain Conversation*, 素问) that the liver is likened to a general in charge of strategy. The main physiological functions of the liver are to govern free flow of qi and store blood. The liver opens into the eyes, controls tendons, and has its outward manifestation on the nails. It is associated with anger in emotions and tear in fluids. The liver meridian and the gallbladder meridian are mutually connected, and more noticeably, the liver and the gallbladder themselves are also connected internally and externally.

The Main Physiological Functions of the Liver

1. The liver governs dredging and ventilating, in other words, it is in charge of the free flow of qi so as to maintain the smooth circulation of the qi all over the body. This function reflects such physiological characteristics of the liver as ascending and moving. It covers the following aspects:

(1) *Regulation of qi activity*

This refers to the ascending, descending, entering and exiting of qi. The dredging and ventilating function of the liver plays a critical role in maintaining the balance of the ascending, descending, entering and exiting of qi. If it is normal, the qi movements will be smooth, the qi and blood will be harmonious, and the physiological activities of the viscera, meridians, and tissues will be normal. On the contrary, if it is abnormal, there will be stagnation of qi activities or malfunction of the ascending, descending, entering and exiting of qi, marked by distension, fullness and pain in the chest, hypochondria, breasts, lower abdomen and external genitalia, or characterized by depression, unhappiness and occasional sighing, etc. If the situation aggravates, it will involve the circulation of blood and body fluid, the secretion and excretion of bile, the ascent of lucidity by the spleen and the descent of turbidity by the stomach, as well as emotional activities, etc. Both the circulation of blood and the distribution of body fluid rely on the ascending, descending, entering and exiting movements of qi. If the liver fails to govern free flow of qi, there will be qi stagnation, irregular blood circulation and even blood stasis, marked by irregular menstruation, difficult menstruation, amenorrhea, or masses and lumps, etc. Besides, the distribution of body fluid will also be hampered, leading to retention of phlegm, edema, superficial nodules and drum belly, etc.

(2) *Promoting the reception and digestion of water and food*

The absorption and distribution of nutrients rely on the coordination between the ascent of lucidity by the spleen and the descent of turbidity by the stomach. If the liver can promote free flow of qi properly, the qi movements will be smooth, and the ascent of lucidity by the spleen and the descent of turbidity by the stomach will also be normal. However, if it is not, the transforming function and the ascending function of the spleen will be impaired, leading to dizziness or diarrhea, etc. The descending function of the stomach may also be involved, resulting in vomiting, belching, distending pain in the gastric and abdominal region, and constipation, etc.

(3) *Regulating emotional activities*

Emotional activities are not only associated with the heart in governing spirit, but also are influenced by the liver in promoting free flow of qi. This is because normal emotional activities rely mainly on the normal circulation of qi and blood. If the liver functions properly to promote free flow of qi, the qi activities will be smooth, and there will harmonious co-existence of qi and blood, as well as a happy, contented state of mind. Otherwise, if the liver fails to function properly, there will be stagnation of liver qi, depression and emotional vulnerability. If the liver is hyperactive in ascending, there will be adverse up-flaming of qi and fire, irascibility and irritability. It is thus clear that the abnormal emotions are often attributed to the dysfunction of the liver in promoting free flow of qi. For this reason, we often treat those with emotional disorders from the perspective of the liver.

(4) *Promoting the smooth excretion of bile*

The gallbladder, located among the hepatic lobules, is connected to the liver. Bile is derived from the liver. It is transformed from the surplus qi of the liver. Therefore, the secretion and excretion of bile also rely on the dredging and ventilating function of the liver. If such a function is abnormal and the liver qi is stagnated, the secretion and excretion of bile will be hampered, leading to distending pain in the hypochondriac region, indigestion of food, bitterness sensation in the mouth, or even jaundice, etc.

(5) *Regulating spermiation and menstruation*

The spermiation and menstruation are closely associated with the dredging and ventilating function of the liver. If it functions properly, the seminal excretion will be smooth and moderate, menstruation will be regular and uninhibited, and ovulation will also be sound and normal. If it functions improperly, there will be unsmooth spermiation and irregular, inhibited, or difficult menstruation.

2. *The liver is in charge of storing blood*

In other words, the liver has the physiological function of storing blood and regulating blood volume. This function is mainly reflected by the fact that there must be adequate yin-blood stored in the liver so as to inhibit the hyperactivity of liver yang, maintain the dredging and ventilating function of the liver, and at the same time prevent blood from flowing out the vessels. Hence, if the liver fails to store blood, there will be insufficiency of liver blood, hyperactivity of liver yang, and different kinds of hemorrhagic tendency. The physiological function of the liver to regulate blood volume refers to that the liver can regulate the blood volume of different parts of the body, especially the peripheral blood volume. Under normal conditions, the blood volume of different parts of the blood is relatively stable. However, with the variation of the amount of physical activity, the fluctuation of emotions as well as the change of weather, the blood volume of different parts of the body also changes. For example, when the body is in an active state, when people are excited, or when the weather becomes warmer, the liver will distribute its stored blood to the peripheral parts of the body; while when people are at rest or in a stable emotional state, or when the weather becomes cold, the amount of physical activity will diminish, and accordingly, the requirement for peripheral blood volume will also decrease; hence the surplus blood may finally return to the liver. It is just because the liver can store and regulate blood, that the physiological activities of different parts of the body are closely associated with the liver. If the liver fails to store blood properly, there will be blood deficiency, bleeding or malnutrition of different parts of the body, such as insufficient liver blood failing to nourish the eyes or tendons, marked by dry, dim-sighted and night-blind eyes, or contraction of tendons, numbness of limbs and inhibited movements of joints, etc. Therefore, in *Su Wen*, it is said, "nourished by blood, the liver (eye) can see, the feet can move, the palm can grasp, and the fingers can pinch." The functions of the liver in storing and regulating blood are also reflected in the menstruation of women. If there is insufficient liver blood, or the liver fails to store blood, there will be scanty or profuse menstrual blood, amenorrhea, or even metrorrhagia and metrostaxis, etc.

The function of the liver to store blood is prerequisite to its regulation of blood volume. Only when there is adequate blood volume and no extravasation, the blood volume can be effectively adjusted. The distribution of stored blood to the peripheral parts is actually attributed to the dredging and ventilating function of the liver in promoting blood circulation. This is just like what is said in *Xue Zheng Lun* written by Tang Zonghai, "the liver pertains to wood, which is characterized by free growth. So when it is uninhibited, the blood circulation will be smooth." In this sense, it is considered that the normal functioning of the liver to regulate blood volume requires a balance between the storage and discharge of blood. If the liver is hyperactive or diminished in the function of blood storage, there will be various kinds of bleeding; if it fails to promote free flow of qi, blood stasis may be present.

The Relationship of the Liver to Emotions, Fluids, Body Constituents and Orifices

1. The liver is associated with anger in emotions, which holds that anger may cause the adverse flowing-up of qi and blood and the ascending and dissipating of yang qi. Because the liver is in charge of free flow of qi, and yang qi, characterized by ascending and dispersing, is used by the liver to perform its functions. That is why it is said that the liver is associated with anger. For example, intense anger may cause excessive ascending and dissipating of yang qi, and ultimately impairs the liver; on the contrary, if the yin-blood of the liver is inadequate, then yang qi of the liver will be uncurbed and may lead to irritability or irascibility.

2. The liver is associated with tear in fluids because the liver opens into the eyes, and tears may occasionally be secreted to moisten and protect the eyes. Under normal circumstances, tears can moisten the eye without

flowing out. However, when there are foreign bodies in the eye, tears may be secreted in large volume to clean the eye and remove the foreign bodies. However, pathologically, there will be abnormal secretion of tears. For example, when the liver yin-blood is insufficient, there will be symptoms such as dry eyes due to inadequate yin-fluid; in the cases of wind-fire red eye or damp-heat in the liver meridian, tears may come out involuntarily if encountered with wind; moreover, when one is extremely sorrowful, he or she will also have profuse tears in the eyes.

3. The liver is associated with tendon, or fascia, which is a kind of tissue adherent to the bones and convenes at the joints. Its main function is to connect joints and muscles, and its contraction and remittence will cause the movements of limbs and joints. In *Su Wen*, it is said, "the liver governs the tendon of the body." This remark emphasizes the nourishment of tendons provided by liver blood. If liver blood is sufficient, the tendons will be well-nourished and movements will be forceful and agile. The energy for physical activities is derived from the liver with the function of storing blood and adjusting blood volume. If the liver blood is deficient, the tendons will be malnourished, marked by feeble tendons, inhibited movements, tremor of hands or feet, body numbness and unsmooth flexion and extension of joints, etc. Nails, including finger nail and toe nail, are an extension to the tendons. The exuberance and decline of liver blood can be manifested on the nail. If the liver blood is sufficient, the nail will be red, firm and shiny; and if the liver blood is inadequate, the nail will be thin, fragile, withered or deformed.

4. The liver is associated with the eye, which is a visual organ. The liver meridian of foot jueyin is connected to the eye, so the dredging-ventilating function and the nourishment of the liver are indispensable to eyesight, that is why it is said that the liver opens into the eyes. In *Ling Shu* (*Miraculous Pivot*, 灵枢), it is said, "all the essential qi from the five zang-organs and six fu-organs shall reach the eye and become its nutrients." So we can see that the eye is inherently associated with all the viscera. Since there is close connection between the liver and the eye, the hepatic function can be revealed from the state of the eye. For instance, if the liver yin-blood is insufficient, there will be dry, blurred, or night-blind eyes; wind-heat in the liver meridian may lead to itching and painful eyes; up-flaming of liver fire may cause red eyes with nephelium; hyperactivity

of liver yang may result in dizziness and blurred vision; and internal stirring of liver wind may give rise to distorted eyes and distracted vision, etc.

Daily Exercises

1. What does it mean to say that the liver governs free flow of qi?
2. What does it mean to say that the liver governs storage of blood?
3. Why it is said that the liver opens into the eye?
4. Why it is said that the liver is associated with tendon in the five body constituents?

The Kidney

The kidney is situated in the lumbar region and beside the spine, each on one side. The kidney stores prenatal essence, which is the root of visceral yin and yang and the source of life. That is why it is called the congenital foundation. The kidney pertains to water in five elements, and its main physiological functions are to store essence, to govern growth, development and reproduction, to manage metabolism of water and fluid, and to control bones and marrow production. Its luster is manifested on the hair, and it opens into the ear and two lower orifices (the anus and external genitalia). It is associated with terror or fright in emotions and saliva in fluids. Its meridian is connected with the meridian of the urinary bladder, so the kidney and urinary bladder are externally and internally related.

The Main Physiological Functions of the Kidney

1. The kidney is in charge of storing essence; in other words, the kidney can receive, store and contain essence, preventing it from unnecessary loss. In *Su Wen*, it is said that the kidney, characterized by hiding, is the foundation for storage and the house of essence. This indicates that the main physiological significance of the kidney to store essence lies in its ability to constantly promote the replenishment of essence in the kidney and to prevent the loss of essence for no reason, thus greatly facilitating the performance of essence within the body. If the kidney's storing ability debilitates, there will be loss of kidney essence such as nocturnal emission

or slipping emission, as well as impaired functions of growth, development and production due to insufficient essence.

2. Essence is the basic substance constituting the human body, and is also the material basis for the growth, development and other functional activities. Thus it is said in *Su Wen* that essence is the foundation of life. The essence stored in the kidney includes prenatal essence and postnatal essence. The former, inherited from the reproductive essence of parents, is the most primitive substance for embryonic development. That is why it is said that the kidney is the prenatal foundation of the body. The latter is obtained after birth from water and food, or from the viscera (the remaining part of a fine substance after metabolism, which is produced during the physiological activities of the viscera). It is just like what is said in *Su Wen*, "The kidney controls water, and receives and stores the essence from the five-zang organs and six fu-organs."

Although the source of prenatal essence and postnatal essence are different, they both pertain to the kidney and are interdependent and interacted. The prenatal essence relies on the nourishment and supplement of the postnatal essence to perform its physiological function, while the postnatal essence depends on the support of prenatal essence for constant replenishment and production. They are combined in the kidney and form renal essence to maintain the growth, development and reproduction of the body. In *Su Wen*, there is a vivid description about the birth, growth, maturity, aging and death of the body, suggesting that the key to this process is the exuberance and decline of kidney qi. After birth, the prenatal essence is constantly nourished by the postnatal essence, so the kidney essence gradually becomes abundant, leading to change of teeth and growth of hair. Later, with the replenishment of kidney essence, a material called "Tiangui" appears, which is closely associated with reproductive function. Influenced by Tiangui, the sexual gland starts to develop and thus adolescence begins. When women have menstruation, and men produce sperms, they will be able to reproduce. When entering into middle age, he or she may experience the gradual decline of productive ability with the decrease or even exhaustion of the kidney essence and Tiangui. And finally the body becomes increasingly feeble, entering into the senile age.

The physiological function of the kidney can be discussed in terms of kidney yin and kidney yang. The former, also called primordial yin or genuine yin, has the function of nourishing and moistening the organs and tissues of the body; the latter, also called primordial yang or genuine yang, can warm the organs and tissues or promote their functions. Both rely on the kidney essence as the material base, and the inter-restriction and inter-coordination between them maintain the relative balance of yin and yang in different viscera. If this balance is broken and fails to be self-restored, deficiency of kidney yin or kidney yang will occur, marked by weak waist and knees, dizziness, tinnitus, insomnia, dreaminess, hectic fever, night sweat, seminal emission, red tongue with scanty fluid, and thin-rapid pulse, etc.; or marked by intolerance of cold, cold limbs, loins and knees with pain, white complexion, depression, impotence, pale tongue with white fur, and sinking-weak pulse, etc. Since both kidney yin and kidney yang are based on the kidney essence, pathologically they are mutually affected. For example, deficiency of kidney yin may involve kidney yang, leading to simultaneous deficiency of both, and vise versa.

3. Kidney governing water and fluid, also called kidney governing water, means that the kidney can manage and regulate the metabolism of water and fluid. In *Su Wen*, it is said that the kidney, a water organ, governs body fluid. The metabolism of water and fluid includes two aspects: one is to transport the body fluid transformed from water and food to different parts of the body so as to continuously replenish the blood volume and nourish the organs and tissues; the other is to discharge the metabolized water and fluid or other metabolic products out of the body in the form of sweat or urine. The qi transformation function of the kidney is involved in the whole process of water and fluid metabolism, and this is because all organs participating in this process should be promoted and propelled by the kidney qi; for example, the qi transformation function of the kidney is indispensable to the reception of the stomach, the transformation of the spleen, the dredging of the triple energizer, and the closing and opening of the urinary bladder, etc. If the kidney is deficient, particularly the kidney yang, other viscera involved in this process of metabolism will also be debilitated for lack of promotion and motivation by the kidney yang, thus hindering the normal distribution and discharging of water and fluid. The qi transformation function of the kidney is also associated with

the production and the excretion of urine, which play a key role in maintaining the balance of the whole process of metabolism. If the qi transformation function of the kidney is abnormal, scanty urine or edema will occur. This is discussed in *Su Wen* that the kidney, a checkpoint for the stomach, if it is abnormal and lets the water unchecked, may lead to edema over the skin which is a disorder due to water accumulation. Furthermore, if such a function is abnormal, there will also be unconsolidated kidney qi, or clear and profuse urine due to qi failing to transform water, etc.

4. The kidney is in charge of reception. In other words, the kidney can receive the clear qi inhaled by the lung so as to prevent shallow breathing. The respiratory function, although controlled by the lung, relies on the receptive function of the kidney. In *Lei Zheng Zhi Cai* written by Lin Peiqin, it is said that the lung is the governor of qi, while the kidney is the root of qi. The exhalation of the lung and the reception of the kidney interact harmoniously to ensure normal respiration. The qi-reception function of the kidney is, as a matter of fact, attributed to the function of the kidney in storing essence. Hence, if the qi-reception function of the kidney is normal, the breath will be even and smooth, and otherwise, the respiration will be shallow, marked by gasping on exertion, or excessive exhalation with inadequate inhalation, etc. This is all due to the kidney failing to receive qi.

The Relationship of the Kidney to Emotions, Fluids, Body Constituents and Orifices

1. The kidney is associated with terror in five emotions. Terror is similar to fright; however, the former is a self-conscious fear while the latter is an unexpected sudden startle. Both of them, to physiological activities of the body, are adverse stimulations. Since they pertain to the kidney, if there is an overreaction of fear, there will be unconsolidated kidney qi which moves downwards, marked by urinary and fecal incontinence, seminal emission or slippery diarrhea, etc.

2. The kidney is associated with saliva in fluids. The thick fluid secreted in the mouth is called saliva, which is transformed from kidney essence. If swallowed and not spitted, it can nourish the kidney essence. Contrarily,

excessive or prolonged spitting of sputum will consume the kidney essence. Hence ancient doctors often made their tongue touch the palate, and after the mouth was full of saliva, they swallowed it to nourish the kidney essence. Besides, saliva is also associated with the stomach and spleen. Hence in *Za Bing Yuan Liu Xi Zhu* written by Shen Jinao, it is said, "saliva is a fluid of the kidney, while the kidney is a checkpoint for the stomach, so if saliva is abnormal in patients with renal diseases, it must also be present in the stomach."

3. The kidney is associated with bones. It is in charge of bones and produces marrow. This aspect of function, as a matter of fact, is attributed to the function of the kidney essence in promoting the growth and development of the body. The growth and development of bones rely on the replenishment and nourishment of marrow, but only when the kidney essence is sufficient, the bone marrow will be adequate. Disorders such as infantile delayed closure of fontanel, fragile and feeble bones, or senile rarefaction of bones, are all due to insufficiency of kidney essence and marrow. Marrows, including bone marrow, spinal marrow and brain marrow, are all transformed from the kidney essence. Therefore the state of kidney is critical not only for the growth and development of bones, but also for the replenishment and development of spinal marrow and brain marrow. The spinal marrow is connected with the brain, and the brain is an accumulation of marrow; hence, the brain is also termed "the sea of marrow." If the kidney essence is adequate for the nourishment of the sea of marrow, the brain will grow and develop soundly, and its functions will come into full play. Otherwise, there will be symptoms of insufficient brain marrow characterized by dizziness, tinnitus, and lassitude, etc. The teeth and bones share the same origin, and the former is also nourished by kidney essence; therefore, there is a saying, "the teeth are the extension of bones." In *Za Bing Yuan Liu Xi Zhu*, it is said that the teeth are the branches of the kidney and root of bones, indicating that the growth and decaying of the teeth are closely related to the exuberance or decline of the kidney essence. If the kidney essence is sufficient, the teeth will be firm and consolidated, and otherwise, they will be loose and apt to fall off. The growth and development of hair rely not only on the nourishment of kidney essence, but also on the supplement of blood; hence it is also called "surplus of blood." During the adolescence and middle age, one's hair is

long and lustrous because of abundant essence and blood, while when he becomes old, the hair will turn white and begin to fall off due to the diminishment of blood and essence.

4. The kidney is associated with the ear and two lower orifices. The sharpness of the hearing sense is closely related to the conditions of the kidney essence. If the kidney essence is abundant, the brain marrow will be nourished and the sense of hearing will be good. Otherwise, if there is depletion of kidney essence, the brain marrow will be malnourished and the sense of hearing will be impaired, leading to tinnitus or even deafness. When people are old, their sense of hearing will degenerate with the decline of renal essence. That is why it is said that the kidney opens into the ear. The two lower orifices, or external genitalia and anus, are organs in charge of urination, reproduction and defecation. The discharging of urine, though controlled by the urinary bladder, relies on the qi transformation function of the kidney as well. Hence frequent urination, enuresis, urinary incontinence and suppression of urine are all attributable to the malfunction of qi transformation. The reproductive function, however, is also dominated by the kidney. And defecation, though pertaining to the large intestine, is also associated with qi transformation. For instance, if the kidney yin is insufficient, there will be constipation due to exhaustion of intestinal fluids; if the kidney yang is deficient, there will be constipation or diarrhea due to dysfunction of qi transformation; if the storing function of the kidney is in disorder, there will be chronic diarrhea or slippery diarrhea; that is why it is said that the kidney opens into the two lower orifices.

Appendix: Mingmen (the Life Gate)

Mingmen, or life gate, means the foundation or the root of life. The position and function of life gate are rather diversified. It is believed to be located in the right kidney, or both of the kidneys, or the region between the kidneys. It is also considered by others to be the motive force between the kidneys. Despite these differences, views on the main physiological function of the kidney are approximately the same. It is deemed that the physiological function of the life gate is, in essence, related to the kidney very closely. Conceiving genuine yin and genuine yang, the kidney is the foundation of the five zang-organs. The viscera yin and yang rely on the kidney yin and yang for nourishment and warmth. Kidney yin is known as "the fire of life gate," and the kidney yang is called "the water of life gate" by Zhang Jingyue. Kidney yin and yang, also called genuine yin and yang, or primordial yin and yang, are very essential to the human body. That is why they are regarded as the gate of life.

Daily Exercises

1. What is refered to as the "fire of life gate"?
2. What does it mean to say that the kidney governs storage of essence?
3. What is Tiangui?
4. What does it mean to say that the kidney controls water and fluid?

Weekly Review

The heart is called "the monarch organ." It has two main functions: controlling blood and vessels and dominating the spirit. The former includes two aspects: control of blood and control of blood vessels. The blood circulates in the vessels and relies on the pumping of the heart to reach all parts of the body, so as to perform its nourishing and moistening functions. The vessels are pathways of blood circulation, the smoothness or obstruction of which directly influences the normal flow of blood. Therefore, among the heart, vessels and blood, a relatively independent system, the heart plays the decisive role. The normal pulsation of the heart depends on the nourishing and moistening functions of the heart blood and heart yin, as well as the warming functions of the heart qi and heart yang. So, only when the cardiac efficiency, rate and rhythm are normal can blood circulate normally to nourish the whole body. Heart governing spirit means that the heart can dominate and control the spiritual, mental and thinking activities of the body. Therefore, normal physiological function of the heart to control spirit will ensure a high spirit, a clear and agile mind, and a sensitive reaction to the external stimulation. However, the abnormal changes of the physiological functions of the heart to govern spirit will bring about symptoms such as insomnia, dreaminess, distraction and even delirium; or slow reaction, amnesia, dispiritedness, and even coma, etc.

The lung is compared to a "canopy" because of the uppermost position among all the viscera. The main physiological functions of the lung are to dominate qi and control respiration, govern ascent, dispersion, purification and descent as well as regulate water passage. It also has regulatory functions because it is associated with various vessels. It controls the general qi throughout the body as well as the air it inhales and exhales. The reason why it controls qi throughout the body is that all kinds of qi ultimately belong to the lung, which is mainly reflected in the process of qi production, particularly the thoracic qi. The lung governing the inhaled and exhaled qi means that the lung is the location where the external air and the internal qi exchange. Both of these two functions of the lung can be ultimately traced back to the respiratory function of the lung. The lung managing ascent and dispersion is mainly reflected in three aspects: a. Discharging the turbid qi within the body by dispersion and qi transformation. b. Distributing the body fluid and essence from water and cereal transformed by the spleen to the whole body as well as the skin and hair in the exterior. c. Diffusing defensive qi to warm and nourish the skin and muscles, to regulate the opening or closing of the skin striae, and to discharge the metabolic products of body fluid by transforming them into sweat. The descent and purification of the lung can also be discussed in three aspects: a. inhaling fresh air from nature; b. dispersing downward the inhaled fresh air as well as the body fluid and essence from water and cereal transformed by the spleen; c. purifying the foreign bodies within the respiratory tract, thus making it clean. The ascent-dispersion and descent-purification of the lung are inseparable. They are a unity of opposites and thus are mutually affected pathologically. The lung is in charge of dredging and regulating waterways. This aspect of the pulmonary function relies on the ascent-dispersion and descent-purification of the lung to regulate the distribution, circulation and discharging of water and fluid. The lung, located above all the other viscera, distributes water and fluid, which are transported to the lung *via* the spleen and stomach, to all parts of the body and at the same time transfers them downwards. That is why it is called "the upper source of water and fluid." The lung opens into various vessels and is in charge of regulation and management. Almost all vessels are convened in the lung which means that all the blood within the body is transported to the lung through different vessels, and after exchange of qi *via* respiration, the fresh blood is sent back to the whole body. It is thus evident that the lung is closely linked to the vessels and blood circulation. The lung is in charge of regulation and management, which means that the lung can manage and regulate the physiological functions of the whole body. It is largely manifested in four aspects: a. The lung controls respiration and, through this process, fresh air is inhaled for physiological activities, and the metabolized turbid qi is exhaled out of the body; b. The respiration of the lung regulates the ascending, descending, entering and exiting of qi; c. The lung propels and regulates blood circulation with the function of managing and controlling qi activities; d. With the function of descent and purification, the lung can manage and regulate the distribution, circulation and excretion of body fluid.

The spleen is the organ of storehouse. Its main physiological functions are to govern transportation and transformation, ascend the lucid substances, and control blood circulation. The spleen is in charge of transformation and transportation; such a function can be divided into two aspects: transportation and transformation of water and cereal; and transportation and transformation of water and fluid. Transportation and transformation of water and cereal refers to the digestion and absorption of water and food and the transmission of nutrients. This function relies greatly on the conditions of spleen qi. If the spleen qi is vigorous, the transportation, transformation, and the absorption of water and cereal will be normal, and so will be the production of qi, blood, body fluid and kidney essence, thus ensuring the adequate nourishment of various organs and tissues of the body and the normal physiological functions of the body. On the contrary, if this function debilitates, the digestion and absorption will become abnormal. Hence it is said that the spleen is the postnatal foundation and the source of qi and blood production. Transportation and transformation of water and fluid refers to the absorption, transmission and dispersion of water and fluid so as to maintain the metabolic balance of water and fluid within the body. If the spleen qi is vigorous, the water and fluid circulation will be normal, and there will be no dampness, phlegm or retained body fluid, etc. On the contrary, if the spleen qi is weak, and the spleen fails to transport properly, there will be dampness, phlegm and fluid retention, etc. The spleen governs the ascent of the lucid substances; in other words, the spleen is characterized by ascending the nutrients from water and cereal upward to the heart, lungs, head and eyes so as to transform into qi and blood and nourish the whole body. Ascent and descent is a pair of opposites in terms of visceral qi activities. The ascent of lucidity by the spleen is often mentioned in relation to the descent of turbidity by the stomach, and only when they are in a dynamic balance will digestion and absorption by the body be normal. Otherwise, the deficient spleen qi will fail to fully ascend the nutrients from water and cereal to the head and eyes. Moreover, the ascent of the spleen can also prevent visceroptosis. The spleen controls blood; in other words, the spleen can govern or control the blood circulation, containing it within the vessel without flowing out. The spleen controlling blood is closely related to the fact that the spleen is the source of qi and blood. Because the spleen governs the ascent of lucid substances and the spleen qi is characterized by ascending, we often attribute hematochezia, blood urine and metrorrhagia and metrostaxis to the spleen failing to control blood.

The liver is likened to a general in charge of strategy. The main physiological functions of the liver are to govern free flow of qi and store blood. The former function is manifested in two aspects: regulation of qi movements and regulation of emotional activities. The dredging and ventilation function of the liver plays a critical role in maintaining the balance of the ascending, descending, entering and exiting movements of qi. If it is normal, the qi movements will be smooth, the qi and blood will be harmonious, and the physiological activities of the viscera, meridians and collaterals, as well as tissues will be normal. On the contrary, if it is abnormal, there will be stagnation of qi movements and malfunction of ascending, descending, entering and exiting of qi, marked by distension, fullness and pain in the chest or hypochondriac region, breasts, lower abdomen or external genitalia. Besides, if the liver fails to promote free flow of qi, the circulation of blood and fluid, the secretion and excretion of bile, and the ascent of the lucid and the descent of the turbid of the spleen will be affected. The spermiation and menstruation are closely associated with the dredging and ventilating function of the liver. The abnormal emotions are often attributed to the dysfunction of the liver in dredging and ventilating. If the liver functions properly to dredge and ventilate, the qi activities will be smooth, and there will harmonious co-existence of qi and blood, as well as a happy, contented state of mind. Otherwise, if the liver fails to function properly, there will be stagnation of liver qi, or depression and sentimental emotion. If the liver is hyperactive in ascending, there will be adverse up-flaming of qi and fire, irascibility and irritability.

The liver is in charge of storing blood; in other words, the liver has the physiological functions of storing blood and regulating blood volume. This function is mainly reflected by the fact that there must be adequate yin-blood stored in the liver so as to inhibit the hyperactivity of liver yang, maintain the dredging and ventilating function of the liver, and at the same time prevent bleeding. The physiological function of the liver to regulate blood volume refers to that the liver can regulate the blood volume of different parts of the body, especially the peripheral blood volume. When the body is in an active state, when people are excited, or when the weather becomes warmer, the liver will distribute its stored blood to the peripheral parts of the body; while when people are at rest or in a stable emotional state, or when the weather becomes cold, the amount of physical activity will diminish, and accordingly, the requirement for peripheral blood volume will also decrease; hence the surplus blood may finally return to the liver. The function of the liver to store blood is prerequisite to the regulation of blood volume. Only when there is adequate blood volume and no extravasation, the blood volume can be effectively adjusted. The distribution of stored blood to the peripheral parts is actually attributed to the dredging and ventilating function of the liver in promoting blood circulation.

The kidney is the congenital foundation. Its main physiological functions are to store essence, to govern growth, development, reproduction and metabolism of water and fluid, and to control bones and marrow production. The kidney is in charge of storing essence; in other words, the kidney can receive, store and seal essence, preventing it from loss for no reason. The essence stored in the kidney includes prenatal essence and postnatal essence. The former, inherited from the reproductive essence of parents, is the most primitive substance for embryonic development. The latter is obtained after birth from water and food or from the viscera (the remaining part of a fine substance after metabolism, which is produced during the visceral physiological functions). Although the source of prenatal essence and postnatal essence are different, they both pertain to the kidney and are interdependent and interacted. They are combined in the kidney and forms renal essence to maintain the growth, development and reproduction of the body. The physiological function of the kidney can be explained in terms of kidney yin and kidney yang. Both of them rely on the kidney essence as the material base, and the inter-restriction and inter-coordination between them maintain the relative balance between yin and yang of different viscera.

Kidney governing water and fluid, also called kidney governing water, means that the kidney is in charge of and regulates the metabolism of water and fluid. The qi transformation function of the kidney is involved in the whole process of water and fluid metabolism, and this is because all organs participating in this process should be promoted and propelled by the kidney qi; for example, the qi transformation function of the kidney is indispensable to the reception of the stomach, the transformation of the spleen, the dredging of the triple energizer, or the closing and opening of the urinary bladder, etc. The qi transformation function of the kidney is also associated with the production and the excretion of urine, which play a key role in maintaining the balance of the whole process of metabolism. If the qi transformation function of the kidney is abnormal, scanty urine or edema will occur.

The kidney is in charge of reception, and in other words, the kidney can receive the clear qi inhaled by the lung so as to prevent shallow breathing. The respiratory function, although controlled by the lung, relies on the receptive function of the kidney. The qi-reception function of the kidney is, as a matter of fact, a concrete manifestation of the function of the kidney to store essence in respiration. Hence, if the qi-reception function of the kidney is normal, the breath will be even and smooth.

Daily Exercises

1. To be familiar with the main physiological functions of each zang-organ.
2. To be familiar with the relationship of the five zang-organs to emotions, fluids, body constituents and orifices.

THE FIFTH WEEK

SECTION 2   THE SIX FU-ORGANS

The six fu-organs, namely gallbladder, stomach, large intestine, small intestine, urinary bladder and triple energizer, are mostly hollow organs with the common physiological function of transporting and transforming food and water. There are two approaches for the six fu-organs to perform their functions: 1. First water and food are taken into the mouth and then into the stomach where they are first digested, and then transported downwards to the small intestine where they are further separated into fine substances and waste; the former are distributed to nourish all over the body *via* the spleen, while the latter, is sent down to the large intestine where it is transported and transformed and eventually discharged out of the body *via* the anus. In this process, the bile is also involved to facilitate food digestion. 2. The body fluid are distributed to nourish and moisten all parts of the body *via* the triple energizer, while the metabolic products are transported to the urinary bladder *via* the lower energizer where they are transformed into urine and discharged out of the body. It is evident that the digestion, absorption and excretion of water and food are processes in which the six fu-organs intimately cooperate and interact; therefore, the disorder of one fu-organ may ultimately involve another, and may further affect the reception, digestion, absorption and excretion of water and food.

The physiological characteristics of the six fu-organs can be classified as "transporting without storing," marked by prompt evacuation of their contents and downward transportation. Hence the six fu-organs are characterized by decent and non-obstruction, or dredging, which are of great significance. During different periods of transporting and transforming water and food, the six fu-organs alternate their state of "fullness" and "emptiness" in succession; while at the period, they are in different states of "fullness" and "emptiness." Meanwhile, there are certain key passes or checkpoints at the entrance or exit of the fu-organs, called the "seven flying portals" in *Nan Jing*. They are responsible for the regulation and coordination of the six fu-organs to ensure the orderly transportation and descent.

For this reason, both excessiveness and inadequateness of decent and dredging are morbid conditions of the six fu-organs. Of the two conditions, the former is more common; in other words, the six fu-organs often fail to "transport without storing," which inevitably leads to accumulation or obstruction of food and waste. Hence the disorders of the six fu-organs are mostly characterized by excess syndromes, such as distending fullness, pain, or tenderness, etc.

The Gallbladder

The gallbladder is the chief of all the fu-organs. It is linked with the liver and appends to the hepatic lobule. Its meridian is connected, interiorly and exteriorly, with the liver meridian. And its main physiological functions are manifested in three aspects:

1. The gallbladder is in charge of storing bile, which is bitter in taste and yellow-green in color. It is transformed from the surplus qi of the liver and accumulates in the gallbladder. When needed, it will flow into the small intestine to facilitate digestion. It is thus clear that the bile is indispensable to the normal performance of the spleen and stomach in transportation and transformation.

2. The gallbladder can excrete bile under the control and regulation of the liver. If the liver functions properly in promoting free flow of qi, the excretion of bile will be smooth and the transportation-transformation of the spleen and stomach will also be normal. Otherwise, if the liver fails to disperse and ventilate, the excretion of bile will be inhibited and the qi movement of the liver and gallbladder will be unsmooth, thus hampering the digesting function of the spleen and stomach, marked by distension, fullness and pain under the costal region, or reduced appetite, abdominal distension and loose stool, etc.; if the bile up-flows or overflows, there will be bitterness sensation in the mouth, vomit of yellow-green fluids, and jaundice, etc.

3. The gallbladder governs decision, which is a mental activity. This function is associated with the liver in governing strategy. The decision-making process is attributable to bile. Under normal circumstances, the bile is abundant, ensuring correct and resolute decisions. Besides, it also reflects the exuberance and decline of healthy qi. Since the healthy qi can resist exogenous pathogenic factors, the state of bile is also a reflection of a person's ability to resist pathogenic factors.

4. Unlike other fu-organs, the gallbladder is an extraordinary fu-organ among the six common fu-organs. There are three reasons: a.

The substance stored in and excreted from the gallbladder is the bile, not foodstuff or waste.

5. The gallbladder itself has no physiological function of transporting and transforming foodstuff. So we can see that there is a big difference between it and the other fu-organs. In this sense, it is called an "extraordinary fu-organ," about which we will discuss later.

The Stomach

The stomach, also called the gastric cavity, is divided into the upper, middle and lower parts. The upper part, or upper epigastrium, includes the carda; the middle part, or middle epigastrium, includes the body of the stomach; and the lower part, or lower epigastrium, includes the pylorus. The stomach, also called sea of water and cereal, is an important organ where food and water are received, digested and absorbed. Because qi and blood originate from water and cereal, the stomach is also termed "sea of water, cereal, qi and blood." The stomach and spleen are interiorly and exteriorly related. The main physiological functions and characteristics of the stomach are indicated in two aspects:

1. The stomach is in charge of reception and digestion; in other words, the stomach receives water and foodstuff and preliminarily decomposes them into chyme. Water and foodstuff are first taken into the mouth, and then into the stomach *via* the esophagus, and after preliminary digestion in the stomach, they are transported to the small intestine and subsequently their essences are transported to all parts of the body after the transformation of the spleen. Thus we can see that the reception and digestion of the stomach should be properly coordinated with the transportation and transformation of the spleen. If there are disorders in reception and digestion of the stomach, there will be anorexia, no feeling of hunger and indigestion of water and food even if they are taken.

2. The stomach is in charge of dredging and descent, or downward transportation of food; in other words, it takes downward transportation of food as the normal functional activities. After reception and digestion of water and foodstuff by the stomach, the small intestine further digests and absorbs them, transforming them into qi, blood and body fluid to nourish the whole body. That is why it is said that the stomach takes dredging and descent as the normal functional activities. This is different from western

medicine and covers a far wider scope, including the transportation of chyme to the small intestine by the stomach and the transportation of residues to the large intestine by the small intestine, as well as the transportation and transformation of the residues by the large intestine. This process, as a matter of fact, covers the functions of the small intestine and some functions of the large intestine in western medicine. The downward transportation of food by the stomach, in contrast to the ascent of the lucid by the spleen, is in essence the descent of the turbid. In this sense, we can see that the digestion and absorption of the spleen and stomach are actually a process of the ascending of lucid by the spleen and the descending of the turbid by the stomach. Besides, the downward transportation of food is prerequisite to further reception. So if the stomach fails to descend, the appetite will be affected, with such signs as foul breath, distending or painful stomach and abdomen, and constipation; and if the stomach qi flows upward, there will be belching, nausea, vomiting, hiccups, etc.

Moreover, during the study of TCM, we often encounter words such as "stomach qi," which covers a wide area encompassing two aspects: one refers to the visceral qi; it is similar to heart qi or kidney qi, and pertains to the gastric body or gastric wall with the function of facilitating the stomach to digest food. The other is the cereal qi in the gastric cavity and the nutrients absorbed for maintaining the normal life activities. They are obtained from normal digestion of water and food by the spleen and stomach, and are indispensable to the maintenance of life activities. The presence or absence of stomach qi is the key to the soundness or even survival of the human body. Hence, it is also called the "postnatal foundation." If the stomach qi is vigorous, the complexion will be rosy and lustrous, and the pulse will be calm and forceful; while if the stomach is depleted, the face will be lusterless and demonstrates its true color, and the pulse will be hastened and feeble, revealing its genuine nature.

The Small Intestine

The small intestine, a long tract organ, is located in the abdomen. Its upper end is connected with the stomach at the pylorus and its lower end with the large intestine at the ileocolic opening. The small intestine and the heart are connected through the meridian and they are in an interior-exterior relationship. It is in charge of the digestion of food, the distribution of nutrients and the transportation of residues. There two main functions of this organ:

1. It is in charge of reception and digestion. Reception means the acceptance of food while digestion refers to the transformation of food into nutrients. The former is the basis of the latter while the latter is a result of the former. Water and food, after preliminary digestion by the stomach, must stay in the small intestine for a period of time so as to be digested completely and be separated into nutrients and residues.

2. The small intestine is in charge of separating the lucid (nutrients) from the turbid (residues). After the small intestine digests water and cereals, it absorbs the nutrients from water and cereals and transports the residues to the large intestine. The small intestine also absorbs large amount of water and fluid when assimilating the nutrients. In this sense it is said that the small intestine governs thick fluid. In ancient medical classics, there are records that the function of separating the lucid from the turbid is realized through the ileocolic opening at the lower end of the small intestine, which is depicted as a paliform organ where chyme is separated into clear water and turbid residues. The former flows into the urinary bladder while the latter goes to the large intestine. So it can be seen that such a function is concerned with the urine volume. If this function is normal, urination and defecation will be normal; otherwise, the stools will become loose and the urine scanty. Moreover, this function also give reasonable explanations for the pathogenesis of heart fire moving downward to the small intestine, marked by red urine with hot and painful sensation.

From the above-mentioned, it can be seen that the functions of the small intestine to receive and digest food and separate the lucid from the turbid are, as a matter of fact, attributable to the ascent of the lucid by the spleen and the decent of the turbid by the stomach. Hence if the small intestine is in disorder, there will be turbid qi failing to descend, with such symptoms as abdominal distension, abdominal pain, vomiting and constipation; or lucid qi failing to ascend, with such signs as loose stool and diarrhea, etc.

Daily Exercises

1. What are the important channels for the performance of the physiological functions of the six fu-organs?
2. What is stomach qi?

The Large Intestine

The large intestine, a tract organ, is located in the abdomen. Its upper end is connected with the small intestine at the ileocolic opening and its lower end with the anus. Its meridian is connected with the lung meridian and they have an interior-exterior relationship. It can absorb the remnant water from the residues and then discharge them out of the body. Its main physiological functions covers two aspects:

1. It is in charge of transporting and transforming residues; in other words, it receives the food residues from the small intestine, absorbs the remnant water, and transforms the residues into feces, which are finally discharged out of the body *via* the anus. If this function fails to work properly, there will be such symptoms as loose stool, diarrhea and constipation, etc.

2. It can absorb the remnant water from the residues transported from the small intestine, thus influencing the discharging of water in some degree. If the residues stay in the large intestine for a relatively shorter time, there will be diarrhea due to less water absorption; on the contrary, if they stay for a longer time, there will be constipation due to excessive water absorption.

The transportation and transformation of the large intestine are actually attributable to the descent of the turbid by the stomach. So if the stomach fails to descend, the large intestine will be involved. Owing to the fact that all the viscera are interrelated, disorders of other viscera may also affect the large intestine. For instance, if the lung fails to descend and purify, or if the kidney fails to transform qi, there will be constipation; if the kidney fails to warm the body, there will be diarrhea. Moreover, the malfunction of the small intestine to separate the lucid from the turbid may also involve the large intestine.

The Urinary Bladder

The urinary bladder, a capsular organ, is located in the center of the lower abdomen. The urinary bladder and the kidney are interiorly and exteriorly connected via their meridians. The main physiological functions of the urinary bladder cover two aspects:

1. It is in charge of storing urine. Under the qi-transformation function of the kidney, the body fluid are changed into urine and stored in the urinary bladder for a period of time. This function relies on the qi-transformation function of the kidney and urinary bladder as well as the consolidation-astringency function of the kidney qi. If the urinary bladder fails to control, or the kidney qi fails to consolidate and astringe, there will be profuse urine at night, enuresis or incontinence of urine, etc.

2. It is in charge of excreting urine. When the volume of urine in the urinary bladder reach a certain degree, the urinary bladder will be full and there will be micturition desire. Under the influence of qi-transformation by the kidney and urinary bladder, the urine will be discharged out of the body. So the function of urinary bladder to discharge urine relies on the qi-transformation by the kidney and urinary bladder. If qi-transformation fails to function properly, there will be unsmooth urination, difficult urination or retention of urine, etc.

The Triple Energizer

The triple energizer, or sanjiao, is a special fu-organ with different concept. The triple energizer is a collective term for the upper energizer, middle energizer and lower energizer. In ancient medical classics, there is no clear description as to the concept of triple energizer. So opinions on its location and function are quite controversial. It has four different meanings: a. As one of the fu-organs, it serves as the passages among different viscera and even among the internal space within a particular organ. In these passages, primordial qi and body fluid circulate. Hence the smoothness of the triple energizer is indispensable to the movements of qi and the distribution or excretion of body fluid. From above, we can infer that it may cover the thoracic cavity and the abdominal cavity. b. It simply refers to different regions; for example, the upper energizer is located above the diaphragm, the middle energizer is between the diaphragm and the umbilicus, and the lower energizer is below the umbilicus. c. It refers to the viscera within the upper, middle or lower energizer. For instance, the upper energizer includes the heart and lung, the middle, the spleen and stomach, and the lower, the liver and kidney. d. It refers to different stages of febrile diseases. For instance, disorders of the upper energizer appear at the early stage, those of the middle energizer, the middle stage, and those of the lower energizer, such as liver and kidney diseases, the late stage.

The Main Functions of the Triple Energizer as One of the Six Fu-Organs

1. It is in charge of all kinds of qi and controls qi activity of the whole body because the triple energizer is both the passage for qi movements and the location for qi transformation. Primordial qi, the fundamental qi within the body, is rooted in the kidney and is distributed to all parts of the body through the triple energizer.

2. It is the waterway for water and fluid. The triple energizer can dredge the waterway for the circulation of water and fluid. Although the metabolism of water and fluid is conducted by the coordination of the lung, spleen, stomach, intestines, kidney and urinary bladder, it must rely on the triple energizer as the passage to ascend, descend, enter and exit normally. Hence in TCM, the balancing function of the triple energizer in the metabolism of water and fluid is called "qi-transforming of triple energizer," which mainly represents the qi-transforming function of other viscera such as the lung, spleen, and kidney.

The aforementioned functions are interconnected. This is because the circulation of water and fluid relies on the ascent, descent, entering and exiting of qi, and qi is attached to blood and body fluid, so the passage for qi movements is certainly the passage for water and fluid; conversely, the passage for fluid circulation is also the pathway for qi.

The Physiological Characteristics of Triple Energizer as a Reference to Location

1. The upper energizer is above the diaphragm, including the heart, lung, head and face, or even the upper limbs. Its main function is to govern the ascent and dispersion of qi; in other words, it disperses the defensive qi and distributes the nutrients all over the body.

2. The middle energizer is located at the upper abdomen between the diaphragm and the umbilicus, including the spleen and stomach.

Its main physiological function is to digest, absorb and distribute the nutrients so as to produce blood, and this process covers the whole transportation-transformation activities of the spleen and stomach. That is why it is said that the middle energizer can process food into residues and distribute body fluid all over the body, serving as the pivot of ascent and descent and the source of qi and blood. Noticeably, the liver, though located in the middle energizer, is classified into the lower energizer, as is exemplified by the theory of warm diseases.

3. The lower energizer is below the umbilicus, including the small intestine, large intestine, kidney and urinary bladder, etc. Its main function is to discharge residues and urine.

Daily Exercises

1. What is the connotation of the triple energizer?
2. What are the physiological functions of the large intestine and urinary bladder?

SECTION 3   THE EXTRAORDINARY FU-ORGANS

"Extraordinary fu-organs" is a collective term for the brain, marrow, bones, vessels, gallbladder, and uterus. Being hollow organs with the function of transporting food and storing essence, the six extraordinary fu-organs are similar both to the fu-organs in morphology and to the zang-organs in function. The extraordinary fu-organs do not have internal-external relationships with other organs, nor do they pertain to any element; the only exception, however, is the gallbladder, which also pertains to the six fu-organs. Since we have discussed about the vessels, marrow, bones and gallbladder previously, we will only introduce the brain and uterus in this section.

The Brain

The brain, being one of the extraordinary fu-organs, is located in the skull and connected with the spinal cord. Since it is actually a collection of marrow, it is termed "the sea of marrow." Its main physiological functions are as follows:

1. Controlling life activities. In *Su Wen*, it is pointed out, "When needling the head, if Naohu (DU 17) is punctured, one will die instantly." And in *Ben Cao Gang Mu* written by Li Shizhen during the Ming Dynasty, it is pointed out that the intelligence and memory come from the brain, not from the heart. This indicates that the ancient doctors have recognized the importance of the brain in human life activities. The vital center is located in the brain which is one of the signs of life activities, so the brain can dominate our life activities.

2. Relating to emotional activities. Emotional activities include consciousness, thinking, sentiment and memory, etc. As early as the period when the visceral theory was formed, the brain functions were unclear to the TCM doctors. They just called them the sea of marrow, and recognized that it is a collection of marrow and is closely associated with the kidney. That is why we ascribe the brain functions to the heart and also attribute them to the five zang-organs, respectively. The heart is in control of consciousness and thinking activities, so it is said that the heart stores the spirit. The spirit, however, is subdivided into ethereal soul, corporeal soul, ideation, will and vitality, which pertain to the five zang-organs respectively. All of them are commanded by the heart. The spirit has a closer relationship with the heart, liver and kidney. Therefore, for emotional or mental disorders, we cannot simply attribute all of them to the dysfunction of the heart in governing spirit and rule out the possibility of other visceral disorders. For brain disorders, we should also not ascribe them simply to the kidney and exclude the possibility of other visceral disorders. This is a brief introduction to the recognition about the brain in traditional Chinese and Western medicine. And such a cultural trait is carried on throughout the ages till today. For example, at the present time we still use the heart to describe the emotional or mental activities in common Chinese language.

3. Governing abilities of hearing, seeing, smelling and speaking. The abilities to hear, see, smell and speak pertain to and is governed by the brain. This is similar to the viewpoint that the brain gathers a variety of vital centers in modern medicine. Meanwhile, TCM also ascribes these functions to different viscera, e.g., the sense of hearing is closely related

to the liver and kidney, seeing to the liver (and sometimes the heart), and smelling to the lung.

The Uterus

The uterus, or the palace of the fetus, is located in the center of the lower abdomen and connected with vagina at the lower end, posterior to the urinary bladder and anterior to the rectum. It resembles an inverted pear when not conceived. The main physiological functions of the uterus are as follows:

1. Governing menstruation. The uterus is an organ where menstruation occurs after the maturity of female reproductive function. A healthy female begins to develop in productivity at the age of 13 to 14 years old, and under the influence of tiangui, the conception vessel will be unobstructed, and the thoroughfare vessel is abundant in qi and blood, and thus menstruation occurs. So the normal functions of the uterus are of great significance to the menstrual onset.

2. Conceiving fetus. After normal menstrual onset, the uterus will be capable of producing and conceiving the fetus. After pregnancy, the menstruation stops, and visceral or meridian qi, blood and body fluid will reach the uterus through the thoroughfare vessel and the conception vessel to nourish the fetus. So the uterus also plays a key role in conceiving the fetus.

The Relationship of the Uterus to Tiangui, Thoroughfare Vessel, Conception Vessel, Heart, Liver and Spleen

The process of the uterus in governing menstruation and pregnancy is very complicated and involves tiangui, thoroughfare vessel and conception vessel, as well as the heart, liver and spleen, which mainly manifests as follows:

1. The functions of tiangui. Tiangui, a substance produced when the kidney essence is abundant to a certain extent, can promote the development and maturity of sexual glands and maintain the female reproductive functions. Hence, promoted by it, the female sexual organs begin to develop and menstruation begins to occur, preparing for conceiving the

fetus. When people are old, however, their renal essence begins to decline and tiangui becomes declined and depleted. It is thus evident that the arrival or discontinuation of tiangui is decisive in triggering the onset of menstruation and the action of thoroughfare vessel and conception vessel.

2. The functions of thoroughfare vessel and conception vessel. The two meridians both start from the uterus. The thoroughfare vessel runs alongside the kidney-meridian and connects with the stomach-meridian. Because the thoroughfare vessel can regulate qi and blood from the 12 meridians, it is called the sea of blood; the conception vessel, connecting with the three yin meridians of foot at the lower abdomen, is in charge of the uterus and can regulate the yin meridians all over the body, therefore it is called the sea of yin meridians. Only when qi and blood from the 12 meridians are abundant can they overflow into the thoroughfare vessel and conception vessel and subsequently into the uterus to promote menstruation. The waxing and waning of qi and blood in the thoroughfare vessel and conception vessel are regulated by tiangui. Before adolescence, the kidney essence is inadequate, tiangui has not come, the conception vessel is obstructed and thoroughfare vessel is not abundant, hence there will be no menstruation; when people become old, tiangui begin to decline, Qi and blood in the thoroughfare vessel and conception vessel begin to wane, and there will be irregular menstruation and eventually menopause. If there are disorders of the thoroughfare vessel and conception vessel, there will be irregular menstruation or even amenorrhea and infertility, etc.

3. The influences of the heart, liver and spleen. The uterus plays a significant role in menstrual onset and cycle as well as fetal conception. All of these functions, however, rely on the abundance of qi and blood and the normal regulation of blood which is dominated by the heart, stored by the liver, and controlled by the spleen. Hence, menstruation is closely associated with the heart, liver and spleen. If the liver fails to store blood or the spleen fails to control blood, there will be profuse menses, shortened menstrual cycle, prolonged menstrual period, or even metrorrhagia and metrostaxis. If the spleen is weak in producing qi and blood, there will be scanty menses, prolonged menstrual cycle or even amenorrhea. If the heart-spirit is impaired or the dispersion-ventilation function of the liver is affected due to emotional disorders, such pathological manifestations as irregular menstruation may also appear.

Daily Exercises

1.   What are extraordinary fu-organs?
2.   What are the main physiological functions of the uterus?

SECTION 4   THE RELATIONSHIPS AMONG THE VISCERA

The human body, a unified organic whole, is composed of many tissues and organs such as the viscera, meridians and collaterals. Their functional activities are not isolated, but a coordinated performance of the whole body. They are physiologically inter-restricted, interdependent and inter-promoted; besides, they also constitute a coordinated, unified organic body aided by the connection of meridians and the circulation of qi, blood and body fluid.

The Relationships Among the Five Zang-Organs

The relationships between the five zang-organs are rather complicated; for instance, the heart is the monarch of the five zang-organs, so the life activities of the five-zang organs are dominated by the heart; the kidney yin and kidney yang are the root of the yin and yang of the five zang-organs and the excess and deficiency of the kidney essence is the key to the exuberance and debilitation of yin and yang of the five zang-organs; the spleen and stomach is the source of qi and blood, so the functions of the spleen and stomach are of great significance to the volume of qi and blood of the five zang-organs. Besides, traditional Chinese medicine also explains their relations in terms of the five elements. The specific relationships between them are introduced as follows:

The Relationships Between the Heart and the Lung

The relationships between the heart and lung are mainly manifested as the coordination between the heart governing blood and the lung governing qi as well as the interaction between the heart governing blood circulation and the lung governing respiration.

1. The coordination between the heart governing blood and the lung governing qi is, as a matter of fact, a specific manifestation of the inter-dependence and inter-promotion between qi and blood, which will be further discussed in the following chapter of qi, blood, fluid, and liquor.

2. The interaction between the heart governing blood circulation and the lung governing respiration can be generalized into "qi commanding blood" and "blood carrying qi." The dispersion-descent function of the lung and the feature of all vessels converging in the lung can facilitate the heart to promote blood circulation; conversely, only when the heart pro-pels blood normally can respiration functions properly. The ancients believed that the key link to blood circulation and respiration is thoracic qi, which permeates throughout the heart vessels and manages respiration, thus reinforcing the coordination and balance between blood circulation and respiration. For this reason, the deficiency of lung qi and the dysfunc-tion of the lung in ascent and descent can both affect blood circulation, leading to chest distress, alteration in heart rate, cyanic lips and purple tongue, etc. Conversely, if the heart qi is deficient, or the heart yang is weak, or the heart vessels are blocked, the respiration function of the lung will be affected, leading to adverse rising of lung qi, with such signs as coughing and panting, etc.

The Relationships Between the Heart and Spleen

The relationships between the heart and spleen can be discussed in terms of blood production and circulation. The heart governs blood while the spleen controls it; besides, the spleen is the source of qi and blood, so the relation between the heart and spleen is very close. If the spleen is normal in transportation and transformation, there will be abundant blood for the heart to govern; and only when the spleen qi is vigorous and controls blood normally without extravasation can the heart perform its function of governing blood. So pathologically, there will be simultaneous deficiency of the heart and spleen. For instance, excessive thinking may both con-sume the heart blood and affect the digesting function of the spleen; weak-ness of spleen qi will lead to insufficiency of qi and blood and then to deficiency of heart blood; moreover, dysfunction of the spleen to control blood will lead to loss of blood and insufficiency of heart blood. Therefore, clinically there will be symptoms of simultaneous deficiency of heart blood and spleen qi, such as dizziness, palpation, insomnia, dreaminess, abdominal pain, poor appetite, lassitude, and pale complexion, etc.

The Relationships Between the Heart and Liver

The relationships between the heart and liver can be discussed in terms of blood circulation and emotional activities.

1. Blood is produced by the spleen, governed by the heart, and stored by the liver. So only when the heart functions properly in blood circulation can the liver has adequate blood to store; if the liver fails to store blood, the heart may have nothing to govern. Therefore, clinically "blood deficiency of both the liver and heart" is very common.

2. The spiritual, mental and emotional activities, though dominated by the heart, are closely associated with the liver in promoting free flow of qi. Emotional disorders may stagnate the liver qi, which eventually transforms into fire and impairs yin-fluid; hence clinically "hyperactive fire of the heart and liver" and "deficient yin of the heart and liver" are very common.

The Relationships Between the Heart and Kidney

The relations between the heart and kidney can be discussed in terms of yin-yang and water-fire. The heart, located above the kidney, pertains to fire and yang, while the kidney, located below the heart, pertains to water and yin. From the ascent-descent theory of yin-yang and water-fire, the heart fire must descend to reach the kidney and the kidney water must ascend to arrive at the heart. Only by doing so can they maintain the balanced physiological functions. That is why we say "coordination between heart and kidney" and "inter-promotion between water and fire." Pathologically, if the heart fire cannot reach the kidney and the kidney water fails to arrive at the heart, there will be imbalanced conditions such as "disharmony between the heart and kidney" and "discordance between water and fire," clinically marked by insomnia, palpation, vexation, weak loins and knees, nocturnal emission in males and dreamed coitus in females, etc.

The Relationships Between the Lung and Spleen

The relations between the lung and spleen can be discussed in terms of the production of qi and the metabolism of body fluid.

1. The lucid qi inhaled by the lung and the cereal nutrients transformed by the spleen and stomach are basic materials for the production of qi. Hence, the production of qi relies chiefly on the respiratory function of the lung and the transportation-transformation function of the spleen and stomach. They are mutually affected. For instance, deficiency of spleen qi often leads to insufficient lung qi; conversely, prolonged lung disease may also involve the spleen, leading to malfunction of transportation and transformation or deficiency of spleen qi.

2. The metabolism of body fluid is actually a coordinated process involving the lung with the functions of dispersion-descent and dredging waterways and the spleen with the function of transporting, transforming and distributing water and fluid. The aforementioned functions of the lung is conducive to the spleen in transporting and transforming water and fluid, thus preventing internal dampness from accumulating in the body; similarly, the function of the spleen in transporting body fluid is the prerequisite to the function of the lung in dredging waterways, and the spleen can also distributes nutrients to the lung, thus providing essential nourishment for the lung.

Daily Exercises

1. Concisely describe the relations between the heart and lung.
2. Concisely describe the relations between the heart and kidney.

The Relationships Among the Five Zang-Organs

The Relationships Between the Lung and Liver

The relationships between the lung and liver are mainly reflected by the regulation of qi activities. The lung is in charge of ascending while the liver is in charge of ascending, the coordination of which is essential to the regulation of qi. If the liver qi ascends excessively or the liver qi descends insufficiently, there will adverse rising of qi and fire, marked by cough with dyspnea or even hemoptysis. This is called "liver fire invading the lung." Conversely, if the lung fails to purify and causes internal heat and dryness, the liver may be involved and becomes stagnated in qi activity, marked by cough, distension and radiating pain in the chest and hypochondria, dizziness, headache, reddened complexion and eyes, etc.

The Relationships Between Lung and Kidney

The relationships between the lung and kidney can be discussed in terms of water metabolism and respiration.

1. The kidney governs water while the lung is the upper source of water. The lung is in charge of dispersing and descending as well as dredging waterways, which are dependent on the steaming and qi-transforming functions of the kidney; conversely, the function of the kidney in governing water also relies on the function of the lung to disperse and descend qi as well as dredge waterways. Pathologically, they are also mutually affected. So if the lung fails to function properly in this regard, the kidney will be involved, leading to edema and scanty urine; if the kidney malfunctions in this respect, water will attack the lung upwardly, leading to coughing, wheezing and panting with inability to lie down calmly.

2. The lung is in charge of exhalation while the kidney is in charge of reception of qi, which are interdependent. So there is a saying that the lung is the governor of qi while the kidney is the root of qi. Only when the kidney qi is sufficient can the inhaled qi be descended by the lung and received by the kidney; otherwise, if the kidney essence is inadequate, there will be adverse rising of qi marked by cough with asthma; or if the lung qi is persistently deficient, the kidney will be involved, leading to failure of the kidney to receive qi manifested as panting on exertion, etc.

Besides, the lung yin and kidney yin are inter-promoted physiologically and inter-affected pathologically. Deficiency of lung yin may involve kidney yin and vice versa. So clinically we often see simultaneous deficiency of lung yin and kidney yin, characterized by rosy cheeks, osteopyrexia with hectic fever, night seating, hoarseness with dry cough, and weak loins and knees, etc.

The Relationships Between the Liver and Spleen

The liver stores blood, and promote free flow of qi, while the spleen controls blood, and governs transportation and transformation; besides, the spleen is also the source for qi and blood. For this reason, the relations between the two viscera can be discussed in the following aspects:

1. The liver governs free flow of qi and the spleen governs transportation and transformation. The latter relies on the former; otherwise, there will be such pathological conditions as "disharmony between the heart and liver," clinically characterized by depression, distension in the chest and hypochondriac region, abdominal distension and pain, and diarrhea with loose stools, etc.

2. The liver and spleen coordinate closely in the process of producing, storing, transporting and controlling of blood. If the spleen functions normally in transforming food into qi and blood, and contains the blood properly within the vessels, the liver will have something to store; otherwise, if the spleen is too weak to produce enough qi and blood, or fails to contain the blood within the vessels, there will insufficient liver blood. Moreover, the function of the liver in storing blood and the function of the spleen in controlling blood are often performed concertedly to prevent bleeding.

3. The spleen and stomach (earth) often invade the liver (wood) when dampness and heat are abundant, leading to lassitude, anorexia, discomfort in the chest and hypochondriac region, and jaundice, etc.

The Relationships Between the Liver and Kidney

The relationships between the liver and kidney are very close, and there is even a saying that the liver and kidney share the same origin. This can be discussed in the following aspects:

1. The liver and kidney share the same origin. The liver stores blood while the kidney stores essence. Essence and blood, however, are inter-promoted and inter-transformed. The production of blood relies on the qi transforming activity of kidney essence while the replenishment of kidney essence depends on the nourishment of blood. So blood and essence are

interchangeable. Pathologically kidney essence and liver blood are also mutually affected.

2. Yin and yang of the liver and kidney are closely associated, inter-restricted and inter-coordinated. Pathologically, insufficiency of kidney yin can lead to deficiency of liver yin, causing hyperactivity of liver yang, also called "water failing to nourish the wood," conversely, insufficiency of liver yin can also lead to depletion of kidney yin, causing hyperactivity or kidney fire.

3. The liver promotes free flow of qi and the kidney stores essence. They are inter-restricted and inter-promoted, and this is mainly manifested in menstruation and seminal emission. If the two are imbalanced, there will be irregular menstrual cycle, profuse menses or amenorrhea in women, as well as nocturnal emission or postcoital protrusion without ejection in men.

The Relationships Between the Spleen and Kidney

The relationships between the spleen and kidney are, in fact, reflected by the coordination between the prenatal foundation and postnatal foundation. The spleen is the postnatal foundation while the kidney is the prenatal foundation. They are inter-supplemented and inter-promoted. The spleen relies on the warmth of the kidney yang to transform food into nutrients, so it is said that the spleen yang is rooted in the kidney yang; On the other hand, the kidney essence also relies on the nourishment of cereal nutrients to accumulate and grow. Pathologically, they are mutually affected. For example, if the kidney yang is too weak to warm the spleen yang, there will be abdominal pain and cold, indigested diarrhea or diarrhea before dawn, and even edema; if the spleen yang is persistently deficient, the kidney yang will be involved, resulting in yang deficiency of both the spleen and kidney.

Daily Exercises

1. Briefly introduce the relation between the kidney and the lung.
2. Briefly introduce the relation between the kidney and the liver.

Weekly Review

In this week, we mainly studied the six fu-organs and the extraordinary fu-organs as well as the interrelation between the five zang-organs. Now we will have a brief review as follows:

1. The six fu-organs refer to the gallbladder, stomach, large intestine, small intestine, urinary bladder and triple energizer. The physiological characteristics of the six fu-organs can be classified as "transporting without storing." Hence the six fu-organs are characterized by decent and non-obstruction. Apart from the triple energizer, all the fu-organs have interior-exterior relationship with the zang-organs, and the anatomical positions of the fu-organs are approximately identical with their counterparts in modern medicine.

The gallbladder is above all the other fu-organs, attached to the liver, and adherent to the hepatic lobule. Its main physiological functions are to store and excrete bile, which can facilitate the digestion of food.

The stomach is also called the "great storehouse," "sea of water and cereal," or "sea of qi and blood." Its main physiological function is reception and digestion of food. It is also in charge of descent and takes downward action as the normal functional tendency.

The small intestine is a relatively long tunnel-shaped organ. It is in charge of reception and transformation of food and separation of the lucid from the turbid.

The main physiological functions of the large intestine are transporting and transforming residues, as well as absorbing remnant water from the residues.

The main physiological functions of the urinary bladder are storing and excreting urine.

The triple energizer is a collective term for the upper energizer, middle energizer and lower energizer. In ancient medical classics, there is no clear description as to the concept of triple energizer. The upper energizer is above the diaphragm, including the heart, lung, head and face, or even the upper limbs. The middle energizer is located at the upper abdomen between the diaphragm and the umbilicus, including the spleen and stomach. The lower energizer is below the umbilicus, including the small intestine, large intestine, kidney and urinary bladder, etc. Its main physiological functions are circulating primordial qi as well as water and fluid.

2. "Extraordinary fu-organs" is a collective term for the brain, marrow, bones, vessels, gallbladder, and uterus. Being hollow organs with the function of transporting food and storing essence, the six extraordinary fu-organs are similar both to the fu-organs in morphology and to the zang-organs in function. That is why they are called the extraordinary fu-organs. The extraordinary fu-organs do not bear internal-external relationships with other organs, nor do they pertain to any element. The only exception, however, is the gallbladder.

The brain is the sea of marrow and the intelligence and memory come from the brain, not from the heart. The brain can dominate life activities, metal activities and emotional activities. In TCM, we ascribe the brain functions to the heart and also attribute them to the five zang-organs, respectively.

The uterus is also called the palace of the fetus. Its main physiological functions are menstruation and conceiving the fetus. The process of the uterus in governing menstruation and pregnancy is very complicated and involves the tiangui, thoroughfare vessel and conception vessel, as well as the heart, liver and spleen.

3. The relationships between the five zang-organs

The relationships between the five zang-organs are called the 10 major relationships. There are 10 which are the most basic ones.

(1) The relationships between the heart and lung are mainly manifested as the coordination between the heart governing blood and the lung governing qi as well as the interaction between the heart governing blood circulation and the lung governing respiration.

(2) The relationships between the heart and spleen can be discussed in terms of blood production and circulation.

(3) The relationships between the heart and liver can be discussed in terms of blood circulation and emotional activities.

(4) The relationships between the heart and kidney can be discussed in terms of yin-yang and water-fire.

(5) The relationships between the lung and spleen can be discussed in terms of the production of qi and the metabolism of body fluid.

(6) The relationships between the lung and liver are mainly reflected by the regulation of qi activities.

(7) The relationships between the lung and kidney can be discussed in terms of water metabolism and respiration.

(8) The relationships between the liver and spleen can be illustrated by the fact that the liver stores blood, and promote free flow of qi, while the spleen controls blood, and governs transportation and transformation; besides, the spleen is also the source for production of qi and blood.

(9) The relationships between the liver and kidney are very close, and there is even a saying that the liver and kidney share the same origin. This can be discussed in the following aspects: a. The liver and kidney share the same origin. b. Yin and yang of the liver and kidney are closely associated, inter-restricted and inter-coordinated. c. The dispersion-ventilation of the liver and the storage function of the kidney are inter-restricted and inter-promoted.

(10) The relationships between the spleen and kidney are, in fact, reflected by the coordination between the prenatal foundation and postnatal foundation.

Daily Exercises

1. What are the definitions and physiological characteristics of the six fu-organs?
2. Describe the physiological functions of the six fu-organs one by one.
3. What are the definitions and physiological characteristics of the extraordinary fu-organs?
4. Describe the physiological functions of the extraordinary fu-organs one by one.
5. Understand the relationships between a zang-organ and another zang-organ, between a zang-organ and a fu-organ, and between a fu-organ and another fu-organ.

THE SIXTH WEEK

The Relationships Among the Six Fu-Organs

The main physiological functions of the six fu-organs are to transport and transform food. Hence the relationships between the six fu-organs are mainly reflected by the interaction and coordination in the process of digesting, absorbing and excreting water and food.

Let us have a glimpse of this process. First, water and food are taken into the stomach where they are decomposed and initially digested, and later they are transported downward to the small intestine where they are further digested and separated into lucid substances (nutrients) and turbid substances (waste); the nutrients are distributed to nourish all parts of the body *via* the spleen. The remnant water is absorbed and then permeates into the urinary bladder to form urine, which is discharged out of the body by qi transforming action. The residues are sent down to the large intestine where they are dried (for further absorption of water); eventually, they are transported downward and discharged out of the body *via* the anus. In this process, the excretion of the bile and qi transforming action of the triple energizer are also involved to facilitate digestion of water and food.

It is a ceaseless process of reception, digestion, transportation and excretion which requires smooth transportation without stagnation. This process is also characterized by alternated fullness and emptiness; in other words, when the stomach is full, the intestines are empty, and when the intestines are full, the stomach is empty. That is why the ancient doctors said, "the six fu-organs take unblocked transmission as its normal functional state," and "the six fu-organs takes purgation as its own way of nourishment."

Pathologically, the six fu-organs are mutually affected. If there is excess-heat in the stomach consuming body fluid, the large intestine will be obstructed, leading to constipation; conversely, dryness in the large intestine may also lead to adverse rising of stomach qi, with such sings as nausea and vomiting, etc. Besides, if the gallbladder fire is hyperactive, the stomach will be involved, leading to adverse rising of stomach qi, marked by vomiting of bitter water; conversely, if there damp-heat in the spleen and stomach, the liver and gallbladder will be involved, leading to leaking of bile and jaundice.

The Relationships Between the Five Zang-Organs and Six Fu-Organs

The zang-organs pertain to yin while fu-organs to yang; the zang-organs belongs to the interior while the fu-organs to the exterior. The five zang-organs and six fu-organs (except for the triple energizer) are coordinated through their yin-yang or interior-exterior relationship and are connected through their meridians and collaterals. Hence, their relationships are, as a matter of fact, the relationship between yin and yang or interior and exterior.

The Relationships Between the Heart and Small Intestine

The meridian of the heart pertains to the heart and connects with the small intestine, while the meridian of the small intestine pertains to the small intestine and connects with the heart. Hence they constitute a relationship of yin-yang and interior-exterior through the connection of meridians. Pathologically, they are mutually affected. For example, heart fire may transmit its heat to the small intestine, leading to scanty urine, red and hot urine, and painful urination; the heat within the small intestine may also go upward to the heart, leading to vexation, red tongue and oral ulcers, etc.

The Relationships Between the Lung and Large Intestine

The lung and large intestine are also associated interiorly and exteriorly through the connection of meridians. Under normal circumstances, the descending of lung qi is conducive to the transportation of the large intestine and *vice versa*. Pathologically, they are mutually affected. For instance, excess-heat may block qi movements in the large intestine, further involving the lung, marked by chest fullness, wheezing and coughing; if the lung fails to descend body fluid to the large intestine, constipation may occur; if the lung qi is too weak to promote bowel movements, constipation due to qi deficiency will be seen.

The Relationships Between the Spleen and Stomach

The spleen and stomach are connected internally and externally through their meridians. The stomach is in charge of reception while the spleen governs transportation and transformation as well as distributes body fluid for the stomach, the coordination of which ensures the successful accomplishment of the digestion, absorption and distribution of water and food so as to nourish the whole body. Meanwhile, the ascent of the spleen and the descent of the stomach are well balanced and cooperated to guarantee the distribution of cereal essence and the downward transportation of water and food as well as residues. Besides, the spleen is fond of dryness and loathes dampness while the stomach is on the contrary. The balance between their propensities is very important to the transportation and transformation of water and food. Pathologically they are mutually affected; for example, the spleen, if encumbered by dampness, may fail to ascend lucid qi and affect the reception and descent of stomach, leading to anorexia, vomiting, nausea and distending pain in the stomach and abdomen, and so on; conversely, improper diet may lead to food retention within the stomach and subsequently failure of the stomach to descend and failure of the spleen to ascend and transform, characterized by abdominal distension or diarrhea, etc.

The Relationships Between the Liver and Gallbladder

The gallbladder is attached to and connected with the liver internally and externally through their meridians. The excretion and functional activities of the bile, which is originated form the surplus qi of the liver, depend on the liver with the function of promoting free flow of qi. Conversely, the liver also relies on the excretion of the bile to promote free flow of qi. Besides, the liver governs strategy while the gallbladder manages decision. These two aspects are closely related because, from the perspective of emotions, decision must be made after strategy while strategy is a prerequisite for decision.

The Relationships Between the Kidney and Bladder

The kidney and urinary bladder are connected internally and externally through their meridians. The urinary bladder relies on the qi transforming action of the kidney to store and excrete urine. In other words, if the kidney is sufficient, the opening and closing of the urinary bladder will be normal and the urine will be discharged properly. Pathologically, however, there will be difficult urination, urinary incontinence, enuresis, or frequent urination due to insufficient kidney resulting in improper opening and closing of the urinary bladder. For example, urinary incontinence and profuse urination in old people are often caused by insufficient kidney qi.

Daily Exercises

1. What are the relationships between the six fu-organs?
2. What are the relationships between the five zang-organs and six fu-organs?

CHAPTER 6

Qi, Blood, and Body Fluid

Qi in TCM refers to a vital fine substance in constant motion; blood refers to the red liquid within the vessels; and body fluid is a collective term for all kinds of normal liquids in the body except for the blood. In terms of yin-yang attribution, qi, with the action of propelling and warming, pertains to yang; while blood and body fluid, both in liquid state and with the function of moistening and nourishing, pertain to yin.

Qi, blood and body fluid are essential substances constituting the human body and also serve as the material foundation for the physiological activities of the viscera, meridians and tissues, etc. Qi, blood and body fluid are produced, stored and dominated by the viscera, meridians and tissues which, in turn, are nourished, activated and coordinated by the former. Moreover, essence, another basic substance constituting the human body, has two connotations: in a broad sense; it refers to all fine substances, encompassing qi, blood, body fluid and cereal nutrients, so it is also called "essence-qi," in a narrow sense it refers to the reproductive essence.

Qi

The Connotation of Qi

Qi, as the most essential substance constituting the human body and sustaining its life activities, is by nature material, invisible, motional, vital and functional. Since it can promote life activities and warm the human body, its movement and variation are often used in TCM to explain the life activities of the human body.

The Production of Qi

Qi within the body is derived from three sources: congenital essence-qi inherited from parents, nutrients from water and cereal, and fresh air inhaled from nature. The production of qi depends on the synthetic actions of the lung, spleen, stomach and kidney, and so on.

(1) Congenital essence-qi is inherited from parents, stored in the kidneys, and nourished by the cereal nutrients so as to maintain its metabolism and adequacy and perform its physiological activities.
(2) The cereal nutrients come from water and food, and are transported and transformed by the spleen and stomach, which play a key role in the production of qi. After birth, cereal nutrients become indispensable to the sustaining of life activities, and only through the reception, transportation and transformation of the spleen and stomach can water and food be digested, absorbed and transformed into cereal nutrients.
(3) Similarly, only through the respiration of the lung can fresh air from nature be inhaled into the body.

Hence, the production of qi is closely associated with the kidney, lung, spleen and stomach apart from innate endowment, postnatal nourishment and natural environment. If any link is in disorder, the production, or physiological functions of qi will be hampered, leading to pathological changes.

The Physiological Functions of Qi

Qi, the most essential substance for maintaining life activities, is indispensable to the human body. At the early stage of TCM theoretical development, all things in the world, including the blood and body fluid, are considered to be a collection of qi. Later on, with the deepening of the recognition about blood and body fluid and in order to facilitate clinical medication, the visible blood and body fluid are separated from invisible qi. Thus, we may classify the functions of qi into the following aspects:

1. *Promoting function*

TCM holds that qi is a vigorous, refined, and constantly motive substance with powerful action. It promotes and stimulates the growth and development of the human body, the physiological activities of the viscera and meridians, the production and circulation of blood, as well as the production, distribution and excretion of body fluid. If qi is too weak to promote or stimulate, there will be subsequent abnormalities such as presenility due to delayed growth and development, debilitated physiological functions of the viscera and meridians, as well as impeded production or circulation of blood and body fluid, marked by blood deficiency, blood stasis and edema.

2. *Warming function*

Qi is the source of heat energy within the body, and this is an essential prerequisite for the maintenance of normal body temperature, the normal performance of physiological functions of the viscera and meridians, and the normal circulation of blood and body fluid. If the warming function of qi fails to work properly, there will be cold manifestations such as preference for heat and intolerance of cold, cold limbs, low temperature, and slow circulation of blood and fluid; if qi stagnates and transforms into heat, there will hot manifestations such as preference for cold and aversion to heat, or fever, and so on.

3. *Defensive function*

Qi can protect the body surface from external invasion by pathogenic factors, which is a reflection of the resistance ability of the body against diseases. If the defensive ability of qi weakens, exogenous pathogenic factors will find their way to attack, leading to malfunction of the body.

4. *Consolidating function*

This function refers mainly to the prevention of blood, body fluid and other liquids from unnecessary loss. It is mainly manifested in two aspects: first, to contain blood within its vessels and prevent it from extravasation. Second, to regulate the secretion and excretion of sweat, urine, saliva, gastric juice, intestine juice or sperm, and to prevent them from unnecessary loss; pathologically, if qi fails to control blood, there will be bleeding; if qi fails to control body fluid, there will be spontaneous sweating, profuse urine, urinary incontinence, drooling, vomiting of clear water, and diarrhea; if qi fails to control sperm, there will be nocturnal emission, slippery emission or premature ejaculation, etc.

What is worth mentioning is that the consolidating function and the promoting function of qi are not contradictory but inter-complementary; the balance between them is essential to the normal circulation, secretion and excretion of liquids within the body, and is also critical for maintaining the normal blood circulation and water metabolism of the body.

5. *Qi-transforming function*

Qi-transformation refers to the various changes produced by activities of qi. To be specific, it refers to the metabolism and mutual transformation of essence, qi, blood and body fluid. Qi-transformation is mainly manifested in the following process: the transformation from water and food to cereal nutrients, and then to qi, blood and body fluid, etc. The transformation of body fluid to sweat and urine after metabolism; and the transformation of food residues into feces, etc. hence, the process of qi-transformation is, as a matter of fact, the course of material metabolism and energy transformation.

Daily Exercises

1. Concisely describe the connotation and composition of qi.
2. Concisely describe the physiological functions of qi.

Qi

The Movements and Motive Patterns of Qi

The movements of qi can be classified into four basic patterns: ascending, descending, exiting and entering.

The viscera and meridians of the body are places where activities of qi take place. Such activities are essential to the life activities, the end of which means the ceasing of life.

The ascending, descending, exiting and entering activities of qi can promote and stimulate various physiological functions of the human body, including those of the viscera and meridians which also embody such movements of qi. In terms of respiration by the lung, exhalation represents exiting of qi, inhalation represents entering of qi, dispersion represents ascending qi and purification represents descending of qi. Take the spleen and stomach for another example, the ascent of the lucid by the spleen and the descent of the turbid by the stomach represent the ascending and descending activities of qi, which is also a generalization of the whole process of digesting, absorbing, distributing and excreting of water and food. Hence, the various physiological activities are, in fact, a concrete manifestation of the ascending, descending, exiting and entering movements of qi.

The ascending-descending and exiting-entering of qi are two pairs of motive pattern that are both contradictory and complementary. As far as the individual organs are concerned, not all of them encompass each pattern of the ascending, descending, exiting and entering movements; instead, each of them lays particular emphasis on a certain pattern. For example, the liver and spleen are characterized by ascending while the lung and stomach are characterized by descending. From the perspective of the whole body, however, ascending and descending as well as exiting and entering must maintain a relative balance so as to sustain normal physiological activities. Such a balance is called in TCM "harmonious flow of qi" whereas its opposite aspect is called "disequilibrium of qi movements." The latter is often manifested as unsmooth flow of qi due to certain reasons, stagnation of qi in local areas, averseness of qi characterized by excessive ascending or insufficient descending, sinking of qi characterized by insufficient ascending or excessive descending, qi prostration characterized by outward escape of qi, and knotting of qi characterized by internal accumulation of qi, as well as depression of qi and blockage of qi in varying degrees, etc.

The Distribution and Classification of Qi

Generally speaking, qi within the body originates from congenital essence qi, cereal nutrients and fresh air, synthesized by the kidney, lung, spleen and stomach, and distributed throughout the body. However, specifically speaking, qi within the body takes different forms and has different actions. According to the different composition, distribution and function, qi can be divided into several types, such as visceral qi represented by heart qi and lung qi. The following is a few special forms of qi:

1. *Primordial qi*

(1) Connotation. Primordial qi, also called "original qi" or "genuine qi," is the most basic and important kind of qi. Encompassing primordial yin and primordial yang, it is regarded as the motive power for life activities.

(2) Composition: It is mainly composed of kidney essence which relies on both congenital essence and postnatal nutrients from water and food. Hence, the excess or deficiency of primordial qi depends not only on congenital endowment but also on postnatal nourishment by cereal nutrients.

(3) Distribution. It is originates from the kidney and distributed through the triple energizer to the viscera internally and to the skin and interstices externally.

(4) Main functions. Being the motive power for life activities, it can promote, warm and stimulate the physiological functions of the viscera and meridians.

2. *Pectoral qi*

(1) Connotation. Pectoral qi refers to qi within the chest. The place where it accumulates is called "sea of qi" or "Danzhong."

(2) Composition. It is composed of fresh air inhaled by the lung from nature and cereal nutrients transformed by the spleen and stomach from water and food. Hence, the respiration of the lung and the transformation of the spleen and stomach play a key role in determining the excess or deficiency of pectoral qi.

(3) Distribution. Pectoral qi is accumulated in the chest and flows into the heart and lung. It flows upward out of the lung, and goes along the throat and air tube; it flows down to the pubic region, infuses into Qijie (ST 30) of the stomach meridian of foot yangming and reaches the foot; part of it flows into the heart and subsequently into the vessels to propel blood circulation.

(4) Main functions. Its functions can be generalized as "flowing into the respiratory tract to facilitate respiration and goes into the heart vessels to promote circulation of qi and blood." Therefore, speech, voice and

respiration are all associated with pectoral qi; moreover, pectoral qi also plays an essential role in the circulation of qi and blood, movements and temperature of the limbs, perceptive ability of visual or aural senses, and strength or rhythm of heartbeat, etc.

3. *Nutrient qi*

(1) Connotation. Nutrient qi flows within the vessel with the function of nourishment. Since nutrient qi and blood flows simultaneously in the vessels and bear a close relationship with each other, they are collectively called nutrient-blood. Nutrient qi, contrary to defensive qi, pertains to yin, so it is also called nutrient-yin.

(2) Composition. Nutrient qi primarily originates from the quintessential part of cereal nutrients transformed by the spleen and stomach.

(3) Distribution. Nutrient qi is distributed inside the vessels, becomes part of blood and flows along the vessel to nourish the whole body.

(4) Main functions. The primary functions of nutrient qi are to nourish the body and produce blood. The main component of it comes from the quintessential part of cereal nutrients which, also being part of blood, are essential to the physiological functions of the viscera and meridians.

4. *Defensive qi*

(1) Connotation. Defensive qi flows outside of the vessels. In contrast to nutrient qi, it pertains to yang, so it is also called "defensive yang."

(2) Composition. Similar to nutrient qi, it also originates from cereal nutrients transformed by the spleen and stomach.

(3) Distribution. It is very active, rapid, and free from the restriction of vessels. It flows between the skin and muscular interstices, warms the membranes and spreads over the chest and abdomen.

(4) Main functions. The physiological functions of defensive qi are as follows: first, to protect the superficies from external invasion by pathogenic factors; second, to warm viscera, muscles, skin and hair, and so on; third, to regulate the opening and closing of skin interstices, the excretion of sweat and the maintenance of normal body temperature, etc.

What worth mentioning here is that in TCM, there are many terms named after qi, such as "water qi," "healthy qi" and "evil qi," etc. All of these are different from the various kinds of qi we discussed in this section which are the most basic substances for constituting the human body.

Daily Exercises

1. What are the motive patterns of qi?
2. What are the common types of qi?

Blood

The Connotation of Blood

Blood, a red liquid circulating inside the vessels, is regarded as one of the most essential substances constituting the body and maintaining its life activities. Its chief functions are to nourish and moisten the human body. Since blood vessels can contain the blood and prevent it from extravasation, it is called the "house of blood," and the blood circulating out of the vessels is called "deviated blood."

The Production of Blood

1. *The material foundation for blood production*

Blood is primarily composed of nutrient qi and body fluid which come mainly from cereal nutrients transformed by the spleen and stomach. Hence cereal nutrients are the most basic substances for production of qi and blood. Besides, essence and blood are also inter-promoted and inter-transformed.

2. *The relationship between blood production and the viscera*

Blood is mainly transformed from nutrient qi and body fluid by the spleen and stomach and cooperated by the heart, lung, liver and kidney, etc. This can be discussed in the following aspects: firstly, the spleen and stomach, as the postnatal foundation and the source of qi and blood, transform water and food into cereal nutrients, the most essential substance for production of blood. So if the spleen and stomach are weak, there will be insufficient cereal nutrients for the production of blood, leading to blood deficiency. Secondly, the heart, which governs blood and vessels, propel blood to all parts of the body for nourishment so as to maintain their normal functional activities; while this, in turn, promotes the production of fresh blood. Thirdly, the lung, with the function of governing qi, absorbs the cereal nutrients transmitted through the spleen and gets rid of the stale qi, and then pours refreshed nutrients into the heart where they are reddened into fresh blood. Fourthly, the liver, which pertains to wood and signifies growth and vitality, can facilitate the spleen, heart and lung to produce blood. Fifthly, the kidney, which stores essence, can produce primordial qi to assist the spleen and stomach to transform food into nutrients. Finally, essence and blood can be inter-transformed, that's why it is said that the essence and blood share the same origin.

The Functions of Blood

The main functions of blood are to nourish and moisten the body. Blood circulates inside the vessels, arriving internally at the viscera and externally at the skin, muscles, tendons and bones. It flows continuously and ceaselessly to nourish and moisten all the organs and tissues, thus maintaining their physiological functions. To be specific, its functions are mainly manifested as follows:

(1) The nourishing and moistening functions of blood are signified by such manifestations as ruddy complexion, well-developed and strong muscles, lustrous skin and hair, keen sensation, nimble and flexible movement, etc. If blood production is insufficient, or blood consumption is excessive without timely supplement, or blood function is weak in moistening and nourishing, general or local pathological manifestations of blood deficiency may occur.

(2) Blood is also the main material basis for mental activities. If blood is sufficient and vessels are smooth and well-regulated, one will be vigorous in spirit, clear in mind, keen in sensation and nimble in movement. Pathologically, blood deficiency or circulative disturbance may lead to mental disorders in varying degrees, such as fright, insomnia and dreaminess when heart blood or liver blood is deficient, and restlessness, absentmindedness or even coma when there is excessive loss of blood.

The Circulation of Blood

The ancient TCM doctors have long recognized that blood circulates continuously and ceaselessly throughout the body inside the relatively close and tight circulatory system made up of the heart, lung and vessels. This system is indispensable to the nourishment of all the organs and tissues of the body.

Compared with qi, blood pertains to yin and is quiet by nature. The normal circulation of blood, therefore, relies on the coordination between the promotion and consolidation of qi. The promoting function of qi is associated with the heart, lung and liver, such as the pulsation of the heart, the dispersion of the lung which opens into all the vessels, and the dispersing and ventilating function of the liver, etc. The consolidating function of qi is associated with the spleen with the function of controlling blood and the liver with the function of storing blood. Furthermore, the velocity of blood circulation is directly influenced by the smoothness of vessels and the conditions of blood such as whether it is cold or hot, etc.

Hence, the normal circulation of blood relies not only on the physiological function of the heart, but also on the balance and coordination among the lung, liver and spleen, etc. If the factors contributing to the propelling or promoting of blood circulation increase, or the factors contributing to the astringing or decelerating of blood circulation decrease, blood circulation will be hastened, leading to extravasation and bleeding; otherwise, blood circulation will become slow and unsmooth, leading to such pathological changes as blood stasis, etc.

Daily Exercises

1. Briefly describe the connotation and production of blood?
2. What are the functions of blood and how does it circulate inside the body?

Body Fluid

The Connotation of Body Fluid

Body fluid is a collective term for all the normal liquids of the body with the exception of blood. This includes various kinds of liquids existing in every organ and tissue of the body as well as the normal liquid excretions, such as gastric juice, internal juice, nasal discharge, tears, etc. Similar to qi and blood, body fluid is also a basic material for constituting the human body and maintaining its life activities.

It is derived from the foodstuff transported and transformed by the spleen and stomach. According to the difference in property, function and distribution, it is subdivided into jin (fluid) and ye (liquid). Generally speaking, the thin fluid, jin, is dilute, more fluidic, and mainly distributed in the body' surface, such as the skin, muscles and pores; it can also permeate into the blood and function to moisten. The thick fluid, ye, is dense, less fluidic, and generally distributed in the bones, joints, viscera, brain and marrow to perform its nourishing function.

Fluid and liquid share the same origin and are of no difference in nature. Physiologically they are mutually complemented and inter-transformed during the process of production, circulation and metabolism of body fluid; while pathologically they are mutually affected. In this sense, they are often collectively called "body fluid." Differentiation between them is needed only when there is impairment of fluid or depletion of liquid.

The Production, Distribution and Excretion of Body Fluid

The production, distribution and excretion of body fluid are a very complicated physiological process involving the coordination of many viscera. In Su Wen, it is said, "After water and food come into the stomach, essence qi will permeate throughout the stomach, and then go upward to the spleen where it is transmitted to the lung; through the waterways, it is sent to bladder, thus making the nutrients distributed all over the body and throughout the meridians." This is a brief introduction to the production, distribution and excretion of body fluid.

1. The production of body fluid

Body fluid originates from water and food. This is a process involving the reception of food by the stomach, the separation of the lucid from the turbid by the small intestine, and the upward transmission of nutrients to the spleen. This process can be divided into the following stages: a. First water and food are taken into the stomach where they are initially digested and absorbed, and later transported to the spleen where the lucid substances are transmitted to the lung, and subsequently to the whole body. b. The water and food initially digested by the stomach are sent downward to the small intestine where they are further digested and separated into nutrients and waste; the former are distributed all over the body *via* the spleen, and the latter, are sent down to urinary bladder and the large intestine. c. In the large intestine, part of the remnant water is reabsorbed and the food residues are dried to form feces, which are discharged out of the body *via* the anus.

2. *The distribution of body fluid*

It is a synthetic process involves the spleen, lung, kidney, liver and triple energizer, etc. a. The spleen can disperse essence and transmit body fluid for the stomach, which is manifested in two aspects: one is the transmission of body fluid to the lung, through the dispersing and ascending actions of which they are distributed all over the body to nourish and moisten the viscera, limbs or orifices, etc.; the other is the transmission of body fluid through the meridians so as to moisten and nourish the whole body. b. The lung governs qi, regulates waterways and serves as the upper source of water. On the one hand, the lung disperses the body fluid transmitted from the spleen to THE upper part and the surface of the body; on the other hand, it descends body fluid to the kidney, urinary bladder and the lower part of the body. c. The kidney governs body fluid, which is manifested in two aspects: for one thing, through the steaming action of the kidney, the distribution of body fluid is promoted, thus providing the motive power for the digestion by the stomach, the dispersion by the spleen, the regulation of waterways by the lung as well as the separation between nutrients and waste by the small intestine; for another, under the qi transforming function of the kidney, the body fluid transported from the lung to the kidney is divided into the lucid part and the turbid part. The former is dispersed all over the body and the latter is transformed into urine and infused into the urinary bladder. d. The liver promotes free flow of qi so as to regulate qi movement and, as a result, to promote the distribution and circulation of body fluid. e. The triple energizer is in charge of dredging and ditching, thus functioning as passages for the distribution and circulation of body fluid inside the body.

3. *The excretion of body fluid*

This process also relies on the coordination between the lung, spleen and kidney, etc. To be specific, there are three channels: a. The lung disperses body fluid to the body surface, skin and hair where it is steamed and transformed into sweat by yang qi and finally discharged out of the body through the pores; besides, by exhalation, the lung also takes away some body fluids. b. Urine, the final metabolic product of fluid metabolism, is closely associated with the kidney, which cooperates with the urinary bladder to form urine and discharge it out of the body. Hence, the kidney plays a key role in maintaining the balance of fluid metabolism. c. The large intestine converts residues into feces. In this process, some body fluids are also taken away. When one develops diarrhea, there may be much water in the feces, and consequently fluid impairment may be caused.

In summary, in the process of the production, distribution and excretion of body fluid, many viscera are involved, particularly the lung, spleen and kidney. The disorders of these viscera may break the balance of fluid metabolism, causing impairment of fluid and depletion of liquid, or leading to internal accumulation or retention of water, dampness, or phlegm, etc.

The Functions of Body Fluid

The functions of body fluid are manifested as follows:

1. *Moistening function*

Body fluid contains water and nutrients with the function of moistening and nourishing the body. So body fluid can moisten and nourish the skin and hair, orifices (eyes, nose and mouth), viscera, joints and marrows (bone marrow or brain marrow).

2. *Constituting blood*

Body fluid and nutrient qi are both transformed from water and food, and if they are combined and transported into vessels, they will become blood. Hence body fluid is a component part of blood, both of which function to moisten and nourish the human body.

3. *Participating in the regulation of yin-yang balance*

The fluid metabolism plays a very important role in maintaining the balance of yin and yang. Body fluid pertains to yin, so if there is abundant body fluid, hyperactive yang can be restricted, thus preserving the balance between yin and yang as well as cold and heat. Besides, body fluid can also be transformed into sweat, thus regulating body temperature through perspiration.

4. *Excreting metabolic products*

In the process of fluid metabolism, the metabolic products from the viscera are carried to the emunctory organs and discharged out of the body, such as excreting sweat through the pores and discharging urine via the urinary bladder, etc. In this way, the normal physiological functions of the viscera are guaranteed.

The Relationships Among Qi, Blood and Body Fluid

Qi, blood and body fluid, though different in characteristics and functions, play an essential role in constituting the human body and maintaining its life activities. Their however, is inseparable from the cereal nutrients transformed by the spleen and stomach. Besides, their physiological functions are inter-dependent, inter-restricted and inter-promoted. Hence, the relationships among them are very close either physiologically or pathologically.

The Relationships Between Qi and Blood

Qi pertains to yang, governs warming and is active by nature; on the contrary, blood pertains to yin, governs moistening and is quiet by nature. Apart from the distinction in terms of property and function, there is another difference between qi and blood: qi is the commander of blood while blood is the mother of qi. Specifically, their relations can be discussed in terms of the following four aspects:

1. *Qi can produce blood*

Qi and its motion and variation, or qi transformation, play a significant role in the production of blood. From the transformation of water and food into cereal nutrients, from the conversion of cereal nutrients to nutrient qi and body fluid, and from the change of nutrient qi and body fluid to red blood, the movements and changes of qi are ubiquitous. Hence, if qi is abundant, blood will be sufficient; otherwise, if qi is inadequate, blood will be insufficient. For this reason, qi-supplementing herbs are often used clinically to treat blood-deficiency disorders in order to promote blood production.

2. *Qi can promote blood circulation*

Since blood pertains to yin and is characterized by quietness, it relies on the promotion of qi to circulate. So if qi stagnates, blood stasis will appear. The circulation of blood depends on the pulsation of heart qi, the dispersion of lung qi and the free flow of liver qi. Pathologically, either qi deficiency or qi stagnation will result in sluggish movement of qi or even blood stasis; adverse rise of qi may lead to reddened complexion and eyes, headache, or even vomiting of blood; sinking of qi will cause sinking and distending sensation in the stomach and abdomen, or even hematockezia and massive vaginal bleeding, etc. For this reason, clinically herbs with the functions of nourishing qi, promoting qi or descending qi can be used to treat disorders of blood circulation.

3. *Qi can control blood*

Qi is capable of containing blood within its vessels without extravasation. This action of qi, as a matter of fact, is attributable to the function of the spleen in controlling blood. Pathologically, if qi fails to control blood, there will be various manifestations of bleeding. So clinically qi-nourishing herbs are often used to stop bleeding.

4. *Blood is the mother of qi*

This means that blood carries qi and provides qi with adequate nourishment. Blood is involved in the entire process of qi production and circulation. Since qi is very active and liable to escape, it must adhere to blood or body fluid so as to exist inside the body. That is why it is called blood is the carrier of qi. Pathologically, blood deficiency and qi deficiency, or blood depletion and qi depletion, are correlated. Clinically, massive bleeding often involves depletion of qi due to its malfunction of carrying qi. Besides, blood can provide continuous supply of nutrients for the production or functional activities of qi. So the exuberance of blood will ensure abundance of qi, and the depletion of blood may lead to deficiency of qi. Clinically, if qi deficiency is caused by insufficiency of blood, simultaneous nourishment of qi and blood should be applied.

The Relationships Between Qi and Body Fluid

The relationships between qi and body fluid are very similar to those between qi and blood

1. *Qi can govern production of body fluid*

Qi is the material foundation and motive power for the production of body fluid. Abundance of qi, especially the spleen qi and stomach qi, ensures the adequate supply of body fluid. Pathologically, if qi is deficient, there will be insufficient body fluid accordingly. So during clinical treatment, qi-nourishing herbs are often used to produce body fluid.

2. *Qi can promote circulation of body fluid*

The movements and changes of qi are the motive power for the distribution and excretion of body fluid. This is a synthetic action involving the dispersing and transmitting function of the spleen, the dispersing and descending function of lung qi, as well as the steaming and transforming function of kidney essence. The coordinated performance of these viscera plays an essential role in promoting the circulation, distribution and excretion of body fluid so as to maintain the balanced metabolism of body fluid. Pathologically, the ascending, descending, entering and exiting of qi interact with the distribution and excretion of body fluid. For example, qi deficiency or qi stagnation may lead to retention of body fluid, call "qi failing to move (transform) water" in TCM; conversely, retention of body fluid may result in disorder of qi movements, called qi stagnation due to water retention. It is thus clear that the two are mutually affected and are responsible for retention of dampness, phlegm, fluid or even edema, etc. Clinically, qi-promoting and water-removing methods are often collectively used.

3. *Qi can control excretion of body fluid*

Under the control of qi, body fluid volume stays at a normal level to meet the requirements of the body. Pathologically, if qi is too weak to control body fluid, there will inevitably be unnecessary loss of body fluid, such as profuse sweating, dripping sweating, excessive urination or urinary incontinence. Clinically qi-supplementing herbs are often used to control fluid excretion.

4. *Fluid can carry qi*

Body fluid is one of the carriers of qi and qi is adherent to body fluid for existence. Pathologically, excessive sweating, vomiting, diarrhea or urination may lead to collapse of qi.

The Relationships Between Blood and Body Fluid

Blood and body fluid are both liquids with the functions of moistening and nourishing the body. In contrast to qi, they pertain to yin. Hence, they are physiologically inter-supplemented and pathologically inter-affected.

Since blood and body fluid are both derived from cereal nutrients, there is a saying in TCM that blood and fluid share the same origin. Physiologically, when body fluid permeates into the vessels, it will become a constituent part of blood. Pathologically, body fluid and blood are mutually affected. For instance, when there is massive bleeding, body fluid may infiltrate into the vessel to increase blood volume; meanwhile, since enormous amount of body fluid flows into the vessels, pathological manifestations such as thirst, scanty urine or dry skin will occur as a result. Conversely, when there is mass consumption of body fluid, it is very likely that not only the body fluid outside the vessels fails to flow into the vessels to increase blood volume, but also the body fluid already inside the vessels may flow out, causing lack of blood and depletion of body fluid, etc. Clinically, sweating therapy should not be used for patients with bleeding. In other words, sweating therapy is inapplicable to patients with frequent epistaxis, or patients suffering from frequent bleeding. For those with profuse sweating or depletion of body fluid, drastic blood-breaking or blood-hastening therapies should not be used unless it is necessary. In this sense, it is said, "patients who have lost profuse blood should not be treated by sweating, and those who have sweated massively should not be treated by drastically consuming blood."

Daily Exercises

1. What is the connotation of body fluid?
2. How is body fluid produced, distributed and excreted?
3. What does "blood and fluid sharing the same origin" mean?

Weekly Review

In this week, we mainly studied the relationship among the six fu-organs and the relationship between the five zang-organs and six fu-organs, as well as some knowledge on qi, blood, and body fluid. Now we will take a brief review as follows:

1. The relationship between the six fu-organs is mainly reflected by the interaction and coordination in the process of digesting, absorbing and excreting water and food. The six fu-organs take unblocked transmission as its normal functional state and purgation as its own way of utilization.

2. The relationship between the five zang-organs and six fu-organs is, as a matter of fact, the relationship between yin and yang or interior and exterior. The channel of the heart is connected with the small intestine and *vice versa*, hence they are mutually affected. The lung and large intestine are also associated interiorly and exteriorly through the connection of channels. Under normal circumstances, the descending of lung qi is conducive to the transportation of the large intestine and *vice versa*. Pathologically, they are mutually affected. The spleen distributes fluids for the stomach, which is actually the coordination between the ascent of the spleen and the descent of the stomach. The relationship between the liver and gallbladder is mainly manifested in the production and excretion of bile and the regulation of emotions. The relationship between the

kidney and the urinary bladder is mainly manifested in the production, storage and excretion of urine.

3. Qi, blood, and body fluid. Qi, blood and body fluid are essential substances constituting the human body and also serve as the material foundation for the physiological activities of the viscera, meridians and tissues, etc.

(1) Qi, as the most essential substance constituting the human body and sustaining its life activities, is characterized as material, invisible, motional, vital and functional. It can promote life activities and warm the human body.

Qi within the body is derived from three sources: congenital essence-qi inherited from parents, nutrients from water and cereal, and fresh air inhaled from nature. The production of qi depends on the synthetic actions of the lung, spleen, stomach and kidney, etc.

Qi can promote, warm and defend the human body. It also has astringing and qi-transforming functions.

The movements of qi are various, but generally they can be classified into four basic patterns: ascending, descending, exiting and entering.

According to the composition, distribution and function of qi, it can be divided into the following types:

Primordial qi, also called original qi or genuine qi, is the most basic and important kind of qi. Encompassing primordial yin and primordial yang, it is considered the motive power for life activities. It is mainly transformed from kidney essence and nourished by cereal nutrients. The primordial qi is distributed through the triple energizers to the viscera internally and to the skin and interstices externally. Being the motive power for life activities, it can promote, warm and stimulate the physiological functions of the viscera and channels.

Pectoral qi refers to qi within the chest. It is composed of fresh air inhaled by the lung from nature and cereal nutrients transformed by the spleen and stomach from water and food. It flows upward out of the lung, and goes along the throat and air tube; it flows down to the pubic region, infuses into Qijie (ST 30) of the stomach meridian of foot yangming. Its functions can be generalized as "flowing into the respiratory tract to facilitate respiration and goes into the heart vessels to promote circulation of qi and blood."

Nutrient qi flows within the vessel and primarily originates from the quintessential part of cereal nutrients transformed by the spleen and stomach. The primary functions of nutrient qi are to nourish the body and produce blood.

Defensive qi, also called "defensive yang," flows outside of the vessels. It also originates from cereal nutrients transformed by the spleen and stomach. Since it is very active, rapid, and free from the restriction of vessels, the defensive qi can flow between the skin and muscular interstices, warm the membranes and distribute over the chest and abdomen. The defensive qi can protect and warm the body, as well as regulate body temperature.

(2) Blood, a red liquid circulating inside the vessels, is regarded as one of the most essential substances constituting the body and maintaining its life activities. Its chief functions are to nourish and moisten the human body. Blood is primarily composed of nutrient qi and body fluid which come mainly from cereal nutrients transformed by the spleen and stomach. That is why it is said that the spleen and stomach is the source for production of qi and blood. The main functions of blood are to nourish and moisten the whole body as well as to serve as the main material foundation for the mental activities of the body. Blood circulates inside the vessels throughout the body, reaching internally to the viscera and externally to the skin, muscles, tendons and bones. The normal circulation of blood relies on the coordination between the promoting action and consolidating action of qi.

(3) Body fluid is a collective term for all the normal liquids of the body with the exception of blood. This includes various kinds of liquids existing in every organ and tissue of the body, as well as the normal liquid excretions. It is also a basic material for constituting the human body and maintaining its life activities. The fluid and liquor are different in texture, function and distribution.

Body fluid originates from water and food. This is a process involving the reception of food by the stomach, the separation of the lucid from the turbid by the small intestine, and the upward transmission of nutrients to the spleen. The distribution and excretion of body fluid is achieved through the transmission of the spleen, the dispersion and descent of the lung, as well as the steaming action of the kidney. In this process, the triple energizers serve as the passage for circulating the body fluid to every part of the body. The body fluid functions mainly to nourish and moisten the body.

(4) The relationship between qi, blood and body fluid. In terms of the relationship between qi and blood, qi is the commander of blood, while blood is the mother of qi. This is indicated by not only that qi can produce, promote and control blood, but also that blood can produce qi. The relationship between qi and body fluid is approximately the same, and the relationship between blood and body fluid is mainly marked by "blood and body fluid sharing the same origin."

Daily Exercises

1. Concisely describe the definitions and physiological functions of qi, blood and body fluid.
2. Concisely describe the concepts and physiological functions of primordial qi, pectoral qi and nutrient qi.
3. What are the relationships among qi, blood and body fluid?

THE SEVENTH WEEK

CHAPTER 7

The Theory of Meridians and Collaterals

Meridians and collaterals, or jing and luo in Chinese, are the most important components of the human body. The circulation of qi, blood and body fluid, the functional activities of the viscera, as well as the coordination of different organs must be realized through the transportation, communication and connection of the meridian system. In this way the human body is made into an organic entirety. The meridian theory, an important component of the basic theories in TCM, studies the composition, distribution, physiological function and pathological variation of the meridian system as well as their relationships with the viscera, body constituents, orifices, qi, blood and body fluid, etc. It is indispensable to the theoretical foundation of TCM. For this reason, there is even a saying by the ancients, "if one does not learn the twelve meridians by heart, he will be prone to errors."

The Connotation of Meridians and Collaterals and the Composition of Meridian System

The Connotation of Meridians and Collaterals

The meridians and collaterals are the pathways in which the qi and blood circulate. Through the meridians and collaterals, the viscera, limbs and orifices are connected, and in such a manner that the upper communicates with the lower and the interior with the exterior.

"Meridians and collaterals" is a collective for jing (meridians) and luo (collaterals). Jing means "path" while luo means "net." The form is the trunk running in the deep portion of the body with fixed courses in an upward-downward fashion; whereas the latter is the branches running in both the superficial region and the deep part all over the body in a fine-meshed network. Together they weave the viscera, body constituents and orifices into a coordinated, unified and inter-communicated organic entirety.

The Composition of the Meridian System

The meridian system includes the meridians and collaterals which communicate the viscera internally and connect the tendons, muscles and skin externally.

1. Meridians and collaterals

There are 12 regular meridians, i.e., three pairs of yin meridians and three pairs of yang meridians of the hand and foot, collectively called the "12 regular meridians." The 12 meridians originate from and terminate at certain areas, lie in certain places and have a fixed sequence in circulation. In other words, there is a definite rule for their distribution. Each connects directly with the viscera and serves as the main passage in which qi and blood circulate.

There are eight extraordinary meridians, namely the governor vessel, conception vessel, thoroughfare vessel, belt vessel, yin heal vessel, yang heel vessel, yin link vessel and yang link vessel. They are different from the 12 regular channels because they have no direct connection with any of the zang-fu organs, nor do they have exterior-interior relationships between them. When qi and blood of the 12 regular meridians are superfluous, they will flow into extraordinary meridians for reservation. The eight extraordinary meridians can command, communicate and coordinate the 12 regular meridians.

The 12 divergent meridians are branches spreading from the 12 meridians, starting from the four extremities, traversing the deep portions of the viscera, and emerging from the superficial regions of the neck and nape. The branches of the yin meridians, after splitting from and running through the interior of the body, meet the divergences of the yang meridians that are internally and externally connected to them. In such a way they reinforce the connection between the meridians that are internally and externally related. Besides, they can also reach the organs and body areas that some regular meridians do not traverse.

The collaterals are the branches of the meridians. Most of them have no fixed courses. They can be divided into three categories: divergent collaterals, superficial collaterals and minute collaterals.

The divergent collaterals are the large and major collaterals. Each of the 12 regular meridians has one divergent collateral, and so do the governor vessel and conception vessel. Together with the major collateral of the spleen, they are collectively called the "15 divergent collaterals." Similar to the 12 divergent meridians, the 15 divergent collaterals can strengthen the connection between every pair of the meridians in exterior and interior relationship.

The superficial collaterals run in the shallow region of the body and are often visible on the surface of the body.

The minute collaterals are the smallest and thinnest ones in the body. It is said in *Su Wen* (*Plain Conversation*, 素问) that they are the places where the unusual pathogens are driven out and the nutrient qi and defensive qi are communicated.

2. *The meridian tendons and skin divisions*

The meridian tendons and skin divisions, in the strict sense are not meridians or collaterals, but the affiliated parts of the 12 meridians. According to the theory of meridian system, the meridian tendons are a system, where qi "retains, accumulates, disperses and connects" in or with the musculature and joints. They are so named because the 12 meridian tendons pertain to the 12 meridians. They can connect the four limbs and various bones and is in charge of the movements of joints. The skin is the region reflecting the functional activities of the 12 meridians and the place where the meridian qi disperses. That is why the skin of the body is divided into 12 parts, which correspond directly to the 12 meridians.

3. *The related viscera*

Meridians and collaterals can connect various organs or tissues of the body, spreading not only over the body surface but also deep inside the body. Each of the 12 meridians may pertain to its entering organ. For instance, the three yin meridians of the hand communicate in the chest, and pertain to the lung, pericardium and heart in the interior; the three yin meridians of the foot communicate in the abdomen, and pertain to the spleen, liver and kidney in the interior; the three yang meridians of the foot pertain to the stomach, gallbladder and urinary bladder in the interior; and the three yang meridians of the hand pertain to the large intestine, triple energizer and small intestine in the interior.

Each of the 12 meridians connects with a certain internal organ which is in interior-exterior relationship with its pertaining organ. All the yang meridians pertain to the fu-organs and connect with the zang-organs, and all the yin meridians pertain to the zang-organs and connect with the fu-organs. For example, the lung meridian of hand taiyin pertains to the lung and connects with the large intestine; and the large intestine meridian of hand yangming pertains to the large intestine and connects with the lung. Other meridians are arranged in the similar fashion.

The yin meridians and yang meridians of the 12 meridians, with their pertaining and connecting organs internally and externally related, are in an interior-exterior relationship, i.e., yangming and taiyin, shaoyang and jueyin, and taiyang and shaoyin.

A simple illustration of the meridian system

The meridian system

The meridians

The 12 regular meridians

The three yin meridians of the hand

The lung meridian of hand taiyin

The pericardium meridian of the hand jueyin

The heart meridian the hand shaoyin

The three yang meridians of the hand

The large intestine meridian of hand yangming

The triple energizer meridian of hand shaoyang

The small intestine meridian of hand taiyang

The three yin meridians of the foot

The spleen meridian of foot taiyin

The liver meridian of foot jueyin

The kidney meridian of foot shaoyin

The three yang meridians of the foot

The stomach meridian of the foot yangming

The gallbladder meridian of the foot shaoyang

The urinary bladder meridian of the foot taiyang

The either extraordinary meridians: the governor vessel, conception vessel, thoroughfare vessel, belt vessel, yin heal vessel, yang heel vessel, yin link vessel and yang link vessel.

The 12 divergent meridians

The collaterals

The 15 divergent collaterals the divergent collaterals of the 12 meridians, the conception vessel, the governor vessel, and the large collateral of the spleen

The fine collaterals

The superficial collaterals

The 12 meridian tendons

The 12 skin divisions

The 12 Meridians

The twelve meridians are the key components of the meridian system. The extraordinary meridians, the divergent meridians and the collaterals are all subsidiary parts of the 12 meridians. They are interconnected and mutually cooperated so as to perform their functions.

Names

The 12 regular channels are symmetrically distributed over both sides of the body, running respectively along the medial or lateral side of the upper or lower limbs. Each meridian pertains to a particular zang-organ or fu-organ, so the 12 regular meridians are named based on such factors as the zang-fu organs they belong to, the limbs of hand or foot they run through, and the medial or lateral aspect of the body they circulate along. The various parts of the body are classified into either yin or yang, e.g., zang pertaining to yin, fu pertaining to yang, medial side pertaining to yin and lateral side pertaining to yang. There are three categories of yin, namely shaoyin, jueyin and taiyin; and there are also three categories of yang, namely shaoyang, yangming and taiyang. The channels circulating through the hand are named "hand channel;" the channels running through the foot are termed "foot channel;" the channels circulating along the medial side of the four limbs are named "yin channel" and pertain to zang; and the channels running along the lateral side of the four limbs are named "yang channel" and pertain to fu.

Classification of the Names of the 12 Meridians

	Yin meridians (pertaining to zang)	Yang meridians (pertaining to fu)	Circulating locations (yin meridians running along the medial side, yang meridians running along the lateral side)	
Hand	Lung meridian Pericardium meridian Heart meridian	Large intestine meridian Triple energizer meridian Small intestine meridian	Upper limbs	Anterior side midline Posterior side
Foot	Spleen meridian Liver meridian Kidney meridian	Stomach meridian Gallbladder meridian Urinary bladder meridian	Lower limbs	Anterior side midline Posterior side

At the lower part of the leg and the dorsum of the foot, the liver meridian runs along the anterior side while the spleen meridian runs along the midline; they cross at a point on the leg eight cun above the medial malleolus, and thus the spleen meridian runs along the anterior side while the liver meridian runs along the midline.

The 12 Meridians

The Direction, Connection, Distribution, Relation and Sequence of the Meridians

1. *Direction and connection*

There is a rule for the direction and connection of the 12 meridians, "Three yin meridians of the hand and foot travel from the viscera to the hand; three yang meridians of the hand from the hand to the head, three yang meridians of the foot from head to the foot; three yin meridians of the foot, from foot to the abdomen." (Miraculous Pivot) In other words, the three yin meridians of the hand run from the chest cavity to the finger-tips, where they join the three yang meridians of the hand; the three yang meridians of the hand run from the fingertips to the head and face were they link with three yang meridians of the foot; the three yang meridians of the foot run from the head and face to the tips of the toes, connecting the three yin meridians of the foot; the three yin meridians of the foot run from the toes to the abdominal and thoracic cavities (and extend to the head), where they join the three yin meridians of the hand. In such a way that the 12 meridians run all over the body in an endless circle connecting both yin and yang. (Miraculous Pivot.)

2. *Distribution*

There is a rule for the distribution of the 12 meridians on the surface: a. In the four limbs, the three yin meridians are distributed over the medial aspect and the three yang meridians over the lateral; roughly the taiyin and yangming meridians lie in the anterior portion, the jueyin and shaoyang meridians run in the middle portion, while the shaoyin and taiyin meridians travel in the posterior portion. However, there is an exception. At the lower part of the leg and the dorsum of the foot, the jueyin meridian of the foot runs anteriorly to the taiyin meridian; they cross at a point on the leg eight cun above the medial malleolus, and thus the jueyin meridian runs between the taiyin and shaoyin meridians. b. Over the head and face, the yangming meridian runs through the face and forehead, the taiyang meridian crosses the cheek, vertex and back of the head, while the shaoyang meridian travels along the lateral side of the head. c. In the trunk, the tree yang meridians of the hand run through the scapular region; among the three yang meridians of the foot, the yangming meridian runs in the front (the chest and abdomen), the taiyang meridian in the back and the shaoyang meridian in the lateral side. The three yin meridians all emerge out of the chest from the armpit. The three yin meridians of the foot run through the abdominal surface. The sequence of the meridians running through the abdominal surface from the interior of the body to the exterior is: the meridian of foot shaoyin, the meridian of foot yangming, the meridian of foot taiyin and the meridian of foot jueyin.

3. *Interior-exterior relationship*

The three yin meridians and the three yang meridians of the hand and foot are interiorly and exteriorly related in six pairs, as is seen in the following table:

Table for interior-exterior relationships between the meridians
Exterior
The large intestine meridian of hand yangming
The triple energizer meridian of hand shaoyang
The small intestine meridian of hand taiyang
The stomach meridians of the foot yangming
The gallbladder meridian of the foot shaoyang
The urinary bladder meridian of the foot taiyang
The lung meridian of hand taiyin
The pericardium meridian of the hand jueyin
The heart meridian of hand shaoyin
The three yang meridians of the hand
The three yin meridians of the foot
The spleen meridian of foot taiyin
The liver meridian of foot jueyin
The kidney meridian of foot shaoyin

The 12 meridians meet at the end of the four limbs and travel along the medial or lateral side of the four limbs. In the body, they may pertain to a certain organ and connect with another organ in interior-exterior relationship, e.g., the urinary bladder meridian of the foot taiyang pertains to the urinary bladder and connects with the kidney.

4. *Sequence*

Qi and blood in the 12 meridians circulate from the lung meridian of hand taiyin to the liver meridian of foot jueyin, and finally return to the lung meridian like a large loop. The sequence is as follows:

The Course

1. *The lung meridian of hand taiyin (L)*

This originates from the middle energizer and runs downward to connect with the large intestine. Turning back, it goes along the orifice of the stomach (the lower orifice, pylorus and the upper orifice, cardia), and passes through the diaphragm to enter the lung. After reaching the throat, it runs transversely to the supralateral chest area (Zhongfu, L1) and emerges from the surface of the body under the clavicle. Descending along the anterior border of the medial aspect of the upper arm, it reaches the cubital fossa. Then, it runs continuously downward along the medial aspect of the forearm and arrives at the medial aspect of the styloid process of the radius above the wrist, where it enters the cunkou section. Passing through the thenar eminence, it ends at the tip of the thumb (Shaoshang, L1 1).

Branch: Emerging from the region posterior to the wrist (Lieque, L7), it runs directly to the radial side of the tip of the index finger (Shangyang, LI 1) to connect with the large intestine meridian of hand yangming (Fig. 3).

2. *The large intestine meridian of hand yangming (LI)*

This starts from the tip of the radial side of the index finger (Shangyang, LI 1), runs upward to Hegu (LI 4), and continues to ascend along the anterior border of the extensor side of the upper arm, and then to the anterior border of the scapular joint. Later, it goes posteriorly to the 7th cervical vertebra (Dazhui, GV 14), and then descends anteriorly to the supraclavicular fossa to enter the thoracic cavity and connects with the lung. It runs downward to pass through the diaphragm and finally emerges into the large intestine, its pertaining organ.

Branch: it runs upward from the supraclavicular fossa, passes through the neck to reach the cheek and enters the gum of the lower teeth. Then, it curves around the lip and crosses to the opposite meridian at the philtrum. From there, the left one goes to the right and the right one to the left, on both sides of the nose (Yingxiang, LI 20), where it links with the stomach meridian of foot yangming (Fig. 4).

Daily Exercises

1. What are the distributive rules of the 12 meridians on the body surface?
2. Explain how to master the running course of the lung meridian of hand taiyin.

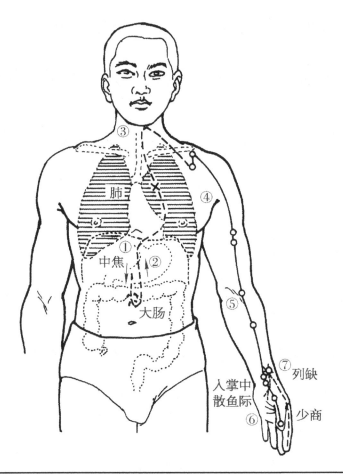

肺	-	Lung
中焦	-	Middle energizer
大肠	-	Large intestine
入掌中，散鱼际	-	Enter the palm and spread over the thenar eminence
列缺	-	*Liè quē* (LU 7)
少商	-	*Shào shāng* (LU 11)

Fig. 3   The lung meridian of hand taiyin.

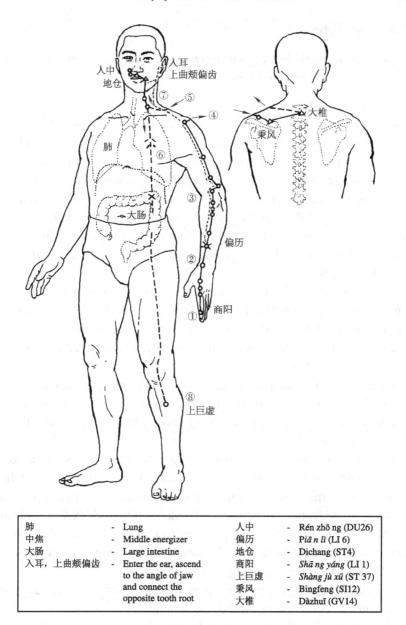

肺	- Lung	人中	- Rén zhōng (DU26)
中焦	- Middle energizer	偏历	- Piān lì (LI 6)
大肠	- Large intestine	地仓	- Dichang (ST4)
入耳，上曲颊偏齿	- Enter the ear, ascend to the angle of jaw and connect the opposite tooth root	商阳	- Shāng yáng (LI 1)
		上巨虚	- Shàng jù xū (ST 37)
		秉风	- Bingfeng (SI12)
		大椎	- Dàzhuī (GV14)

Fig. 4 Large intestine meridian of hand yangming.

The 12 Meridians

3. *The stomach meridian of foot yangming originates from the lateral side of ala nasi (Yingxiang, LI 20)*

It ascends to the bridge of the nose, where it meets the urinary bladder meridian of foot taiyang (Jingming, B 1). Turning downward along the lateral side of the nose (Chengqi, S 1), it enters the upper gum. Then it curves around the lips and runs downward to meet the conception vessel at the mentolabial groove (Chengjiang, CV 24). Subsequently it goes posteriorly across the lower portion of the cheek at Daying (S 5). Winding along the angle of the mandibular region (Jiache, S6), it ascends in front of the ear and traverses Shangguan (G 30) of the gallbladder meridian of foot shaoyang. Then it follows the anterior hairline and reaches the forehead (Touwei, S 8).

The cheek branch: It emerges in front of Daying (S 5), and runs downward to Renying (S 9). From there it goes along the throat and enters the supraclavicular fossa. It further descends and passes through the diaphragm, and then enters its pertaining organ, the stomach, and connects to the spleen, its related organ.

The direct branch: It arises from the supraclavicular fossa, and descends and passes through the nipple. It then reaches the lateral side of the umbilicus (two cun lateral to the anterior midline of the chest), and reaches Qijie (S 30) on the inguinal groove.

The branch of the abdomen: It starts from the lower orifice of the stomach, descends inside the abdomen, and reaches the inguinal groove, where it merges with the previous branch of the channel. From there, it further descends to the front of the coax joint, reaches the quadriceps muscle and enters the knee. From the knee, it goes further down along the anterior border of the lateral aspect of the tibia to the dorsum of the foot and reaches the lateral side of the tip of the second toe (GV 27).

The tibial branch: It emerges from Zusanli (S 36), 3 cun below the knee, and enters the lateral side of the middle toe.

The branch from the dorsal foot: It arises from Chongyang (S 42) and terminates at the medial side of the tip of the big toe (Yinbai, Sp 1) where it links with the spleen meridian of foot taiyin (Fig. 5).

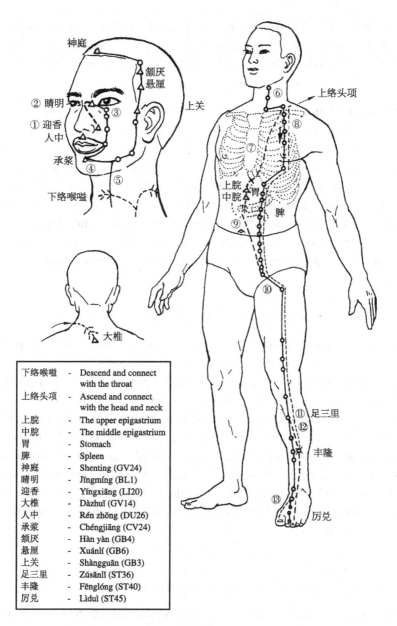

下络喉嗌	-	Descend and connect with the throat
上络头项	-	Ascend and connect with the head and neck
上脘	-	The upper epigastrium
中脘	-	The middle epigastrium
胃	-	Stomach
脾	-	Spleen
神庭	-	Shenting (GV24)
睛明	-	Jīngmíng (BL1)
迎香	-	Yíngxiāng (LI20)
大椎	-	Dàzhuī (GV14)
人中	-	Rén zhōng (DU26)
承浆	-	Chéngjiāng (CV24)
颔厌	-	Hàn yàn (GB4)
悬厘	-	Xuánlí (GB6)
上关	-	Shàngguān (GB3)
足三里	-	Zúsānlǐ (ST36)
丰隆	-	Fēnglóng (ST40)
厉兑	-	Lìduì (ST45)

Fig. 5

4. *Starting from the tip of the big toe (Yinbai, Sp 1), the spleen meridian of foot taiyin runs along the medial aspect of the foot at the junction of the "pinkish and pale skin" ascends in front of the medial malleolus up to the leg, and passes Shangyang (LI 1)*

It follows midline of the medial side of the shank, crosses at a point on the leg 8 cun above the medial malleolus and goes in front of the liver meridian of foot jueyin. Passing through the anterior side of the medial aspect of the knee and thigh, it enters the abdomen, then the spleen, its pertaining organ and connects with the stomach. From there, it ascends, traversing the diaphragm and running alongside the esophagus. When it reaches the root of the tongue, it spreads over the lower surface of the tongue.

The branch from the stomach: It goes upward through the diaphragm and flows into the heart to link with the heart meridian of hand shaoyin (Fig. 6).

5. *The heart meridian of hand shaoyin originates from the heart*

Emerging, it spreads over the "heart connector." Descending, it passes through the diaphragm to connect with the small intestine.

The ascending branch: Splitting from the heart connector, it runs alongside the esophagus to connect with the ocular connection.

The direct branch: Splitting from the heart connector, it goes upward to the lung, then runs downward and emerges from the axilla. From there it goes along the posterior border of the medial aspect of the upper arm down to the cubital fossa of the forearm, to the wrist, and to the pisiform region proximal to the palm. Then, it follows the medial aspect of the little finger to its tip (Shaochong, H 9) and links with the small intestine meridian of hand taiyin (Fig. 7).

6. *The small intestine meridian of hand taiyang starts from the ulnar side of the tip of the little finger (Shaoze, SI 1)*

Following the ulnar side of the dorsal hand and the anterior aspect of the upper limbs, it ascends and passes through the elbow. Emerging from Jianzhen (SI 9) posterior to the shoulder joint, it circles around the scapular region and crosses the conception vessel at Dazhui (GV 14). Then, going forward to the supraclavicular fossa, it connects with the heart. From there

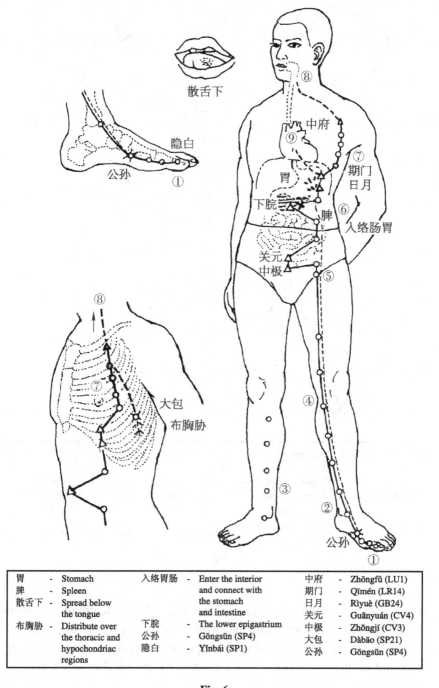

胃	-	Stomach	入络胃肠	-	Enter the interior	中府	-	Zhōngfǔ (LU1)
脾	-	Spleen			and connect with	期门	-	Qīmén (LR14)
散舌下	-	Spread below			the stomach	日月	-	Rìyuè (GB24)
		the tongue			and intestine	关元	-	Guānyuán (CV4)
布胸胁	-	Distribute over	下脘	-	The lower epigastrium	中极	-	Zhōngjí (CV3)
		the thoracic and	公孙	-	Gōngsūn (SP4)	大包	-	Dàbāo (SP21)
		hypochondriac	隐白	-	Yǐnbái (SP1)	公孙	-	Gōngsūn (SP4)
		regions						

Fig. 6

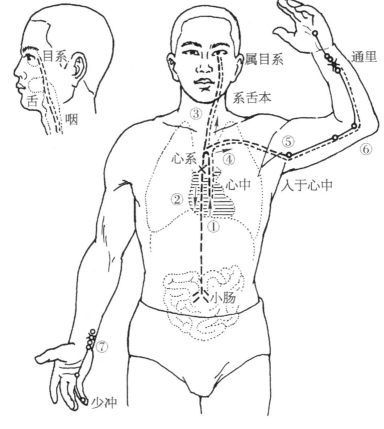

目系	-	Eye connector	舌	-	Tongue
属目系	-	Belong to the eye connector	咽	-	Pharynx
系舌本	-	Connect with the tongue root	小肠	-	Small intestine
心系	-	Heart connector	少冲	-	Shàochōng (HT9)
心中	-	Heart center	通里	-	Tōnglǐ (HT5)
入于心中	-	Enter the heart center			

Fig. 7

it descends along the esophagus, passes through the diaphragm, reaches the stomach, and finally enters the small intestine, its pertaining organ.

The first branch: Splitting from the supraclavicular fossa, it ascends to the neck and further to the cheek. Then it enters the ear via the outer canthus.

The second branch: Splitting from the cheek, it runs upward to the infraorbital region and the inner canthus (Jingming, B 1) to connect with the bladder meridian of foot taiyang (Fig. 8).

7. *The bladder meridian of foot taiyang: It originates from the inner canthus (Jingming, B 1)*

Ascending to the forehead, it joins the governor vessel at the vertex (Baihui, GV 20).

The branch from the vertex: Splitting from the vertex, it reaches the superior angle of the ear.

The direct branch: Splitting from the vertex, it goes posteriorly to the occipital region, enters and communicates with the brain. It then emerges and descends to the neck (Tianzhu, BL 10). After crossing at Dazhui (GV 14), it bifurcates into two lines running down alongside the medial aspect of the scapular region and parallel to the vertebral column. It then reaches the lumbar region (Shenshu, BL 23), where it enters the abdominal cavity *via* the paravertebral muscle to connect with the kidney and joins its pertaining organ, the bladder.

The branch of the lumbar region: it bifurcates into two lines running down alongside the spinal column from the lumbar region. It runs through the hip, and enters the popliteal fossa of the knees along the posterio-lateral side of the thigh (Weizhong, BL 40).

The branch from the posterior aspect of the neck: After splitting from the neck, it runs straight downward along the medial border of the scapula, crosses the hip joint, and then descends along the posterio-lateral aspect of the thigh to meet with the previous branch of the channel in the popliteal fossa. From there, it descends through the gastrocnemius muscle, emerges posterior to the lateral malleolus, and follows along the fifth metatarsal bone to the lateral side of the tip of the little toe (Zhiyin, B 67), where it communicates with the kidney meridian of foot shaoyin (Fig. 9).

Daily Exercises

1. Understand the running course of the stomach meridian of foot yangming.
2. Understand the running course of the lung meridian of hand taiyin.

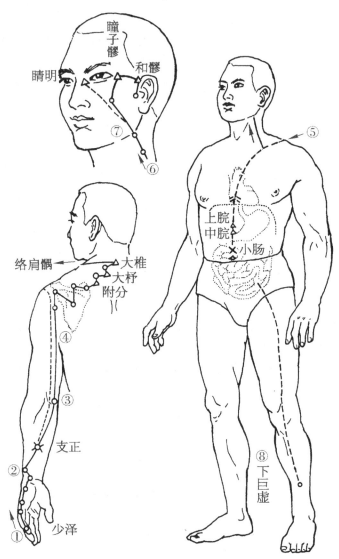

络肩髃	-	Connect with Jiānyú (LI 15)	大椎	-	Dàzhuī (GV14)
上脘	-	The upper epigastrium	大杼	-	Dàzhù (BL11)
中脘	-	The middle epigastrium	附分	-	Fùfēn (BL41)
小肠	-	Small intestine	支正	-	Zhīzhèng (SI7)
瞳子髎	-	Tóngzǐliáo (GB1)	少泽	-	Shàozé (SI1)
和髎	-	Hé liáo (SJ22)	下巨虚	-	Xiàjùxū (ST39)
睛明	-	Jīngmíng (BL1)			

Fig. 8

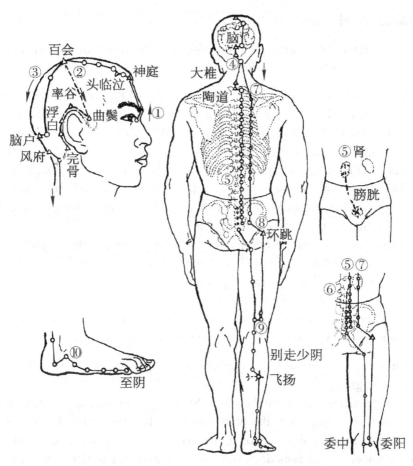

脑	-	Brain	风府	-	Fēngfǔ (GV16)
肾	-	Kidney	完骨	-	Wángǔ (GB12)
膀胱	-	Urinary bladder	曲鬓	-	Qūbìn (GB7)
别走少阴	-	Diverge and run toward the kidney channel of foot shaoyin	至阴	-	Zhìyīn (BL67)
神庭	-	Shenting (DU24)	大椎	-	Dàzhuī (GV14)
头临泣	-	Tóulínqì (GB15)	陶道	-	Táodào (GV13)
百会	-	Bǎihuì (GV20)	环跳	-	Huantiao (GB30)
率谷	-	Shuàigǔ (GB8)	飞扬	-	Feiyang (BL 58)
浮白	-	Fúbái (GB10)	委阳	-	Wěiyáng (BL39)
脑户	-	Nǎohù (GV17)	委中	-	Weizhong (BL40)

Fig. 9

The 12 Meridians

8. *The kidney meridian of foot shaoyin starts from the inferior aspect of the small toe and runs obliquely towards the sole (Yongquan, K 1)*

Emerging from the lower aspect of the tuberosity of the navicular bone and running behind the medial malleolus, it enters the heel. Then it ascends along the medial side of the leg, and goes upward along the posteromedial aspect of the thigh towards the coccyx (Changqiang, G V1). Going through the spinal column, it enters the kidney and connects with the urinary bladder.

The direct branch: Starting from the kidney, it ascends and passes through the liver and diaphragm, enters the lung, and runs along the throat and terminates at the root of the tongue.

The branch springing from the lung: Splitting from the lung, it joins the heart and flows into the chest (Danzhong CV `17) to link with the pericardium meridian of hand jueyin (Fig. 10).

9. *The pericardium meridian of hand jueyin originates from the chest, and enters its pertaining organ, the pericardium*

Then, it descends through the diaphragm to the abdomen, connecting with triple energizer.

The branch arising from the chest: Splitting from the chest, it emerges from the costal region at the point three cun below the anterior axillary fold (Tianchi, P 1) and ascends to the axilla. Following the medial aspect of the upper arm, it runs downward to the cubital fossa along the medial midline of the upper limb, passes through the wrist and enters the palm (Laogong, PC 8). From there it runs along the radial side of the middle finger down to its tip (Zhongchong, P 9).

The branch arises from the palm: Splitting from the palm at Laogong (P 8), it runs along the ulnar side of the ring finger to its tip (Guanchong, TE 1), and links with the triple energizer meridian of hand shaoyang (Fig. 11).

10. *The triple energizer meridian of hand shaoyang starts from the ulnar side of the tip of the ring finger (Guanchong, TE 1), running upward between the fourth and fifth metacarpal bones along the dorsal aspect of the wrist to the lateral aspect of the forearm between the radius and ulna*

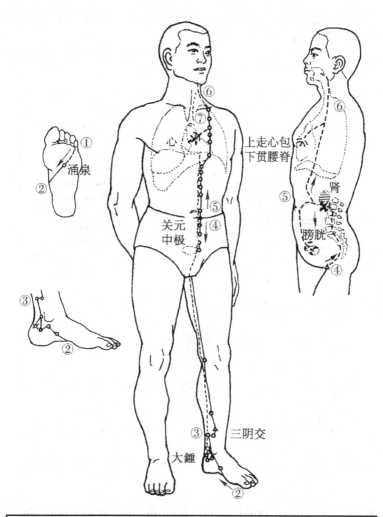

上走心包	-	Ascend and run through the pericardium	心	-	Heart
下贯腰脊	-	Descend and run through the lumbar vertebrae	涌泉	-	Yongquan (KI1)
			关元	-	Guānyuán (CV4)
肾	-	Kidney	中极	-	Chung chi (CV3)
膀胱	-	Urinary bladder	大钟	-	Càzhōng (KI4)
			三阴交	-	Sanyinjiao (SP 6)

Fig. 10

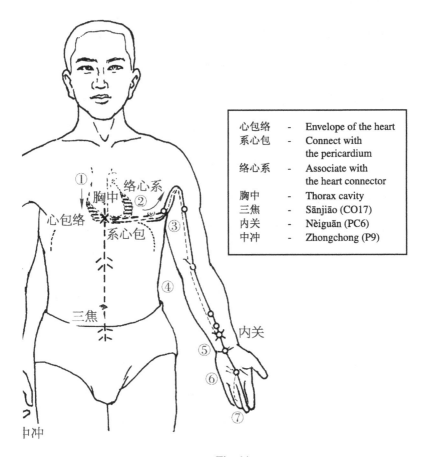

心包络	-	Envelope of the heart
系心包	-	Connect with the pericardium
络心系	-	Associate with the heart connector
胸中	-	Thorax cavity
三焦	-	Sānjiāo (CO17)
内关	-	Nèiguān (PC6)
中冲	-	Zhongchong (P9)

Fig. 11

Passing through the olecranion and along the lateral aspect of the upper arm, it reaches the shoulder region. Winding over to the supraclavicular fossa, it spreads in the chest to connect with the pericardium. Then it descends through the diaphragm down to the abdomen and joins its pertaining organ, the triple energizer.

The branch originating from the chest: Spitting from the chest, or (Danzhong CV 17), it emerges from the supraclavicular fossa, reaches the shoulder and crosses at Dazhui (GV 14). From there it ascends to the neck, running along the posterior border of the ear (Yingfeng TE 17), and further to the superior aspect of the ear. It then turns downward to the cheek and terminates in the infraorbital region.

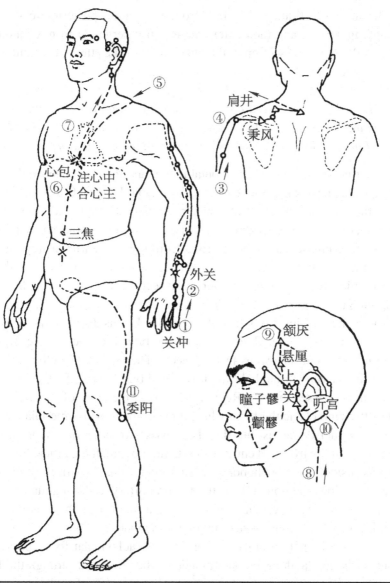

心包	-	Pericardium	三焦	-	Sānjiāo (CO17)	悬厘	-	XuánLí (GB6)
注心中	-	Infuse into the heart	委阳	-	Wěiyáng (BL39)	瞳子髎	-	Tóngzǐliáo (GB1)
合心主	-	Meet the heart channel of hand shaoyin	肩井	-	Jianjing (GB 21)	上关	-	Shàngguān (GB3)
			外关	-	Wangguan (TE5)	听宫	-	Tīnggōng (SI 19)
			中冲	-	Zhongchong (P9)	颧髎	-	Quán liáo (SI 18)
			颔厌	-	Hanyan (GB4)			

Fig. 12

The auricular branch: It arises from the region posterior to the ear (Yingfeng TE 17) and then enters the ear. It emerges in front of the ear, crosses the previous section at the cheek and reaches the outer canthus to link with the gallbladder meridian of foot shaoyang.

11. *The gallbladder median of foot shaoyang originates from the outer canthus (Tongziliao, G 1), ascends to the corner of the forehead (Hanyan, G 4), then descends to the posterior region of the ear*

It further curves upward to the frontal region and the region above the eyebrow, and then returns to the retroauricular region (Fengchi GB 20). Running along the side of the neck to the shoulder, it crosses the triple energizer meridian of hand shaoyang at Dazhui (GV 14) and enters the supraclavicular fossa.

The retroauricular branch. It arises from the retroauricular region and enters the ear via Yifeng (TE 17), then comes out and passes through the preauricular region to the posterior aspect of the outer canthus via Tinggong (SI 19).

The branch arising from the outer canthus: It runs downward to Daying (S 5) on the lower mandible and meets the branch of the triple energizer meridian of hand shaoyang in the cheek. Then, running below the eye socket and passing through the angle of mandible (Jiache ST 6), it descends to the neck, passes through Renying (ST 9) in the front of the neck, and enters the supraclavicular fossa where it meets the previous meridian. From there it further descends into the chest, passes through the diaphragm to connect with the liver and enters its pertaining organ, the gallbladder. Then it turns inside the hypochondriac region, and comes out from the lateral side of the lower abdomen near the femoral artery at the inguinal region. Form there it runs superficially along the margin of the pubic margin. And then it transversely goes to the hip joint (Huantiao, G 30).

The direct branch: it emerges from the supraclavicular fossa, passes in front of the axilla along the lateral side of the chest and through the free end of the floating rib to the hip region (Huantaio GB 30) where it meets the previous section. Then it descends along the lateral aspect of the thigh to the lateral side of the knee. Going further downward along the anterior aspect of the bibula all the way to its lower end, it reaches the anterior aspect of the external malleolus. It then follows the dorsal foot to the lateral side of the tip of the 4th toe (Fig. 13).

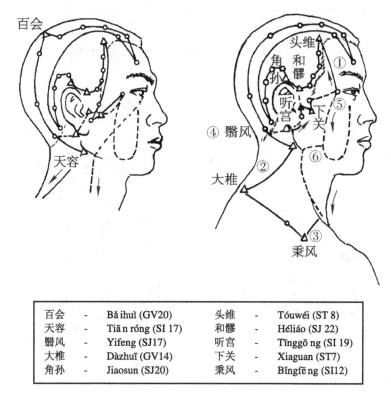

百会	-	Bǎihuì (GV20)	头维	-	Tóuwéi (ST 8)
天容	-	Tiān róng (SI 17)	和髎	-	Héliáo (SJ 22)
翳风	-	Yifeng (SJ17)	听宫	-	Tīnggōng (SI 19)
大椎	-	Dàzhuī (GV14)	下关	-	Xiaguan (ST7)
角孙	-	Jiaosun (SJ20)	秉风	-	Bǐngfēng (SI12)

Fig. 13a

12. *The liver meridian of foot jueyin originates from the dorsal hairy region of the big toe (Dadun, Liv 1)*

Running upward along the dorsal foot, it passes through Zhongfeng (Liv 4) 1 cun in front of the medial malleolus, and ascends to the area 8 cun above the medial malleolus where it crosses behind the spleen meridian of foot taiyin. Then, it runs further upward to the medial side of the knee along the medial aspect of the thigh to the pubic margin, where it curves around the external genitalia and goes up to the lower abdomen. It then runs upward and curves around the stomach to enter the liver, its pertaining organ, and connects with the gallbladder. From there it continues to spread, passing through the diaphragm, and branching out in the costal and hypochondriac region. Then it ascends along the posterior aspect of the throat to the nasopharynx and

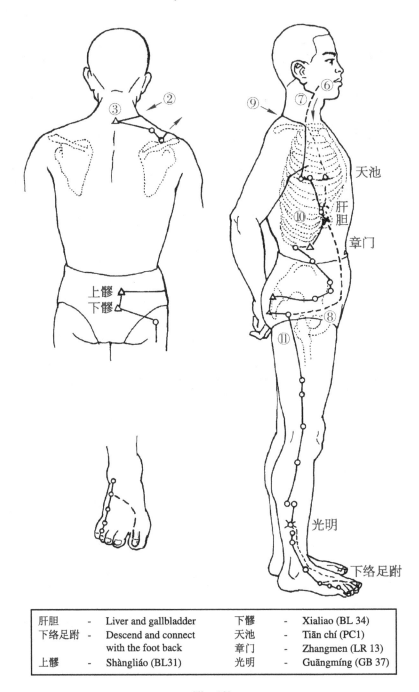

肝胆	-	Liver and gallbladder	下髎	-	Xialiao (BL 34)
下络足跗	-	Descend and connect with the foot back	天池	-	Tiān chí (PC1)
			章门	-	Zhangmen (LR 13)
上髎	-	Shàngliáo (BL31)	光明	-	Guāngmíng (GB 37)

Fig. 13b

connects with the ocular connection. Running further upward, it emerges from the forehead and meets the governor vessel at the vertex (Baihui GV 20).

The branch splitting from the ocular connection: it descends to the cheek and curves around the lips.

The branch arising from the liver: It passes through the diaphragm, flows into the lung and links with the lung meridian of hand taiyin (Fig. 14).

Daily Exercises

1. Understand the running course of the kidney meridian of foot shaoyin.
2. Understand the running course of the liver meridian of foot jueyin.

The Eight Extraordinary Meridians

There are eight extraordinary meridians, namely the governor vessel, conception vessel, thoroughfare vessel, belt vessel, yin heal vessel, yang heel vessel, yin link vessel and yang link vessel. They were sporadically discussed in *Huang Di Nei Jing* (*The Yellow Emperor's Canon of Medicine*, 黄帝内经) and did not have the name of "eight extraordinary meridians" until the appearance of Nan Jing. Different from the 12 regular channels, they are not distributed all over the body. For example, there are no such meridians over the upper limbs. All the extraordinary meridians ascend either from the lower limbs or from the lower abdomen except that the belt vessel circles around the waist and a branch of the thoroughfare vessel goes downward. They have no direct connection with any of the zang-fu organs, nor do they have exterior-interior relationships between them. Only a few extraordinary meridians are connected with the zang-fu organs, e.g., the governor vessel enters the brain, its pertaining organ, and connects with the heart; the thoroughfare vessel, the conception vessel and the governor vessel are all associated with the uterus. These differences are the reason why they are called the "eight extraordinary meridians."

The Functions of the Eight Extraordinary Meridians

1. Further strengthening the connection of the 12 meridians, e.g., "The yang link vessel connects with yang," combing all the yang meridians; while "the yin link vessel connects with yin," combining all the yin

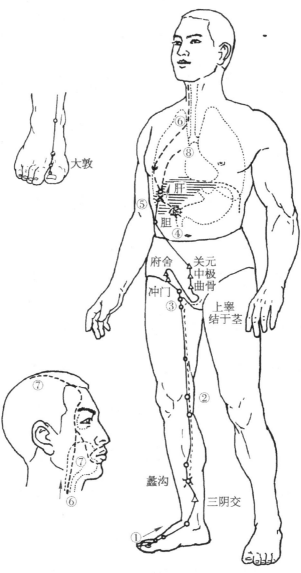

肝	-	Liver	冲门	-	Chōng mén (SP 12)
胆	-	Gallbladder	关元	-	Guānyuán (RN4)
上睾	-	Ascend to the testicle	中极	-	Zhōngjí (CV3)
结于茎	-	Gather at the penis	曲骨	-	Qūgǔ (RN2)
大敦	-	Dàdūn (LR 1)	蠡沟	-	Lìgōu (LR 5)
府舍	-	Fù shě (SP13)	三阴交	-	Sanyinjiao (SP 6)

Fig. 14

meridians; the governor vessel "governs all the yang meridians" whereas the conception vessel is "the sea of all yin meridians;" the thoroughfare vessel passes up and down, irrigating the three yin meridians and the three yang meridians; and the belt vessel "binding all the meridians." Both arising from the ankle, the yin vessels and yang vessels can coordinate the yang meridians and yin meridians in the lower limbs.

2. Regulating qi and blood in the 12 meridians. When qi and blood are in excess, they flow into and are stored in the eight extra meridians. When the 12 meridians lack qi and blood, they can be recharged from the eight extra meridians.

3. They are inter-related as well as closely related with the liver, kidney, uterus, brain and marrow physiologically and pathologically.

The Governor Vessel

1. *The course*

The governor vessel starts from the uterus. Descending, it emerges at the perineum. Then it ascends posteriorly along the spinal column to Fengfu (GV 16) at the nape, where it enters the brain. It further ascends to the vertex and winds along the midline of the forehead to the columella of the nose.

The first branch: It splits from the inside of the spinal column and merges into the kidney.

The second branch: It ascends directly from the inner abdomen and passes through the umbilicus and then through the heart to the throat. Then it ascends to the lower mandible, curves around the lips, and reaches the central region below the eyes (Fig. 15).

2. *Main functions*

To govern means to control or command, so the governor vessel has the functions as follows:

(1) Regulating the qi and blood in the yang meridians. It runs along the posterior midline of the back and frequently joins the three yang meridians of the hand and foot and the yang link meridian, so it can

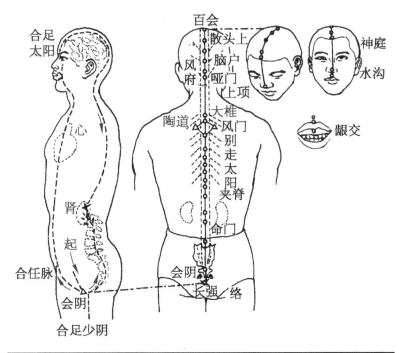

合足太阳	-	Meet the channel of foot taiyang	风府	-	Fēngfu (DU16)
心肾起	-	Start from the heart and kidney	哑门	-	Yamen (DU15)
合任脉	-	Meet the Conception vessel	大椎	-	Dàzhuī (GV14)
合足少阴	-	Meet the channel of foot shaoyin	陶道	-	Táodào (GV13)
散头上	-	Spread over the head	风门	-	Fengmen (BL12)
上项	-	Ascend to the head	夹脊	-	Jiájǐ (EX-B2)
别走太阳	-	Diverge and run toward the channel of foot taiyang	命门	-	Mìngmén (GV4)
			长强	-	Changqiang (DU1)
会阴	-	Huì yīn (RN1)	神庭	-	Shenting (DU24)
百会	-	Bǎihuì (GV20)	水沟	-	Shuǐ gōu (DU26)
脑户	-	Naohù (DU17)	龈交	-	Yín jiāo (DU28)

Fig. 15

control and regulate all the yang meridians of the body. That why it is called "the sea of yang meridians."

(2) Reflection the functions of the brain, marrow and kidney. As it traverses the spinal column, runs upward to enter the brain and merges into the kidneys after splitting from the spinal column, it is closely related to the brain, marrow and kidney.

3. Indications

Diseases or disorders of the brain, five sensory organs, spinal cord and the four limbs, such as head-wind syndrome, headache, stiff neck, heavy head, spinning sensation, tinnitus, dizziness, blurring vision, lethargy, mania, stiff and painful lumbar vertebra, inhibited bending and stretching, sore and weak limbs, as well as spasm, tremor, convulsion, numbness of the foot and hand and speechlessness due to stroke.

The Conception Vessel

1. *The course*

The conception vessel starts from the uterus and emerges from the perineum. It runs anteriorly to the pubic region and ascends along the midline of the abdomen and chest to the throat and lower mandible. Running further upward, it curves around the lips, passes through the cheek and enters the infraorbital regions.

Branch: Starting from the uterus, it runs posteriorly and then goes along with the thoroughfare vessel before the spinal column (Fig. 16).

2. *Main functions*

Conception means assumption of a responsibility or pregnancy.

(1) Regulating the qi and blood of the yin meridians. As the conception vessel runs along the anterior midline of the abdomen, frequently crosses the three yin meridians of the foot and the yin link vessel, it can coordinate the yin meridians and regulate the qi and blood in the yin meridians. For this reason, it is also called the "sea of yin meridians".
(2) Governing the uterus and pregnancy. The conception vessel starts from the uterus, so it is concerned with the uterus and fetus. It can regulate menstruation, promote female reproductive functions and is related to pregnancy. In this sense, it is said that the conception vessel governs the uterus and pregnancy.

3. *Indications*

Mainly disorders of the lower abdomen, male or female genitals, and the throat such as hernia, pudendum swelling and pain, masses, accumulation,

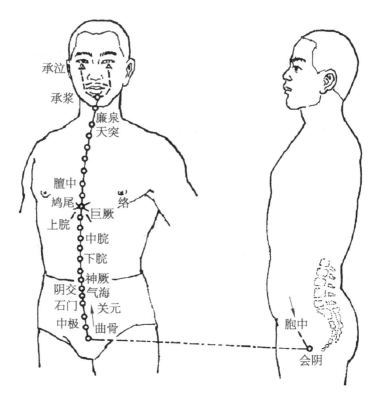

胞中	-	Uterus	巨阙	-	Jùquè (RN 14)
上脘	-	The upper epigastrium	神阙	-	Shénquē (CV8）
中脘	-	The middle epigastrium	阴交	-	Yinjiao (SP 6)
下脘	-	The lower epigastrium	气海	-	Qìhǎi (CV6)
承泣	-	Chéngqì (ST 1)	石门	-	Shí mén (RN5)
承浆	-	Chéngjiāng (CV24)	关元	-	Guānyuán (CV4)
廉泉	-	Liánquán (CV23)	中极	-	Zhōngjí (CV3)
天突	-	Tiān tū (RN22)	曲骨	-	Qūgǔ(RN2)
膻中	-	Dàn zhōng (RN17)	会阴	-	huì yīn (RN1)
鸠尾	-	Jiūwěi (CV15)			

Fig. 16

inhibited urination, bed-wetting, and hemorrhoids, etc. If there is qi adverseness, dry and unsmooth throat can be seen because the meridian circulates through this region. Other disorders include diarrhea, dysentery, coughing, pharyngeal swelling, diaphragm coldness, gastric pain and postpartum disorders.

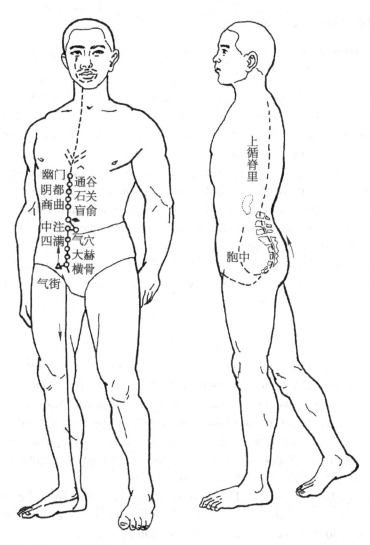

上循脊里	-	Ascend before the spinal column	盲俞	-	Mangshu (KI 16)
胞中	-	Uterus	中注	-	Zhongzhu (KI 15)
幽门	-	Yōu mén (KI21)	四满	-	Sì mǎn (KI14)
通谷	-	Tōng gǔ (KI20)	气穴	-	Qixue (KI 13)
阴都	-	Yīn dōu (K19)	大赫	-	Dahe (KI 12)
石关	-	Shiguan (KI 18)	横骨	-	Hénggǔ (KI11)
商曲	-	Shāngqū (KI 17)	气街	-	Qijie (ST30)

Fig. 17

The Thoroughfare Vessel

1. *The course*

The thoroughfare vessel originates from the uterus. Descending, it emerges from the perineum. Then it coincides with the kidney meridian of foot shaoyin from the region of qi passage. Passing by the umbilicus, it spreads over the chest. It further runs up to the throat, curves around the lips and reaches the region below the eye socket.

The first branch: Starting from the region of qi passage, it enters the popliteal fossa along the medial aspect of the thigh, and then travels downward to the sole along the medial border of the tibia; another section splits from the posterior and medial malleolus and runs anteriorly, entering the dorsal foot and big toe.

The second branch: Originating from the uterus, it ascends before the spinal column, and goes posteriorly to communicate with the governor vessel.

2. *Main functions*

(1) Regulating the qi and blood of the 12 meridians. As it ascends to reach the head and descends to reach the foot, it can receive qi and blood of the 12 meridians and become the key pass of qi and blood of all the meridians. When qi and blood from the viscera or meridians are in excess or in deficiency, the thoroughfare vessel will regulate the volume of qi and blood of the 12 meridians by storage or irrigation. So it is also called the "sea of 12 meridians."

(2) Being the sea of blood. The thoroughfare vessel starts from the uterus, so it is also called the "sea of blood." It can promote reproduction and has a close connection with menstruation in women.

3. *Indications*

Mainly disorders in the lower abdomen, such as pain in the lower abdomen, qi adverseness, heartache, vexation, chest distress, hypochondriac distension, abdominal discomfort, unsmooth urination and defection, hernia, bed-wetting, and incontinence of feces. Since the thoroughfare vessel and conception vessel are related, so it can also treat male or female infertility, metrorrhagia and metrostaxis, menstrual disorders and postpartum diseases.

The Belt Vessel

1. *The course*

It starts from the hypochondriac region, descends obliquely to reach Weidao (G 28), and then surrounds the body in a circle. The section in the abdominal surface descends to the lower abdomen (Fig. 18).

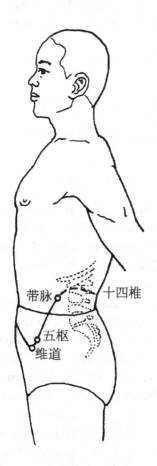

十四椎	-	The second lumbar vertebrae
带脉	-	Daimai (GB 26)
五枢	-	Wushu (GB27)
维道	-	Weidao (GB28)

Fig. 18

2. *Main functions*

It curves around the waist like a belt and can control all the meridians traversing vertically. It can regulate the meridian qi and prevent qi of the vertical meridians from sinking. It also governs vaginal discharge.

3. *Indications*

Mainly soreness and flaccidity in the waist, abdominal distension, abdominal pain involving the lumbar vertebrae, inhibited movements of the lower limbs, and male or female genital disorders including impotence, nocturnal emission, irregular menstruation, metrorrhagia and metrostaxis, morbid leucorrhea, contraction of the lower abdomen, and sinking sensation caused by hernia, etc.

Daily Exercises

1. What are the eight extraordinary meridians?
2. What are the functions of the eight extraordinary meridians?

Weekly Review

In this week, we discussed meridians. The meridian theory in TCM, with an early beginning, is formulated into a complete set of unique theories on physiology, pathology and therapeutics. Some aspects are parallel to the visceral theory, such as the therapeutic significance of the meridians and the therapeutic significance of the viscera.

Meridians and collaterals, or jing and luo in Chinese, are the most important components of the human body. The circulation of qi, blood and body fluid, the functional activities of the viscera, as well as the coordination of different organs must be realized through the transportation, communication and connection of the meridian system, making the human body into an organic entirety. The meridian theory, an important component of the basic theories in TCM, studies the composition, distribution, physiological function and pathological variation of the meridian system as well as their relationships with the viscera, body constituents, orifices, qi, blood and body fluid, etc. It is indispensable to the theoretical foundation of TCM and there is a saying by the ancients, "if one does not learn the 12 meridians by heart, he will be prone to error."

The meridians are divided into 12 regular meridians, eight extraordinary meridians and 12 divergent meridians, etc.

1. There are 12 regular meridians, i.e., three pairs of yin meridians and three pairs of yang meridians of the hand and foot, collectively called the "12 regular meridians." The three yin meridians of the hand: The lung meridians of hand taiyin, the pericardium meridian of the hand jueyin, the heart meridian the hand shaoyin; The three yang meridians of the hand: The large intestine meridian of hand yangming, the triple energizer meridian of hand shaoyang, the small intestine meridian of hand taiyang; The three yin meridians of the foot: The spleen meridian of foot taiyin, the liver meridian of foot jueyin, the kidney meridian of foot shaoyin; The three yang meridians of the foot: The stomach meridians of the foot yangming, the gallbladder meridian of the foot shaoyang, the urinary bladder meridian of the foot taiyang.

The 12 meridians originate from and terminate at certain areas, lie in certain places and have a fixed sequence in circulation. In other words, there is a definite rule for their distribution over and passing through the body. Each connects directly with the viscera and serves as the main passage in which qi and blood circulate. Each of the 12 meridians may pertain to its entering organ or connect with another organ that is interiorly and exteriorly related with the former one. The yin meridians and yang meridians of 12 meridians, with their pertaining and connecting organs internally and externally related, are in an interior-exterior relationship, i.e., yangming and taiyin, shaoyang and jueyin, and taiyang and shaoyin.

There is a rule for the direction and connection of the 12 meridians, "Three yin meridians of the hand and foot travel from the viscera to the hand; three yang meridians of the hand from the hand to the head, three yang meridians of the foot from the head to the foot; three yin meridians of the foot, from the foot to the abdomen." (Miraculous Pivot.) In other words, the three yin meridians of the hand run from the chest cavity to the fingertips, where they join the three yang meridians of the hand; the three yang meridians of the hand run from the fingertips to the head and face were they link with three yang meridians of the foot; the three yang meridians of the foot run from the head and face to the tips of the toes, connecting the three yin meridians of the foot; the three yin meridians of the foot run from the toes to the abdominal and thoracic cavities (and extend to the head), where they join the three yin meridians of the hand. In such a way the 12 meridians run all over the body in an endless circle connecting both yin and yang. (Miraculous Pivot.)

There is a rule for the distribution of the 12 meridians on the surface: a. In the four limbs, the three yin meridians are distributed over the medial aspect and the three yang meridians over the lateral side; roughly the tai-yin and yangming meridians lie in the anterior portion, the jueyin and shaoyang meridians run in the middle portion, while the shaoyin and tai-yin meridians travel in the posterior portion. However, there is an exception. At the lower part of the leg and the dorsum of the foot, the jueyin meridian of the foot runs anteriorly to the taiyin meridian; they cross at a point on the leg 8 cun above the medial malleolus, and thus the jueyin meridian runs between the taiyin and shaoyin meridians. b. Over the head and face, the yangming meridian runs through the face and forehead, the taiyang meridian crosses the cheek, vertex and back of the head, while the shaoyang meridian travels along the lateral side of the head. c. In the trunk, the three yang meridians of the hand run through the scapular region; among the three yang meridians of the foot, the yangming meridian runs in the front (the chest and abdomen), the taiyang meridian in the back and the shaoyang meridian in the lateral side. The three yin meridians all emerge out of the chest from the armpit. The three yin meridians of the foot run through the abdominal surface. The sequence of the meridians running through the abdominal surface from the interior of the body to the exterior is: the meridian of foot shaoyin, the meridian of foot yangming, the meridian of foot taiyin and the meridian of foot jueyin.

Qi and blood in the 12 meridians circulate from the lung meridians of hand taiyin to the liver meridian of foot jueyin, and finally return to the lung meridian like a large loop. The sequence is as follows: The lung meridian of hand taiyin

- The large intestine meridian of hand yangming
- The stomach meridian of the foot yangming
- The spleen meridian of foot taiyin
- The heart meridian the hand shaoyin

- The small intestine meridian of hand taiyang
- The urinary bladder meridian of the foot taiyang
- The kidney meridian of foot shaoyin
- The pericardium meridian of the hand jueyin
- The triple energizer meridian of hand shaoyang
- The gallbladder meridian of the foot shaoyang
- The liver meridian of foot jueyin
- The lung meridian of hand taiyin.

The above-mentioned 12 meridians should be memorized because they are the most commonly used ones in the clinic.

2. There are eight extraordinary meridians, namely the governor vessel, conception vessel, thoroughfare vessel, belt vessel, yin heal vessel, yang heel vessel, yin link vessel and yang link vessel. The extraordinary meridian can mainly command, communicate and coordinate the 12 meridians.

Different from the 12 regular meridians, they are not distributed all over the body. For example, there are not many meridians over the upper limbs. All the extraordinary meridians ascend either from the lower limbs or from the lower abdomen except that the belt vessel circles around the waist and a branch of the thoroughfare vessel goes downward. They have no direct connection with any of the zang-fu organs, nor do they have exterior-interior relationships between them. Only a few of the meridians are connected with the zango-fu organs, e.g., the governor vessel enters the brain, its pertaining organ, and connects with the heart; the thoroughfare vessel, the conception vessel and the governor vessel are all associated with the uterus. The functions of the eight extraordinary meridians: a. Further strengthening the connection of the 12 meridians b. Regulating qi and blood in the 12 meridians c. They are closely related with the liver, kidney, uterus, brain and marrow physiologically and pathologically.

The governor vessel ascends posteriorly along the spinal column, and is called "the sea of yang meridians." The conception vessel ascends along the midline of the abdomen and chest and is called the "sea of yin meridians" and the "governor of uterus and fetus." The thoroughfare vessel is called the "sea of blood" and the "sea of 12 meridians" These are also commonly used clinically.

3. The 12 divergent meridians are branches spreading from the 12 meridians, starting from the four extremities, traversing the deep portions of the viscera, and emerging from the superficial regions of the neck and nape. The branches of the yin meridians, after splitting from and running through the interior of the body, meet the divergences of the yang meridians that are internally and externally connected to them. In such a way they reinforce the connection between the meridians that are internally and externally related. Besides, they can also reach the organs and body areas that some regular meridians do not traverse.

4. The collaterals are the branches of the meridians. Most of them have no fixed courses. They can be divided into three categories: divergent collaterals, superficial collaterals and minute collaterals.

The divergent collaterals are the large and major collaterals. Each of the 12 regular meridians has one divergent collateral, and so do the governor vessel and conception vessel. Together with the large spleen collateral, they are collectively called the "15 divergent collaterals." Similar to the 12 divergent meridians, the 15 divergent collaterals can strengthen the connection between every pair of the meridians in exterior and interior relationship.

The superficial collaterals run in the shallow region of the body and are often visible on the surface of the body.

The fine collaterals are the smallest and thinnest ones in the body. It is said in *Su Wen* (*Plain Conversation*, 素问) that they are the places where the extraordinary pathogens are driven out and the nutrient qi and defensive qi are communicated.

5. The meridian tendons and skin divisions, in the strict sense, are not meridians or collaterals, but the affiliated parts of the 12 meridians. According to the theory of meridian system, the meridian tendons are a system, where qi "retains, accumulates, disperses and connects" in or with the musculature and joints. They are so named because the 12 meridian tendons pertain to the 12 meridians. They can connect the four limbs and various bones and is in charge of the movements of joints. The skin is the region reflecting the functional activities of the 12 meridians and the place where the meridian qi disperses. That is why the skin of the body is divided into 12 parts, which correspond directly to the 12 meridians.

Daily Exercises

1. Master the connotation of meridians and the composition of the meridian system.
2. Understand the name, direction, and course of the 12 meridians.
3. Describe the distributing rule of the 12 meridians and sequence of qi and blood flowing inside them.
4. What are the concepts and main functions of the eight extraordinary meridians?

THE EIGHTH WEEK

The Eight Extraordinary Meridians

The Yin Heel Vessel and the Yang Heel Vessel

1. *The course*

The heel vessels are a pair of meridians on the left and right sides of the body. Both start from the area below the malleolus.

The yin heel vessel splits from Zhaohai (K 6) below the malleolus, ascends along the posterior side of the malleolus and goes directly along the medial aspect of the lower limb, then enters the supraclavicular fossa *via* the external genitalia, abdomen and chest, and then emerges anteriorly from Renying (S 9) to reach the inner canthus *via* the side of the nose, joining the taiyang meridians of the hand and foot and the yang heel vessel (Fig. 19).

After splitting from Shenmai (B 62) below the lateral malleolus, the yang heel vessel ascends along the posterior side of the lateral malleolus, passes through the abdomen, continuously ascends along the posterior-lateral side of the chest, scapular region, and lateral aspect of the neck to the corner of the mouth, then reaches the inner canthus to connect with the taiyang meridians of the hand and foot and the yin heel vessel. Then it runs further upward to the hairline, runs downward to the posterior ear and meets with the gallbladder meridian of foot shaoyang at the posterior nape (Fig. 20).

2. *Main functions*

"Heel" here refers to mobility and agility.

(1) Governing movements of the limbs. Both the yin heel vessel and the yang heel vessel ascend from the medial and lateral aspects to the head and face, so they can communicate the yin qi and yang qi of the whole body and are capable of regulating the muscular movements. Their main function is to make the movements of the lower limbs agile and nimble.
(2) Controlling the movements of the eyelids. Since the yin heel vessel and yang heel vessel join at the inner canthus, they have the action of nourishing the eyes and controlling the movements of the eyelids.

3. *Indications*

Eye pain, insomnia, lethargy, lassitude and epilepsy, etc.

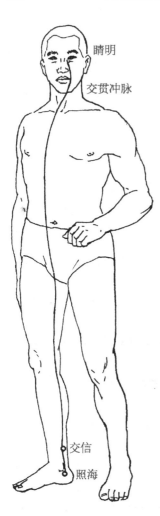

睛明

交贯冲脉

交信

照海

交贯冲脉	-	Connect with the thoroughfare vessel
睛明	-	Jīngmíng (BL1)
交信	-	Jiāo xìn (KI8)
照海	-	Zhàohǎi (KI6)

Fig. 19

The Yin Link Vessel and Yang Link Vessel

1. *The course*

The yin link vessel originates from the medial aspect of the leg where the three yin meridians meet, then ascends along the medial aspect of the lower limb to the abdomen. Ascending together with the spleen meridian of foot taiyin to reach the hypochondriac region, it meets the liver

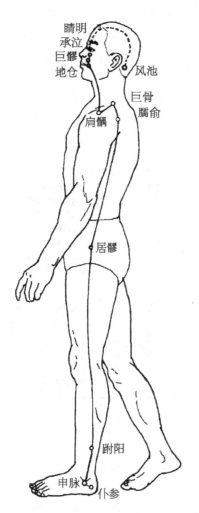

睛明	-	Jīngmíng (BL1)
承泣	-	Chéngqì (ST 1)
巨髎	-	Jùliáo (ST 3)
地仓	-	Dì cāng (ST4)
风池	-	Fēngchí (GB20)
巨骨	-	Jùgǔ (LI 16)
臑俞	-	Nào shū (SI10)
肩髃	-	Jiānyú (LI 15)
居髎	-	Jūliáo (GB29)
跗阳	-	Fuyang (BL 59)
仆参	-	Pú cān (BL 61)
申脉	-	ShēnMài (BL 62)

Fig. 20

meridian of foot jueyin and then runs upward to reach the throat, connecting with the conception vessel (Fig. 21).

Yang link vessel starts from the area below the lateral malleolus, runs upward parallel to the gallbladder meridian of foot shaoyang, and then ascends along the lateral aspect of the lower limb. It further passes through the posterior aspect of the trunk, goes upward to reach the shoulder, and then runs anteriorly to the forehead *via* the neck and the posterior ear,

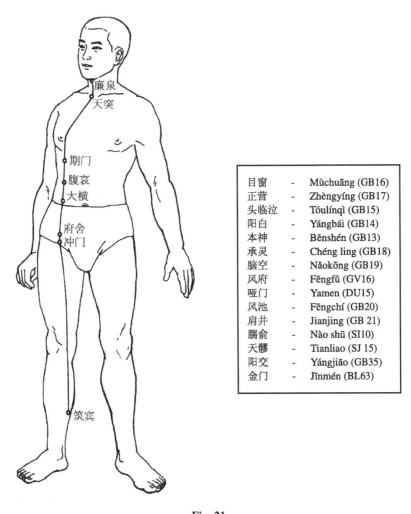

目窗	-	Mùchuāng (GB16)
正营	-	Zhèngyíng (GB17)
头临泣	-	Tóulínqì (GB15)
阳白	-	Yángbái (GB14)
本神	-	Běnshén (GB13)
承灵	-	Chéng ling (GB18)
脑空	-	Nǎokōng (GB19)
风府	-	Fēngfǔ (GV16)
哑门	-	Yamen (DU15)
风池	-	Fēngchí (GB20)
肩井	-	Jianjing (GB 21)
臑俞	-	Nào shū (SI10)
天髎	-	Tianliao (SJ 15)
阳交	-	Yángjiāo (GB35)
金门	-	Jīnmén (BL63)

Fig. 21

spreads over the lateral head and the posterior neck where it joins the governor vessel (Fig. 22).

2. *Main functions*

"Link" here means to connect or coordinate. The yin link vessel and yang link vessel have the functions of connecting and coordinating the actions

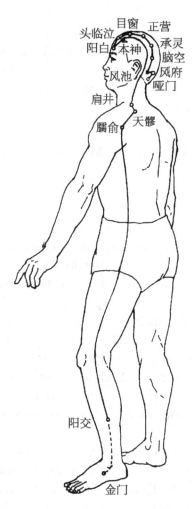

廉泉	-	Liánquán (CV23)
天突	-	Tiān tū (RN22)
期门	-	Qīmén (LR14)
腹哀	-	Fù āi (SP16)
大横	-	Dà héng (SP15)
府舍	-	Fù shě (SP13)
冲门	-	Chōngmén (SP 12)
筑宾	-	Zhùbīn (KI 9)

Fig. 22

of the yin meridians and yang meridians of the whole body. Under normal circumstances, the yin link vessel and yang link vessel are mutually coordinated, and together they regulate the volume of qi and blood by storing or irrigating them. However, they are not involved in the process of qi and blood circulation.

3. *Indications*

Yang syndrome and exterior syndrome such as fever, cold, headache and dizziness if the yang link vessel fails to coordinate; yin syndrome and interior syndrome, such as cardiac and abdominal pain or hypochondriac pain if the yin link vessel fail to coordinate.

The Divergent Meridian, Divergent Collateral, Meridian Tendon and Skin Division

The Divergent Meridian

Divergent meridians are the important branches that split from the 12 regular meridians, traverse deep into the trunk and pass through the chest, abdomen and heat. All of them "split" from the four extremities where the 12 meridians traverse (usually the portion above the elbow and knee) and "enter" the deep part of the internal organ, then "emerge" from the body surface to run upward to the head and face, and finally the branches of the yin meridians "merges" into those of the yang meridians in interior-exterior relationship with the former. So the circulation of the 12 meridians is characterized by "split, merge, emerge and enter." Each pair of meridians in interior-exterior relationship is called a pair of "combination." The three yin meridians and three yang meridians constitute "six pairs of combination."

Although the 12 divergent meridians are only the branches of the 12 regular meridians, they distribute over a relatively wider area and traverse at points the 12 meridians do not go through. Thus they can be used physiologically, pathologically and therapeutically. The main actions are as follows.

1. *Strengthening the connection between the two interiorly and exteriorly related meridians among the 12 meridians within the body*

After the 12 branches of meridians enter the body cavity, the two meridians in interior-exterior relationship coincide with each other and pass through the viscera that are also interiorly and exteriorly related. When they emerge from the body surface, the branch of the yin meridian connects with that of the yang meridian, and together they merge into the yang meridians on the body surface. In such a way the 12 divergent meridians strengthen the intrinsic association between the two interiorly and exteriorly related meridians or viscera.

2. *Strengthening the centripetal connection between the superficial and deep parts of the body, or between the four extremities and trunk*

The branches of the 12 meridians split from the sections of the 12 meridians in the four extremities and traverse centripetally after entering the body. This plays an important role in widening the body's connection with the meridians and in transmitting messages from the exterior to the interior of the body.

3. *Strengthening the connection between the 12 meridians with the head and face*

The meridians covering the head and face are mainly the six yang meridians. However, among the 12 divergent meridians, not only the branches of the six yang meridians traverse the head and face, but also those of the six yin meridians reach the head. The branches of the three yin meridians of the foot reach the head after merging into the branches of yang meridians. While the branches of the three yin meridians of the hand meet at the head and face *via* the throat. This is the foundation for the theory that "qi and blood in the 12 meridians and the 365 collaterals run upward to reach the face and pass through the sensory organs." (Miraculous Pivot.)

4. *Widening the range of indications of the 12 meridians*

As the branches of the 12 meridians distribute themselves over the area where the 12 meridians do not reach, the range of indications of the acupoints are widened correspondingly. For example, although the meridian of foot taiyang does not reach the anus, its branch enters the anus so that the acupoints, such as Chengshan (B 57) and Chengjin (B 56) of the meridian may be chosen for treating anal disorders.

5. *Strengthening the connection between the heart and the three yin meridians and three yang meridians of the foot*

As the branches of the three yin and yang meridians of the foot ascend to pass through the abdomen and chest, they are connected with the heart in the chest cavity and make the connection of the viscera in the abdominal cavity closer. Therefore, the branches of the 12 meridians are important to the analysis of the physiological and pathological connection between the viscera in the abdominal cavity and the heart.

The Divergent Collaterals

Divergent collaterals are also branches splitting from the main meridians, most of which are distributed over the body surface. There are 15 divergent collaterals: 12 of them are branches splitting from the 12 meridians, two of them are branches splitting from the conception vessel and governor vessel, and the rest one is the major collateral of the spleen. If the collateral of the stomach is added, there will be 16 divergent collaterals.

They are the major ones among the collaterals, playing a leading role among the numerous fine collaterals. The fine collaterals splitting from the large ones are called the "minute collaterals;" those that are distributed over the body surface are called the "the superficial collaterals."

The main physiological functions of the divergent collaterals are given below.

1. *Strengthening the connection between the two interiorly and exteriorly related meridians among the 12 meridians*

They strengthen the connection between the two interiorly and exteriorly related meridians in the trunk and limbs because the divergent collateral of the yin meridian connects with the yang meridian, and that of the yang meridian with the yin meridian. Although certain divergent collaterals enter the thoracic and abdominal cavities and connect with the viscera, there is no definite relation between the collaterals and the viscera.

2. *Controlling other collaterals and strengthening the connection between the anterior, posterior and lateral sides of the body*

As the divergent collateral of the conception vessel is distributed over the abdomen, that of the governor vessel over the back, and the major collateral of the spleen over the thoracic and hypochondriac region, the integral unity of the anterior, posterior and lateral portions of the body are strengthened.

3. *Irrigating and nourishing the body with qi and blood*

The minute and superficial collaterals split from the divergent collaterals and spread all over the body like a network which contacts the tissues of the entire body. Though such a network, qi and blood flow in the main meridians in a linear way can spread to every direction and reach every destination so as to nourish the whole body.

The Meridian Tendons

The meridian tendons are a system of tendons and muscles connecting to the 12 meridians. Their functions are based on qi and blood in the meridians and regulated by the 12 meridians. That is why they are classified into the "12 meridian tendons."

Their main function is to control the bones and promote the flexion and extension of the joints. So the meridian tendons can connect the limbs and the bones as well as govern the movement of the joints.

The Skin Divisions

The skin division refers to the regions divided according to the distribution of meridians. To be specific, the skin surface of the body is divided into various areas according to the distribution of the twelve meridians and their collaterals. Hence the skin of the body is divided into 12 areas, called the 12 skin divisions. The skin divisions are not only the regions where the twelve meridians and their collaterals go through, but also the places where the meridian qi spread over.

Daily Exercises

1. Familiarize yourself with the courses of the yin heel vessel and yang heel vessel.
2. Familiarize yourself with the courses of the yin link vessel and yang link vessel.

The Physiological Functions of Meridians and the Application of Meridian Theory

The Physiological Functions

The physiological functions of the meridians are chiefly to promote qi and blood circulation for nourishing the viscera and tissues, to connect the viscera and organs for communicating the exterior with the interior and the upper with the lower, and to receive and conduct messages for regulating the functions of various parts of the body.

1. *Promoting qi and blood circulation and nourishing*
   the viscera and tissues

The meridians can promote qi and blood so as to nourish yin and yang, moisten the tendons and bones, and lubricate the joints. (Miraculous Pivot.). So qi and blood rely on the meridians for their circulation in the body, so as to nourish the viscera internally and moisten the interstitial spaces externally, and maintain the normal life activities of the body.

The 12 meridians are the core of the meridian system and the main passage for the circulation of qi and blood. If the functional activities of the meridians are normal, the circulation of qi and blood is smooth, and the functions of the viscera are vigorous, the exogenous pathogenic factors will be resisted and disease can be prevented; otherwise, if the meridians function improperly, or the meridian qi becomes inhibited, the exogenous pathogenic factors will find their ways to invade the body and cause diseases.

2. *Connecting the viscera and organs, and communicating the exterior*
   with the interior, the upper with the lower

The human body is a complex organism composed of the five zang-organs, six fu-organs, five sensory organs, nine orifices, four extremities, and various bones. Although the meridians have different physiological functions, they jointly carry on their functions to keep the harmony of different parts of the body. Such a coordination is achieved mainly by the communicating action of the meridians. The 12 meridians and their collaterals form a network that merges at the interior of the body and emerges from the exterior. They also pertain to or connect with certain viscera and the limbs. The eight extraordinary meridians coordinate the 12 regular meridians and regulate the volume of qi and blood inside them. Consequently, various viscera, tissues and organs are linked to form a unity. In this way the exterior and interior, upper and lower, or left and right portions of the body are closely connected and coordinated.

The connection and coordination of all the viscera, tissues and organs by meridians are manifested as follows.

(1) The connection between the viscera and limbs. The connection between the viscera and peripheral limbs is established through the 12 meridians. The 12 meridians are connected with the five zang-organs and six fu-organs, and their qi is spread over and accumulates in the meridian tendons and the skin divisions.

(2) The connection between the viscera and the five sensory organs and nine orifices. The eyes, ears, nose, mouth, tongue, external genitalia and anus are the areas where the meridians go through. Since the meridians mostly pertain to the internal organ, the five sensory organs and nine orifices are connected with the viscera through the meridians. For example, the heart meridian of hand shaoyin pertains to the heart, connects with the small intestine and links with the "eye connector." Its divergent collateral connects with the "root of the tongue."

(3) The connection between the five zang-organs and six fu-organs. Each of the 12 meridians connects with and pertains to a zang-organ or a fu-organ respectively, thus establishing the interior-exterior connection between the zang-organ and fu-organ. A meridian may connect with several viscera, and a viscus may be linked by several meridians. For example, the liver meridian of foot jueyin pertains to the liver, connects with the stomach, curves around the stomach, and enters the lung. The kidney meridian of foot shaoyin pertains to the kidney, connects with the bladder, goes through the liver, enters the lung, and links with the heart; the meridian pertains to the lung is the lung meridian of hand taiyin while the meridian connects with the lung is the large intestine meridian of hand yangming, etc.

(4) The connection between the meridians. The 12 meridians have a certain link and sequence in terms of the flow of qi and blood. The crisscross network of the 12 regular meridians and eight extraordinary meridians, and the interconnection of the eight extraordinary meridians, form multiple connections among the meridians. For example, the three yang meridians of the hand and foot all join at Dazhui (GV 14) of the governor vessel, and the yang heel vessel and the governor vessel meets at Fengfu (GV 16), so the governor vessel is termed the "sea of yang meridians;" the three yin meridians of the foot, the yin link vessel, and the thoroughfare vessel all connect with the conception vessel, and the three yin meridians of the foot ascend to link with the three yin meridians of the hand. So the conception vessel is said to be the "sea of yin meridians;" the thoroughfare coincides with the conception vessel in the chest, and the posterior branch communicates with the governor vessel. The conception vessel and governor vessel connect with the 12 meridians whereas the thoroughfare vessel can receive qi and blood from the 12 meridians. That is why the thoroughfare vessel is known as the "sea of the 12 meridians;" the governor vessel, the conception vessel and the thoroughfare vessel all originate from the uterus. Such a multi-faceted and multi-leveled connection makes the meridians into a complete regulative system.

(5) Inducing and conducting messages and regulating the balance of the body. The automatic regulation of the body is achieved mainly through the meridian system and the qi and blood circulating inside it. As the network for information transmission of the body, the meridian system can receive various messages from the internal and external environments of the body. According to their nature, characteristic, volume or degree, the messages are transmitted to different viscera, tissues, five sensory organs, nine orifices, four limbs and all the bones correspondingly so as to reflect or regulate their functional conditions.

The Application of the Meridian Theory

1. To elucidate pathological changes

Under normal circumstances, the meridian promotes qi and blood circulation through its transmitting and conducting actions. If diseases occur, it will become the pathway to transmit the pathogenic factors and a sign of the ailment. Through the meridians, disease can transfer from one viscus to another. For example, the liver meridian of foot jueyin curves around the stomach and enters the lung, so liver disease may easily be transmitted to the stomach or the lung; the kidney meridian of foot shaoyin enters the lung and connects with heart, so kidney water may be apt to attack the heart and invade the lung; the zang-organs and fu-organs are often mutually affected pathologically because they are either connected by the same meridian or by two meridians that are interiorly and exteriorly related. For instance, the heart fire may transmit downward to the small intestine; obstruction of qi in the fu-organs may cause unsmooth flow of lung qi, characterized by chest distress, wheezing and cough, etc.

Besides, the meridians are also the channels through which the viscera and superficies are mutually affected under pathological conditions. For example, distension and pain in the hypochondria and lower abdomen are frequently seen in the syndrome of stagnant liver qi because the liver meridian of foot jueyin reaches the lower abdomen and distributes itself over the hypochondria; real cardiac pain (angina pectoris) is not only manifested as a precordia pain, but also pain in the ulnar border of the medial aspect of the upper limbs because the heart meridian of hand shaoyin runs through the posterior border of the medial aspect of the upper limb.

2. *Directing diagnosis*

Since a meridian has a fixed course, connects with or pertains to a certain viscus, it is of diagnostic significance to the analysis of the symptoms and signs at a certain region. For example, hypochondriac pain indicates disorders of the liver and gallbladder. Pain in the supraclavicular fossa is often ascribed to a pathological process of the lung. Take headache for another example, pain in the forehead is usually concerned with the yangming meridian; bilateral headache, the shaoyang meridian; pain in the occipital region and nape, the taiyang meridian; and pain in the vertex, the jueyin meridian. Syndrome differentiation with the acupoints is a method for determining the location of disease by examining and analyzing the abnormal manifestations of the acupoints pertaining to a certain meridian. For instance, a tenderness point may be found at Zusanli (ST 36) or Diji

(SP 8) in patients with gastrointestinal diseases, and tenderness point, irritability or subcutaneous nodule at Feishu (BL 13) and Zhongfu (LU 1) in patients with lung diseases. In recent years, a variety of instruments have been applied to examine the human acupoints. To some extend, these tools can reveal the disorders of the meridians, viscera, tissues and organs so as to facilitate diagnosis. The meridian theory is not only unique in principles and methods for analyzing the clinical symptoms and signs and generalizing them into a certain pattern, but also significant in providing essential theoretical foundations for tongue examination, pulse examination and infantile fingerprint examination, which is characteristic to and widely used in TCM.

3. *Guiding clinical treatment*

The meridian theory has been widely used in various clinical branches of TCM. When the human body is in disorder, various methods such as acupuncture, moxibustion, or daoyin (qi exercise) can be used to stimulate certain acupoints properly to activate the automatic regulative functions of the meridians on the basis of analyzing the specific conditions, such as imbalance between qi and blood, and relative exuberance or debilitation of yin and yang. In this way, "the excess is reduced and the deficiency is reinforced, ensuring the balance between yin and yang" (*Li Shu, Miraculous Pivot*). It is confirmed in clinical practice that, according to the principle of "selection of acupoints along the meridians," the visceral functions can be regulated by needling certain acupoints to induce the arrival of qi or to promote the flow of qi, so that the hyperactive is subdued and the depressive is activated. It is thus evident that the meridian theory is of great significance to guiding the practical application of acupuncture, moxibustion, and tuina.

As for the herbal treatment, medicinal substances can reach the affected area only *via* the meridians that transport them so as to perform their therapeutic functions. On the basis of long-term clinical practice, the ancient medical experts established the theories of "meridian tropism" and "herb-guidance" according to selective action of some herbs on a certain meridian or viscus. Xingren (Apricot Seed) and Jiegeng (Platycodon Root), pertaining to the lung meridian, can treat chest oppression, wheezing and cough; Zhusha (Cinnabar) and Zaoren (Semen Ziziphi Spinosae), pertaining to the heart meridian, can treat palpation and insomnia; for headache due to disorders in the meridian of taiyang, Qianghuo (Incised Notoptetygium Rhizome or Root) may be prescribed; and for headache due to yangming, Baizhi (Dahurian Angelica Root) can be used. It is thus clear that the herbs, if selected properly under the direction of meridian theory, can target at the affected region and perform more efficiently their therapeutic effects or actions on regulating the functional activities of the human body.

Daily Exercises

1. What are the physiological functions of the meridians and collaterals?
2. How do meridians and collaterals communicate with the viscera, tissues and organs of the whole body?

CHAPTER 8

Body Constituents, Sensory Organs and Orifices

"Body constituents" refer to the skin, muscles, tendons, bones and vessels, which are collectively called the "five body constituents." "Sensory organs and orifices" refer to the ears, eyes, nose, mouth, tongue, throat, external genitalia and anus. They are connected with the viscera through the meridians, and thus associated closely with the viscera in physiology and pathology. Nevertheless, each body constituent, sensory organ or orifice is relatively independent in functions.

The Body Constituents

The concept of "body constituents" has two different meanings. In a broad sense it refers to all the tissues or organs with certain shape or structure, including the head, limbs, five zang-organs and six fu-organs. In a narrow sense it refers to the skin, vessels, tendons, bones and muscles with specified meanings. They are essential to constituting the human body. The body constituents are connected with the viscera through the meridians, in which the qi, blood and body circulate. The nutrient blood flows inside the meridians or vessels, whereas the defensive qi and body fluid flow outside them, spreading over and permeating through the skin, muscles, tendons, bones, viscera and membranes.

The five zang-organs can produce essence, qi, blood and body fluid and transport them to different body constituents, facilitating the physiological functions of the body constituents by nourishing, promoting, warming and qi-transforming. Besides, the five zang-organs are associated with the body constituents in certain ways, e.g., the liver is associated with tendon, heart with vessel, spleen with muscle, kidney with bone, and lung with skin.

The Skin

The skin covers the surface of the body and includes the hair and sweat pores. It can resist exogenous pathogenic factors, regulate body temperature and fluid metabolism, and assist the lung in respiration. The skin is most closely related to the lung, and also associated with the 12 meridians extensively.

1. *The structure and function of the skin*

The skin covers the surface of the body and there is hair on it with the exception of the palm and sole. The texture and muscular striae of the skin are collectively called the muscular interstices. There are many sweat pores in the skin, called "qi opening" or "mysterious house" in TCM. It is the porous channel for excreting sweat. The main physiological functions of the skin are as follows.

(1) Resist exogenous pathogenic factors. The skin is the largest protective tissue on the body surface and the main barrier for resisting the exogenous pathogenic factors. If the skin is compact, the pathogenic factors will find no way to invade; otherwise, if the skin is loose and the defensive qi is insufficient, pathogenic factors will invade the body and cause diseases.

(2) Regulating fluid metabolism. Sweat is transformed from body fluid, so sweating is a way of excreting body fluid. If the skin is loose and the sweat pores are open, there will be copious sweat; otherwise, there will be less sweat. Hence, the compactness of the skin plays a decisive role in regulating the excretion of body fluid.

(3) Regulating body temperature. The body relies on defensive qi for warmth. Most defensive yang is stored in body fluid. When exogenous pathogenic factors invade the body, the sweat pores will be closed and there will be no sweat. For this reason the defensive yang is obstructed inside the body, eventually causing stagnant heat. In this case, herbs for relieving the exterior and promoting perspiration can be used to open the sweat pores, let out the sweat and defensive yang, and subdue the fever. Nevertheless, sweating cannot be induced excessively in case of yang loss.

(4) Assisting respiration. Although respiration is mainly controlled by the lung, the opening and closing of sweat pores can also facilitate respiration in that they are associated with the lung.

2. *The relationship between the skin and lung is very close*

In *Su Wen*, it is said that the lung governs the skin and hair. The lung is related to the skin and hair in the following aspects.

(1) The lung distributes essence qi to nourish the skin. The lung distributes the cereal nutrients to the skin and hair so as to make the skin moistened and the hair lustrous.
(2) The lung disperses the defensive qi over the skin. The action of the defensive qi on the skin is threefold, i.e., to warm and nourish the skin, to assist the skin to resist exogenous pathogenic factors, and to control the opening and closing of the sweat pores. If the lung is deficient and the defensive qi is insufficient, the patient may has the symptoms such as muscular coldness, intolerance of cold, excessive sweating, poor resistibility, and susceptibility to exogenous pathogenic factors. If exogenous pathogenic factors invade the lung, the defensive qi may be stagnated inside the body and the sweat pores will be obstructed, leading to absence of sweat. So herbs with the function of dispersing lung qi are also capable of promoting sweating.
(3) Exogenous pathogenic factors often invade the lung through the skin. It is already familiar to all of us that when one feels cold in the skin, he or she may show such symptoms related to the lung meridian as sneezing, nasal discharging, and coughing.

3. *The relationship between the skin and meridians*

According to the distribution of the 12 meridians on the body surface, the skin is divided into 12 areas, called the 12 skin divisions. Each meridian is in charge of nourishing one division. The disorders of a certain meridian can also be reflected by the division it goes through. Moreover, the invasion of pathogenic factors may begin with the collaterals in a certain region, then into the meridian to which this region belongs, and finally into the viscera.

4. *Muscular interstices*

"Muscular interstices," or "cou li' in Chinese, is an ancient concept that refers to the texture of the muscles and skin. "Cou" means the texture of the muscles or interstices between the muscles, and "Li" means the texture of the skin, or interstices of the skin. It is considered that the interstices of the muscles and skin, collectively called the muscular interstices, are interconnected.

The muscular interstices are connected with the triple energizer. The primordial qi and body fluid within the triple energizer can flow outwardly to the muscular interstices so as to moisten and nourish the skin as well as maintain the interchange of qi and fluid between the interior and exterior of the body.

The sweat pores open into the skin. So the compactness of the muscular interstices may affect the opening and closing of the sweat pores as well as the excreting of sweat. Compactness of muscular interstices will lead to closure of the sweat pores and absence of sweat; whereas looseness of the muscular interstices may result in opening of the sweat pores and excretion of sweat. For this reason, it is deemed that the muscular interstices can regulate the body temperature and the fluid metabolism.

The beard, eyebrow, and armpit hair are also associated with the qi and blood inside the meridians and can indicate the exuberance or debilitation of qi and blood of the meridians.

Daily Exercises

1. What are the relationships between the skin and the lung or the meridians?
2. What is the connotation of muscular interstices?

The Body Constituents

The Muscles

Muscles, or fleshes, include the muscular tissues, fat and subcutaneous tissues in modern medicine. The muscles in modern medicine are referred to as "fenrou" in the ancient Chinese medical classics. Muscles can protect the viscera, resist pathogenic factors and perform exercises. They are most closely related to the spleen.

1. *The structure and function of the muscles*

The muscles are located beneath the skin, and adherent to the bones and joints. The texture of fenrou is called muscular striae, and together with the texture of the skin, they are called muscular interstices. The depression between fenrou is called "xi gu;" the smaller one is called "xi" and the larger one is called "gu." Xi gu is mostly the area where the acupoints locate at and the qi of the body accumulates in. The main physiological functions of the muscles are as follows.

(1) Protecting the viscera. The muscles surround the viscera and tendons to protect them, especially those in the chest and abdomen. So the muscles are compared to the wall in *Ling Shu* (*Miraculous Pivot*, 灵枢).

(2) Resisting exogenous pathogenic factors. The texture of the muscle and skin is called muscular interstice, which is the gateway for the exogenous pathogenic factors to invade the body. If the muscular interstice is compact, the pathogenic factors will find no way to invade; otherwise, if the muscular interstice is loose, pathogenic factors will invade the body and cause diseases.

(3) Performing exercises. When one enters into adolescence, his muscles may become gradually strong and the motion will become increasingly agile. However, if qi and blood are insufficient and the tendons and muscles are malnourished, there will be flaccidity, atrophy or even paralysis of the limbs.

2. *The relationship between the muscles and spleen*

The muscles and spleen are closely related. In *Su Wen* (*Plain Conversation*, 素问), it is said that the spleen dominates the muscles of the body. The relationship between the muscles and spleen is manifested mainly as follows.

(1) The spleen transforms essence to nourish the muscles. The spleen is in charge of transforming water and food into essence so as to produce and nourish the muscles; that is why it is said the spleen dominates

the muscles. If the spleen and stomach are active, one will have a good appetite and become well nourished; if the spleen and stomach are weak, he or she will have a poor appetite and become skinny.

(2) The muscular disorders may eventually involve the spleen. The disorders of the muscle, if not treated for a long time, may transmit inwardly to the spleen, causing malfunction of the spleen.

The Tendons

Tendons include sinew, ligament and fascia in modern medicine, which can connect and control the bones and joints as well as govern movements and protect the viscera, etc. Among the five elements, the liver is the organ most closely related to the tendons. The 12 meridians also have a wide connection with the tendons.

1. *The structure and function of the tendons*

The tendons are adherent to the bones and accumulated at the joints, especially the knee joint, which is called the "house of tendons." The tendons of the whole body are classified into 12 meridian tendons according to the three yin meridians and three yang meridians of the hand and foot. The main physiological functions of the tendons are as follows.

(1) Connecting and controlling the bones and joints. The tendons are adherent to the bones and the bones are connected by the bones. The region where the bones are connected may be wrapped by tendons, thus forming the joints and ensuring the movement of limbs.

(2) Controlling movements. The ancients attributed the function of muscles in modern medicine to that of the tendons, and deemed that the reason why the joints are flexible in various movements lies in the contraction and relaxation of the tendons. A series of related therapeutic methods are thus formulated in this regard. And such an understanding is still reflected in today's language, such as "someone's tendons and bones are very good" which means that he has a sound body constitution, especially the motor system.

(3) Protecting the viscera. The tendons, bones, muscles and skin constitute the body collectively which house the five zang-organs and six

fu-organs. In this way the viscera is protected and prevented from unnecessary injury.

2. *The relationship between the tendons and the liver*

The relationship between the tendons and the liver is very close. In *Su Wen*, it is said, "the liver governs the tendons." Their relations are mainly manifested as follows.

(1) The liver qi and blood can nourish the tendons. The essence received by the liver from the stomach may be distributed to the tendons so as to perform its nourishing function. If the liver qi and blood is insufficient, the tendons will be inadequately nourished, leading to disorders.
(2) Prolonged liver disease may cause various disorders of the tendons. In Su Wen, it is said, "Heat in the liver may lead to excretion of bile, bitterness sensation in the mouth, and dryness of the tendons and membranes, eventually leading to spasm or flaccidity of the tendons."
(3) Disorder of the tendons can involve the liver. Prolonged tendon diseases, such as the tendon bi-syndrome, may transmit interiorly to the liver.

3. *The relationship between tendons and meridians*

The tendons of the whole body are classified into 12 parts according to the distribution of the 12 meridians. Each part is nourished by the qi and blood from a certain meridian. The meridian qi "accumulates in, gathers at, disperses over and connects with" this part, making it a "meridian tendon" of this meridian. For instance, the tendon nourished by the qi and blood from the lung meridian of hand taiyin are known as the tendon of the hand taiyin; and the tendon by the stomach meridian of foot yangming, the tendon of foot yangming. These tendons nourished by qi and blood from the 12 meridians are collectively called the 12 meridian tendons.

The Bones

Bones constitute the framework of the body which is made up of cartilages and hard bones and connected by tendons and muscles. The cartilage is a soft bone while the hard bone is strong enough to support the body. The bones can support the body, protect the viscera and perform exercises. They are closely related to the kidney.

1. *The construction and function of the bones*

The bone is a hollow structure with marrows inside, so it is called the "house of marrow." Connected by the joints, the bones form into a skeletal system. The physiological functions of the bones are mainly as follows.

(1) Supporting the human body. The bones located in the posterior mid-line, such as the cervical vertebra, thoracic vertebra, lumbar vertebra, sacral bone and coccyx, are connected by the spinal tendons and formed into the back of the body.
(2) Protecting the viscera. The bones of the head, such as the parietal bone, temporal bone, frontal bone and occipital bone, are connected into a skull which protects the brain. Another case in point is that the thoracic bone is connected with the costal bone, collectively making up the thoracic cage which protects the heart and lung.
(3) Performing exercises. The region where the bones are connected may be wrapped by tendons, thus forming into the joints. The joints connect all the bones. Through the contraction and relaxation of the tendons, the joints may perform such movements as extension, flexion, and rotation.

2. *The relationships between the bones and kidney*

The relationships between the bones and kidney are very close. In *Su Wen*, it is said, "The kidney controls the bones." Their relationships are mainly manifested as follows.

(1) The kidney governs the bones and produces marrow. The bone marrow is transformed from the kidney essence, and the growth, development and repair of bones are all dependent on the nourishment of the kidney. If the kidney essence is adequate, the bone marrow will be sufficient, the bones will be strong, and the body will be agile and forceful in movements; otherwise, if the kidney essence is inadequate, the bone marrow will be insufficient, and there will be underdevelopment of the bones such as retarded closure of the infantile fontanel

and flaccidity due to weak bones. When people get old, the kidney qi will decline and the bones may be malnourished, resulting in fragile bones liable to fracture, which is hard to heal.

(2) The tooth is the branch of the kidney. "The tooth is the surplus of the bone," and both the tooth and the bone share the same source for nutrition, the kidney essence. So it is said in Zá Bìng Yuán Liú Xī Zhú (Wondrous Lantern for Peering into the Origin and Development of Miscellaneous Diseases, 杂病源流犀烛), "The tooth is the branch of the kidney and the foundation of the bone." Clinically the retarded development of infantile teeth and the early decaying or loosening of teeth in adults are often caused by insufficiency of kidney essence. According to the theory of "kidney governing bones," some bone diseases or dental disorders are often treated by nourishing the kidney, which is very effective in most cases.

Daily Exercises

1. What are the relationships between the muscles and spleen?
2. What are the relationships between the tendons and liver?
3. What are the relationships between the bones and kidney?

The Organs and Orifices

Organs and orifices are different in concept. Organs are functionally specified, like the ear, eye, mouth, nose and throat; while the orifices are the openings connecting the viscera to the external environment. In ancient times, they were generally referred to as the "five sensory organs," "seven orifices" or "nine orifices." The five sensory organs refer to the ear, eye, mouth, nose and throat; the seven orifices refer to one mouth, two nostrils, two eyes and two ears; nine orifices are actually the seven orifices plus the external genitalia and the anus. The five sensory organs are habitually called "orifices," whereas the external genitalia and the anus are only named "orifices" rather than "organs."

Each orifice is an organ with specified functions. It connects outwardly to the external environment, and communicates inwardly with the internal organs through the meridian. Each orifice is associated with a certain zang-organ in a certain way. In *Ling Shu* (*Miraculous Pivot*, 灵枢), it is said, "the nose is the organ of the lung; the eyes, the liver; the mouth and lips, the spleen; the tongue, the heart; and the ears, the kidney." The external environmental changes can affect the internal organs through the orifices, and the functional conditions of the viscera can also be reflected by the orifices. In *Ling Shu*, it is also pointed out, "The lung qi is connected to the nose, that is why the nose can differentiate aroma from odor if the lung function is normal; the heart qi to the tongue, that is why the tongue can taste the five flavors if the heart function is harmonious; the liver qi to the eyes, that is why the eyes can discern the five colors if the liver function is sound; the spleen qi to the mouth, that is why the mouth can take the five cereals if the spleen function is vigorous; the kidney qi to the ears, that is why the ears can hear the five sounds if the kidney function is proper. Disorders of the five zang-organs will lead to the obstruction of the seven orifices." Organs and orifices are mostly the gateway for material exchanges between the body and nature. For example, the body needs air, water and food, so it takes them through the mouth and nose; the physiological functions produce metabolic products (feces, urine or other wastes), so they are discharged *via* the external genitalia and the anus.

The Ear

The main physiologic function of the ear is the sense of hearing. Being one of the upper orifices, it is the region where the clear-yang qi arrives. The ear is closely associated with the kidney and heart, and also connected to the triple energizer meridian of hand shaoyang, gallbladder meridian of foot shaoyang and small intestine meridian of hand taiyang.

1. *The relationship between the ear and the viscera*

(1) The kidney opens into the ear. The ear is the external orifice of the kidney. If the kidney essence is sufficient, the sense of hearing will be keen and the reaction will be quick. If the kidney essence is insufficient, there will be tinnitus, deafness, dizziness, slow reaction and instability. In senile people, kidney essence is gradually declining, so their senses of hearing are mostly poor.

(2) The ear serves as the orifice of the heart. The heart is physiologically associated with the ear in a certain way. The heart opens into the

tongue, which is an organ rather than an orifice, so the ear severs as the orifice of the heart as well as the kidney. The kidney opens into the ear, which is also the orifice of the heart. Because the heart pertains to fire and the kidney to water, if the heart fire and kidney water are inter-promoted, the ear will receive the clear, pure and quintessential qi and become sensitive to hearing. If not, there will be loss of hearing. Clinically hyperactivity of heart fire or insufficiency of kidney yin often manifests itself as fural fullness, tinnitus, and poor sense of hearing, etc. Sudden deafness may also be caused by tension or stress.

(3) The relationship between the ear and the liver, gallbladder and spleen. If the liver well-functions in governing free flow of qi, the clear yang can ascend to nourish the upper orifices; if it ascends excessively, there will be averseness of qi movements and obstruction of the upper orifices. The gallbladder is interiorly and exteriorly related to the liver, and the gallbladder meridian of foot shaoyang runs before, behind, and into the ear. Clinically the adverseness of liver qi and gallbladder qi may go upward along the meridian to affect the ear, leading to headache or deafness. The spleen is in charge of transforming food and ascending the lucid, so if the spleen is deficient, the lucid yang and the cereal essence may fail to ascend to nourish the upper orifices, affecting the sense of hearing, too.

2. *The relationship between the ear and meridian*

The ear is the place where the ancestral meridians accumulate. Three meridians enter the ear, i.e., the gallbladder meridian of foot shaoyang and triple energizer meridian of hand shaoyang enter the ear from the posterior region of the ear and then goes before the ear; the small intestine meridian of hand taiyang enter the ear from the outer canthus of the eye. If the three meridians are invaded by pathogenic wind-heat or dampness, there may be redness, swelling, pain, pus discharge and poor hearing of the ear. Since both the meridians of hand shaoyang and foot shaoyang enter the ear, tinnitus and deafness may appear when there is shaoyang disorder. Meanwhile, the ear is associated with nearly all the parts of the body *via* the meridians, and this provides the foundation for curing disease with ear acupuncture.

The Eye

The eye controls sense of sight and is associated with the five zang-organs and six fu-organs, particularly the liver. It also has an extensive contact with the meridians.

1. *The structure and function of the eye*

The white part of the eyeball is called the "Bai Yan (white eye)" while the black part is called the "Hei Yan (black eye);" the pupil is located in the center of the black eye, the inner canthus is in the inner angle of the eye, and the outer canthus, the outer angle of the eye. The upper and lower lids are called "Yue Su (constraint)," and the fasciculation connecting the eye to the brain is called the "eye connector."

The eye controls sense of sight. There is a concise description about its functions, "The eye can see all things, and differentiate black from white as well as short from long." (*Su Wen, Plain Conversation*).

2. *The relationship between the eye and the viscera*

(1) The liver opens into the eye. The liver stores blood, and provides nourishment for the eye to perform it function of vision. So the eye is related to the liver physiologically and pathologically.

(2) The eye is associated with the five zang-organs and the brain. The eye is related to the viscera. The essence of the viscera goes upward to the eye. The kidney (bone) essence forms the pupil of the eye, the liver (tendon) essence forms the black part of the eye, the heart (blood) essence forms the venules of the eye, the lung (qi) essence forms the white part of the eye, and the spleen (muscle) essence forms the connector of the eye, which transports all the essences into the brain alongside the meridian (*Ling Shu, Miraculous Pivot*, 灵枢). It is thus evident that the eye is closely associated with the five zang-organs and the brain.

3. *The relationship between the eye and the meridian*

The connection between the eye and the viscera is mainly achieved by the connection of the meridians, which not only transport the visceral essence to the eye, but also coordinate the activities of the eye with those of the body so as to perform its normal physiological functions. The meridians connected to the eye are: the bladder meridian of foot taiyang starting from Jingming (BL1) at the inner canthus; the gallbladder meridian of foot shaoyang starting from Tongziliao (GB1) at the outer canthus; the branch of the heart meridian of hand shaoyin linking to the eye connector; the liver meridian of foot jueyin linking to the eye connector; the branch of the triple energizer of hand shaoyang reaching the outer canthus; the small intestine meridian of hand taiyang terminating at the inner canthus; the branch of the governor vessel meeting the bladder meridian of foot taiyang at the inner canthus; the conception vessel arriving at the region below the eye socket; the yin heel vessel linking to Jingming (BL1) at the inner canthus; and the yang heel vessel linking to the inner canthus. It can be seen that there are more than 10 meridians reaching the eye. So it is said that all the meridians pertain to the eye (*Su Wen*).

The Nose

The nose is the portal for the inhaled and exhaled qi. It governs the sense of smelling, helps vocalization, and serves as the orifice of the lung. The nose is most closely related to the lung, and also has some connections with the spleen, liver and gallbladder. Moreover, the nose is extensively associated with the meridians.

1. The structure of the nose

The nose is also named "Shan Gen (Mountain Root)" or "Wang Gong (Royal Palace); the lower end, or the tip of the nose, is named "apex of the nose," or "Mian Wang (Facial King)." Its bilateral eminent parts, round in shape, are known as "wings of nose;" and the back of nose is called "Tian Zhu (Celestial Pillar)."

2. The main functions of the nose

(1) The nose is the portal for air exchange. The lung governs respiration, while the nose is the place where the breathing qi is connected to the external environment.

(2) The nose governs sense of smelling. In *Ling Shu* (*Miraculous Pivot*, 灵枢), it is pointed out, "The lung qi is connected to the nose, that is why the nose can differentiate aroma from odor if the lung function is normal." This is a concise description about the function of the nose in smelling.

(3) The nose helps vocalization. Although the voice comes out from the throat, but the nose provides a resonant effect, so it can influence the clearness and quality of the voice.

3. *The relationship between the nose and viscera*

(1) The lung opens into the nose. The nose, connected to the lung, is the portal for the inhaled and exhaled qi. That is why it is called the orifice of the lung. The functions of the nose in respiration and smelling must be realized through the lung. On the other hand, lung diseases are mostly caused by exogenous pathogenic factors invading through the mouth and nose.

(2) The apex of the nose belongs to the spleen. The apex of the nose is closely associated with the spleen and stomach, which pertain to earth and are situated in the middle; because the nose is also located in the middle of the face, it is said that the nose is the external manifestation of the spleen and stomach. That is why it is said in *Su Wen*, "Heat in the spleen is firstly manifested as a red nose."

(3) The liver fire and gallbladder fire often invade the nose. The liver governs ascending, pertaining to wind in nature and wood in the five elements. The liver qi is liable to transform into fire which, if fanned by wind, may aggravate the lung dryness and lead to symptoms such as dry nasal cavity and nasal bleeding. The gallbladder is the fu-organ containing essence and connecting to the brain and nose. So when gallbladder heat transfers into the brain, it may also involve the nose, leading to persistent discharging of turbid nasal excreta.

4. *The relationship between the nose and meridians*

The stomach meridian of foot yangming starts from Yingxiang (LI 20) beside the nasal wing, and ascends to the bridge of the nose. Turning downward along the lateral side of the nose, it enters the upper gum. The large intestine meridian of hand yangming terminates at Yingxiang (LI20) beside the nasal wing. Its branch curves around the lip, crosses to the opposite meridian at the philtrum, and distributes itself at both sides of the nose. The small intestine meridian of hand taiyang ends at Jingming (BL 1) at both sides of the nasal root. The bladder meridian of foot taiyang starts from Jingming (BL 1). The governor vessel travels along the mid-line down to the nasal column, then to the tip of the nose, and finally to the philtrum. From the above, we can see that the nose is physiologically and pathologically associated with the aforementioned meridians.

Daily Exercises

1. What is the relationship between the ear and the viscera?
2. What is the relationship between the eye and the viscera?
3. What is the relationship between the nose and the viscera?

Weekly Review

For this week, we will continue to study the meridian theory.

The yin heel meridian, yang heel meridian, yin link meridian and yang link meridian, belonging to the eight extraordinary meridians, are not used as widely as other extraordinary meridians such as the governor vessel, the conception vessel, the thoroughfare vessel and the belt vessel. However, they can treat some peculiar and refractory diseases.

Divergent meridians are the important branches that split from the 12 regular meridians, traverses deep into the trunk and passes through the chest, abdomen and head. All of them "split" from the four extremities where the twelve meridians traverse (usually the portion above the elbow and knee) and "enter" the deep part of the internal organ, then "emerge" from the body surface to run upward to the head and face, and finally the branches of the yin meridians "merges" into those of the yang meridians in interior-exterior relationship with the former. So the circulation of the 12 meridians is characterized by "splitting, merging, emerging and enter-ing." Each pair of meridians in interior-exterior relationship is called a pair of "combination." The three yin meridians and three yang meridians constitute "six pairs of combination."

Their main actions are as follows: a. Strengthening the connection between the two interiorly and exteriorly related meridians among the 12 meridians. b. Strengthening the centripetal connection between the superficial and deep parts of the body, or between the four extremities and trunk. c. Strengthening the connection between the 12 meridians and the head and face. d. Widening the range of indications of the 12 meridians e. Strengthening the connection between the heart and the three yin meridians and three yang meridians of the foot.

Divergent collaterals are also branches splitting from the main meridians, most of which are distributed over the body surface. There are 15 divergent collaterals: 12 of them are branches splitting from the 12 meridians, two of them are branches splitting from the conception vessel and governor vessel, and the rest one is the major collateral of the spleen. If the collateral of the stomach is added, there will be 16 divergent collaterals.

They are the major ones among the collaterals, playing a leading role among the numerous fine collaterals. The fine collaterals splitting from the large ones are called the "minute collaterals;" those distributed over the body surface are called the "the superficial collaterals."

The main physiological functions of the divergent collaterals: a. Strengthening the connection between the two interiorly and exteriorly related meridians among the 12 meridians. b. Controlling other collaterals and strengthening the connection among the anterior, posterior and lateral sides of the body. C. Irrigating and nourishing the body with qi and blood.

The meridian tendons are a system of tendons and muscles connecting to the 12 meridians. Their functions are based on qi and blood in the meridians and regulated by the 12 meridians. That is why they are classified into the "12 meridian tendons." Their main functions are to control the bones and promote the flexion and extension of the joints.

The skin division refers to the regions divided according to the distribution of meridians.

The physiological functions of the meridians are mainly to promote qi and blood circulation for nourishing the viscera and tissues, to connect the viscera and organs for communicating the exterior of the body with the interior and the upper with the lower, and to receive and conduct messages for regulating the functions of various parts of the body.

The connection and coordination of all the viscera, tissues and organs by meridians are manifested as follows: a. The connection between the viscera and limbs. b. The connection between the viscera and the five sensory organs and nine orifices. c. The connection between the five zang-organs and six fu-organs. d. The connection between the meridians. e. The induction and conduction of messages and the regulation of the balance of the body.

The application of the meridian theory: a. To elucidate pathological changes; For instance, the heart fire may transmit downward to the small intestine. b. Directing diagnosis: Since a meridian has a certain course, connects with or pertains to a certain viscus, it is of diagnostic significance to the analysis of the symptoms and signs at a certain region. For example, tenderness point, irritability or subcutaneous nodule may be found at Feishu (BL 13) and Zhongfu (LU 1) in patients with lung diseases. c. Guiding clinical treatment. It is confirmed in clinical practice that, according to the principle of "selection of acupoints along the meridians," the visceral functions can be regulated by needling certain acupoints to induce the arrival of qi or to promote the flow of qi, so that the hyperactive is subdued and the depressive is activated. In this way, "the excess is reduced and the deficiency is reinforced, ensuring the balance between yin and yang" (Li Shu, Miraculous Pivot). Besides, On the basis of long-term clinical practice, the ancient medical experts established the theories of "meridian tropism" and "herb-guidance" according to selective action of some herbs on a certain meridian or viscus.

Since Wednesday, we began to introduce the body constituents, sensory organs and orifices.

The concept of "body constituents" has two different meanings. In a broad sense it refers to all the tissues or organs with certain shape or structure, including the head, limbs, five zang-organs and six fu-organs. In a narrow sense it refers to the skin, vessel, tendon, bone and muscle with specified meanings. They are essential to constituting the human body.

There are many sweat pores in the skin, called "qi opening" or "mysterious house" in TCM. It is the porous channel for excreting sweat. The main physiological functions of the skin are as follows: a. Resisting exogenous pathogenic factors. b. Regulating fluid metabolism. c. Regulating body temperature. d. Assisting respiration.

The relationship between the skin and lung is very close. In *Su Wen*, it is said that the lung governs the skin and hair. The lung is related to the skin and hair in the following aspects: a. The lung distributes essence qi to nourish the skin. b. The lung disperses the defensive qi over the skin. c. Exogenous pathogenic factors often invade the lung through the skin.

"Muscular interstices," or "Cou Li" in Chinese, is an ancient concept that refers to the texture of the muscles and skin. "Cou" means the texture of the muscles or interstices between the muscles, and "Li" means the texture of the skin, or interstices of the skin. It is considered that the interstices of the muscles and skin are interconnected. The muscular interstices are connected with the triple energizer. The primordial qi and body fluid within the triple energizer can flow outwardly to the muscular interstices so as to moisten and nourish the skin as well as maintain the interchange of qi and fluid between the interior and exterior of the body.

Muscles, or fleshes, include the muscular tissues, fat and subcutaneous tissues in modern medicine. The main physiological functions of the muscles are as follows: a. Protecting the viscera. b. Resisting exogenous pathogenic factors. c. Performing exercises.

The muscles and spleen are closely related. In *Su Wen* (*Plain Conversation*, 素问), it is said that the spleen dominates the muscles of the body. The relationship between the muscles and spleen is manifested mainly as follows: a. The spleen transforms essence to nourish the muscles. b. The muscular disorders may eventually involve the spleen.

Tendons include sinew, ligament and fascia in modern medicine. The main physiological functions of the tendons are as follows: a. Connecting and controlling the bones and joints. b. Controlling movements. c. Protecting the viscera.

The relationship between the tendons and the liver is very close. In *Su Wen*, it is said, "The liver governs the tendons." Their relationships are mainly manifested as follows: a. The liver qi and blood can nourish the tendons. b. Prolonged liver disease may cause various disorders of the tendons. c. Disorder of the tendons can involve the liver.

Bones constitute the framework of the body which is made-up of cartilages and hard bones and connected by tendons and muscles. The physiological functions of the bones are mainly as follows: a. Supporting the human body. b. Protecting the viscera. c. Performing exercises.

The relationship between the bone and kidney is very close. In *Su Wen*, it is said, "The kidney controls the bone." Their relationships are mainly as follows: a. The kidney governs the bone and produces marrow. b. The tooth is the branch of the kidney, and the tooth is the surplus of the bone.

Organs and orifices are different in concept. The organs are functionally specific, like the ear, eye, mouth, nose and throat; while the orifices are the openings connecting the viscera to the external environment. In ancient times, they were generally referred to as the "five sensory organs," "seven orifices" or "nine orifices." The five sensory organs refer to the ear, eye, mouth, nose and throat; the seven orifices refer to one mouth, two nostrils, two eyes and two ears; nine orifices are actually the seven orifices plus the external genitalia and the anus. The five sensory organs are habitually called "orifices," whereas the external genitalia and the anus are only named "orifices" rather than "organs."

The main physiological function of the ear is the sense of hearing. It is one of the upper orifices where the clear-yang qi arrives. The ear is closely associated with the kidney and heart. The kidney opens into the ear, which is also the orifice of the ear. The ear is connected to the triple energizer meridian of the hand shaoyang, gallbladder meridian of the foot shaoyang and small intestine meridian of the hand taiyang. Hearing disorder is ascribed to the liver and gallbladder if it is an excess syndrome and to the kidney if it is deficient.

The eye controls the sense of sight and is associated with the five zang-organs and six fu-organs, particularly the liver. The liver stores blood, and provides nourishment for the eye to perform its function of vision. So the eye is related to the liver physiologically and pathologically. Besides, the eye is also associated with the five zang-organs and the brain. The essence of the viscera goes upward to the eye. The kidney (bone) essence forms the pupil of the eye, the liver (tendon) essence forms the black part of the eye, the heart (blood) essence forms the venules of the eye, the lung (qi) essence forms the white part of the eye, and the spleen (muscle) essence forms the connector of the eye, which transports all the essences into the brain alongside the meridian (*Ling Shu, Miraculous Pivot*, 灵枢). The five-wheel theory for the treatment of eye disorders is thus created.

The nose is the portal for the inhaled and exhaled qi. It governs the sense of smelling, helps vocalization, and serves as the orifice of the lung.

The nose is most closely related to the lung, and also has some connections with the spleen, liver and gallbladder. Moreover, the nose is extensively associated with the meridians.

Daily Exercises

1. What are the main physiological functions of the yin heel vessel, yang heel vessel, yin link vessel and yang link vessel?
2. What are the concepts and functions of the 12 divergent meridians, divergent collaterals, meridian tendons, and skin divisions?
3. Familiarize yourself with the physiological functions and application of the meridians.
4. What are the concepts and functions of the body constituents and five sensory organs?
5. What are the definitions and main physiological functions of the organs and orifices?

THE NINTH WEEK

The Organs and Orifices

The Mouth, Tooth and Tongue

The mouth, tooth and tongue are the organs responsible for taking food, discerning flavors, secreting saliva, facilitating digestion, grinding food, and assisting vocalization. They are connected with the viscera through the meridians, particularly the spleen, stomach, heart and kidney.

1. *The structure and function of the mouth, tooth and tongue*

The lips are referred to as "Fei Men (flying portal)" in *Nan Jing*. The mouth and lips are the starting section from which the food and water enter the digestive tract. Besides, the mouth and lips can facilitate vocalization.

The teeth are the hardest organ of the human body. They are embedded into the tooth socket of the upper and lower jaws and make-up the upper dental arch and the lower dental arch which may bite, tear up, or grind food and facilitate vocalization. So it is called "Hu Men (the first entrance for passing food)" in *Nan Jing*.

The tongue is the most flexible organ inside the mouth. It is located at the bottom of the mouth cavity, and can sense flavors, assist chewing and swallowing, and facilitate sound production, etc.

2. *The relationship between the viscera and the mouth, tooth and tongue*

(1) The spleen opens into the mouth. The mouth coordinates with the spleen and stomach physiologically so as to complete the task of digestion, absorption and distribution of cereal nutrients. Pathologically, the disorders of the spleen and stomach often involve the mouth.

(2) The kidney governs the bone, and the tooth is the surplus of the bone. The physiological functions and pathological changes of the tooth are closely associated with the excess and deficiency of the kidney essence. The growth, development, decaying and falling off of the tooth are influenced by the kidney essence. Meanwhile, renal diseases may also affect the tooth, e.g., kidney heat can lead to black and withering teeth (*Su Wen*).

(3) The tongue is the sprout-organ of the heart. The heart qi is associated with the tongue, so if the heart is normal in function, the tongue can taste the five flavors. So we can see that the tongue is physiologically related to the heart. Pathologically, heart diseases may involve the tongue, e.g., heart heat can lead to ulcers and fissures on the tongue (Wài Tái Mì Yào, Arcane Essentials from the Imperial Library, 外台秘要). However, although the tongue is governed by the heart, it is related to other viscera and visceral diseases can be reflected in the tongue. This is the theoretical foundation of tongue examination in TCM.

3. *The relationship between the meridians and the mouth, tooth and tongue*

There are eight meridians reaching the mouth, tooth and tongue. The stomach meridian of foot yangming curves around the mouth and enters the upper teeth; the large intestine meridian of hand yangming curves around the mouth and enters the lower teeth; the kidney meridian of foot shaoyin and the spleen meridian of foot taiyin arrive at the root of the tongue; the governor vessel reaches the gum crossing; and the liver meridian of foot jueyin, conception vessel and thoroughfare vessel circulate around the mouth and lips. The disorders of these meridians may affect the mouth, tooth and tongue. On the other hand, the acupoints of these meridians can also treat diseases of the mouth, tooth and tongue.

The Throat

The throat is the passage connecting the mouth and nose with the lung and stomach. Its main functions are to assist respiration, vocalization, and reception of food. The throat is closely associated with the viscera such as the lung, stomach, spleen, kidney and liver, as well as the meridians.

1. *The structure of the throat*

The pharynx is connected to the nose anteriorly and superiorly. It is linked with the root of the tongue and connected to the mouth. The throat, separated by the epiglottis posteriorly and connected to the air tube anteriorly, includes the glottis. Its posterior side is linked with the esophagus which goes directly to the stomach. As the passage of the gastric cavity, it pertains to the stomach. The pendulous palate is located in the pharynx and serves as the passage for voice and sound.

2. *The main functions of the throat*

(1) Assisting respiration and vocalization. The throat is the gateway where the turbid qi and lucid qi exchange, and it is also the main organ responsible for producing sound.

(2) Assisting reception of water and food. The throat is the passage for water and cereal. This is because when water and cereal are taken into the mouth, they are first moistened and softened by the saliva secreted from "jingjing" (gold fluid) and "yuye" (jade liquor), then swallowed into the throat, and finally sent down to the stomach along the esophagus.

3. *The relationship between the throat and the viscera*

(1) The relationship between the throat and the lung, stomach and spleen. The throat pertains to the lung and is the main passage for exchange of qi. Therefore, the functional state of the lung affects the throat significantly. For instance, when the lung is obstructed by the exogenous pathogenic factors or phlegmatic fire, the throat will fail to make a sound. Clinically this is called "a solid bell (metal) cannot ring;" if the lung is deficient, the throat will also be involved, leading to loss of voice. This is called "a broken bell (metal) cannot ring." The pharynx pertains to the stomach, and serves as the passage for the stomach qi as well as water and food. The spleen is interiorly and exteriorly related to the stomach. The spleen meridian of foot taiyin curves around the stomach, spreads over the throat, and linked to the root of the tongue. The disorders of the spleen and stomach are mostly reflected in the throat and pharynx.

(2) The relationship between the throat and kidney. The kidney meridian of foot shaoyin starts from the lung, passes along the throat, and arrives at the root of the tongue. The kidney essence goes upward along the meridian to nourish the throat. If the kidney yin is insufficient, the deficient fire will rise along the meridian, marked by dry and painful throat.

(3) The relationship between the throat and liver. The liver meridian of foot jueyin passes the throat and goes upward to enter the nasopharynx. If the liver fails to govern the free flow of qi, there will be fluid retention and phlegm accumulation due to qi stagnancy. When there is emotional depression, phlegm and qi will be mixed and cause obstruction in the throat, leading to "globus hysteritis."

4. *The relationship between the throat and meridians*

The throat is the key region where most meridians traverse. The branches of hand taiyin and hand yangming passes along the throat; the branch of foot yangming runs downward, passes Renying (ST 9) and goes along the throat; the meridian of foot taiyin passes the throat and connects with the root of the tongue; the branch of the hand shaoyin ascends to reach the throat; the meridian of hand taiyang goes along the pharynx and descends to reach the diaphragm; the direct branch of foot shaoyin goes along the throat; the divergent meridian of hand jueyin goes upward to reach the throat; the divergent meridian of foot shaoyang goes upward to reach the throat; the meridian of foot jueyin goes along the throat, and enters the nasopharynx. The governor vessel starts from the lower abdomen and ascends directly to the throat; the conception vessel arrives at the throat; the ascending branch of the thoroughfare vessel emerges from the upper throat and nasal tract; the yin heel vessel reaches the throat and interconnects with the thoroughfare vessel. Hence, once these meridians are in disorder, the throat will be involved. Meanwhile, the disorders of the throat can also be treated by acupoints on these meridians.

The External Genitalia

The external genitalia include male and female external genitals and the urethral orifices where urination, spermiation, menstruation and expulsion take place. The external genitalia are associated with the five zang-organs and six fu-organs, particularly the kidney, urinary bladder, liver and spleen. It is also related to the liver meridian and the conception vessel.

1. *The structure and function of the external genitalia*

The male external genitalia include the penis, scrotum and testis. It is the place where the ancestral tendons accumulate, and has the functions of urination and reproduction. It also closely associated with the secondary sex characters in males. The female external genitalia include the urethral orifice and vaginal orifices, with the functions of excreting urine, discharging menses, and delivering a baby.

2. *The relationship between the external genitalia and the viscera*

(1) The external genitalia are the orifice of the kidney. The kidney opens into the external genitalia, which has a certain effect on reproduction and urination. The kidney governs reproduction, and when the kidney essence is sufficient enough to produce tiangui, it will significantly promote the sexual maturity and maintain the reproductive function. If the kidney essence is deficient, there will be bed-wetting in children; underdeveloped external genitalia and defective reproduction in young people; reduced sexual function, impotence, or even presenility in middle-aged people, and urinary incontinence in senile people. The urinary canal is connected with the urinary bladder upwardly, so they are physiologically interrelated and pathologically inter-affected, e.g., when the urinary bladder is invaded by damp-heat, there will be disorders in urination, marked by frequent urination, urgent urination, and burning pain in the urinary canal.

(2) The relationship between the external genitalia and the liver. The liver promotes free flow of qi and stores blood, both exert a certain influence on the reproduction in male or female. The liver and the kidney must be coordinated in promoting free flow of qi and storing essence so as to ensure the normal reproductive activities of the external genitalia. If the liver fails to promote free flow of qi, there will be blockage of the seminal passage and unsmooth ejaculation in males, or irregular menstruation, unsmooth menstruation and difficult menstruation in females. If the liver is hyperactive in this regard, there will be exuberance of kidney fire and insufficient storage of kidney essence, leading to premature ejaculation and nocturnal emission in males, or profuse menstruation in females, etc.

(3) The relationship between the external genitalia and the spleen. The spleen is in charge of transporting and transforming water and fluid. So if the spleen fails to transport and transform properly, water and fluid will accumulate into dampness which tends to attack downwardly the external genitalia, leading to profuse leucorrhea in women or scrotal edema (when dampness pours into the scrotum) in men. If the spleen fails to ascend the lucid, there will be metroptosis and even prolapse of the uterus in females or hernia (when the small intestine sinks into the scrotum) in males.

3. *The relationship between the external genitalia and the meridians*

(1) The relationship between the external genitalia and the liver meridian of foot jueyin. The liver meridian of foot jueyin "runs along the inner side of the thigh, enters the pubic region, passes the external genitalia, and reaches the lower abdomen......" So when the liver meridian is invaded, the external genitalia will be in disorder, e.g., downward invasion of damp-heat into the liver meridian may cause symptoms such as flushed and itching scrotum with scorching pain, or swelling and painful testicle in males; and itching external genitalia, or yellowish and thick leucorrhea, or smelly leucorrhea like washing water of rice, or yin sore in females.

(2) The relationship between the external genitalia and the conception vessel. The conception vessel passes from the posterior to the anterior through the external genitalia, so the disorder of the conception vessel often involves the external genitalia, leading to seven kinds of hernias in men and abnormal leucorrhea or abdominal masses in women (*Su Wen*).

The Anus

The anus is an organ for excreting feces. Since it discharges exclusively the residues of water and cereal, it is also called the "doorway for dregs." It is the lower end of the large intestine which is interiorly and exteriorly related to the lung where the corporeal soul is stored. For this reason, it has another name, the "doorway of corporeal soul." The anus is closely associated with the large intestine, lung, kidney and spleen. It is also connected with the bladder meridian of foot taiyang.

1. *The relationship between the anus and the viscera*

(1) The relationship between the large intestine and the lung. The anus is the lower opening of the large intestine. They are mutually connected and coordinated to fulfill the task of defecation. The disorders of the anus and those of the large intestine are not only mutually affected, but also inter-transmitted. Interiorly and exteriorly the lung is connected with the large intestine, so the descent of lung qi is conducive to the downward transmission of food residues and, for the same reason, to the defecating activity of the anus.

(2) The anus is the orifice of the kidney. The kidney opens into the anus. That is why it is said in *Su Wen*, "In the five colors, the north pertains to black; in the five zang-organs, to the kidney, which opens into the external genitalia and the anus." The kidney stores essence, thus serving as the foundation for storage. Such a function is essential to the controlling of the defecating activity. Meanwhile, the kidney is the foundation for yin and yang of the whole body. So the deficiency or excess of the kidney yin determines the dryness or moistening of the viscera, e.g., deficiency of kidney yin may lead to dry stools and fissured anus.

(3) The relationship between the anus and the spleen. The spleen transports and transforms water and cereal, and is in charge of ascending the lucid. The former may directly affect the volume of water contained in the feces while the latter, if it is normal, can maintain the original position of the anus and the intestines; however, if the spleen qi is too weak to ascend, there may be anal prolapse due to sinking of the rectum.

2. *The relationship between the anus and the meridians*

The divergent meridian of foot taiyang passes through the anus, so the acupoints on the bladder meridian of foot taiyang can be used to treat anal disorders.

Daily Exercises

1. What are the relationships between the mouth, tooth, tongue and the viscera?
2. What are the relationships between the throat and the viscera?
3. What are the relationships between the external genitalia, anus and the viscera?

CHAPTER 9

Etiology and Nosogenesis

Etiology refers to the causes of disease, and nosogenesis means the ocrrence of disease, i.e., the breaking of equilibrium inside the human body by pathogenic factors, thus triggering off diseases.

SECTION 1 ETIOLOGY

Pathogenic factors can be various, such as abnormal changes of weather, emotional stimulation, improper diet, overstrain, trauma, and insect or animal bites, etc. All of these, concluded by ancient doctors through massive clinical practice, bear a close relationship with traditional Chinese therapeutics and play a significant role in guiding clinical medication and treatment.

The records on etiology are rather abundant, and as early as thousands of years ago, in *Nei Jing*, the pathological factors were already classified to facilitate study and treatment. In *Su Wen*, for example, it is said, "The pathogenic factors originate either from yin or from yang. Those from yang are caused by wind, rain, cold and summer-heat, while those from yin are caused by improper diet or living conditions, sexual overindulgence and emotional changes." We can see that different causes of disease are generalized into either yin or yang. Yang refers to the external climatic changes, while yin refers to the social and environmental changes and improper diet. In this way the characteristics of the disease causes become clear and the treatment can be well-guided.

Since etiology is multi-faceted and can be further complicated by the development of disease, there are other influential classifications by the medical scholars of different times. For instance, in the Eastern Han Dynasty, Zhang Zhongjing summarized pathogenic factors into three kinds, "Diseases are exclusively caused by three kinds of pathogenic factors. The first group is endogenous ones caused by invasion of exogenous pathogenic factors into the viscera from the meridians; the second group is the ones attacking the skin and stagnating the vessels that connect the four limbs and nine orifices; and the third group is the injuries caused by sexual overindulgence, incised wound, or insect and animal bites." In the Song Dynasty, Chen Wuze also summarized the causes of diseases into three categories, namely "internal causes, external causes and causes neither internal nor external." This classification is still widely used by modern TCM doctors.

Another noteworthy point is determining causes through syndrome differentiation; in other words, the disease causes are not revealed by the patient's chief complaint, but by the syndrome differentiation of the doctors.

Normally, determination of causes through syndrome differentiation is conducted in the following situations: a. Patients with unknown or unclear causes; b. Patients with inability to speak or convey clearly the inducing factors, such as patient in critical conditions or children; c. Pathological products turning into new pathogenic factors, which is characteristic to TCM etiology. To be specific, during the development of disease, some pathological products at one stage may become new pathogenic factors at another, thus further complicating and aggravating the diseases. For instance, phlegm, blood stasis or fluid retention, as a result of dysfunction of the viscera, qi and blood, may become the inducing factors of other diseases. If we do not know the causes, we will find no way to approach the diseases. In this sense, the importance of determining disease causes through syndrome differentiation can never be overemphasized.

The Six Abnormal Climatic Factors

The six abnormal climatic factors are the general designation of pathogenic wind, cold, summer-heat, dampness, dryness and fire. By contrast, there are six normal climatic changes of wind, cold, summer-heat, dampness, dryness and fire. The latter is normal, while the former is abnormal and characterized by excessiveness. For this reason, they are also called six excesses.

The ancient TCM doctors in the Yellow River Valley believed that under normal conditions, there are six climatic changes indispensable to the growth of all living things in nature, including the human beings. However, when they are excessive or insufficient, or when they do not take place at due time, the six normal climatic changes will become pathogenic factors. Sometimes when the body resistance is weak, the six climatic factors can still invade the human body and make people fall ill even if the climatic changes are within normal scope. In these cases, they are still viewed as pathogenic factors from the perspective of etiology.

1. *Common characteristics of the six abnormal climatic factors*

The reason why the six abnormal climatic factors are grouped together is because they have the following three common characteristics:

(1) The diseases caused by six abnormal climatic factors have an obvious relationship with season and locality: For example, there are often wind diseases in spring, summer-heat diseases in summer, dampness diseases in long summer and early autumn (rainy season in the Yellow River Valley), dryness diseases in middle and late autumn, and cold diseases in winter; besides, there are often dampness diseases in low-lying areas, etc.
(2) The six abnormal climatic factors are featured by sudden invasion, new contraction and short course of diseases.
(3) The six abnormal climatic factors are characterized by invading the body from the superficies to the internal organs through the skin and muscle or mouth and nose, so they are also named as exogenous pathogenic factors. In this sense, expelling pathogenic factors becomes the primary principle of treatment at the early stage of a disease.

Moreover, there are also two noteworthy points. One is that all of the six abnormal climatic factors can invade people either alone or in a combination of two or more, like simultaneous invasion by wind-heat or wind-cold-dampness. The other is that after invading the body, they may change their nature according to the strength of the pathogenic factors, the constitution of the patients, or the intervention of the treatments; for example, pathogenic cold may transform into heat. Such a transformation, however, is based on the prerequisite that the six pathogenic factors should invade the body first.

2. *There are two points worth mentioning*

(1) Clinically, there are also five endogenous pathogenic factors in contrast to the six exogenous ones. They are internal wind, internal heat (fire), internal dampness, internal dryness and internal cold caused by dysfunction of the viscera which brings on symptoms similar to the ones caused by invasion of external climatic pathogenic factors. Since they are not caused by the six exogenous pathogenic factors, their treatment should be different from that of the six excesses. But on top of this, the correct differentiation between the two similar groups of pathogens should be carried out first.

(2) From the perspective of western medicine, the six exogenous climatic factors are actually microorganisms as well as other physical or chemical factors. The ancient TCM doctors have long recognized the role played by pathogenic microorganisms in the occurrence of disease; however, they still use the six climatic factors to represent them. The reason lies in the frequent and wide application of the six excesses theory in clinical treatment. Currently it is held that different diseases may be caused by different microorganisms. However, if the two separate diseases are considered to be caused by the same causative factor according to TCM syndrome differentiation, they can be treated with similar method and this approach often turns out to be effective. That is why the theory of six excesses is still popular today.

Wind

Wind is predominant in spring, so diseases caused by wind are common in spring.

There are four characteristics of pathogenic wind.

1. Wind, a yang pathogen, is characterized by ventilating, dispersing, moving, ascending, and exiting. It is also prone to invade the yang sites of the body. The ventilating and dispersing ability means wind can easily loosen the interstices, leading to sweating and intolerance of wind. The

yang sites refer to the upper parts of the body (i.e., the head and face), yang meridians, and the superficies of the body.

2. Wind is swift and changeable. "Swift" means that wind is active and movable without fixed location, which is also the feature of clinical manifestations due to wind. For example, wandering arthralgia, characterized by migration with unfixed location, is attributed to wind pathogen. "Changeable" refers to irregular changes of disease with a quick onset, such as wheal (urticaria), marked by skin pruritus with unfixed location.

3. Wind is the leading pathogen responsible for nearly all the diseases. Wind is often combined with other pathogens to invade the body, such as wind-cold, wind-heat, and wind-dampness. So it is often regarded as the first pathogen for all exogenous diseases.

4. Wind tends to move. "Move" means that wind excels at migration and variation. For example, tetanic convulsion is often caused by wind.

The above-mentioned are characteristics of pathogenic wind. So if the same symptoms or signs occur, it can be inferred that the wind is responsible for them.

Daily Exercises

1. What are the common etiological factors?
2. What are the characteristics of pathogenic wind?

The Six Abnormal Climatic Factors

Cold

Cold is predominant in winter, so diseases caused by cold are often seen in winter. However, in other seasons, when weather becomes cold, or when one works or lives in cold environment, pathogenic cold will attack the body even if it is in summer.

There are three characteristics of pathogenic cold

1. *Cold, a yin pathogen, is prone to damage yang qi*

Cold is the manifestation of yin exuberance, so when cold pathogen invades the body, yang qi will become malfunctioned or even impaired, leading to hypofunction of the body. In *Nei Jing*, it is often said that predominant yin leads to coldness or yang diseases. For example, when pathogenic cold invades the skin and muscles, yang qi will be stagnated, leading to aversion to cold and absence of sweat; when pathogenic cold directly attack the spleen and stomach, spleen yang will be restrained, leading to cold and pain in the stomach and abdomen, and diarrhea; when pathogenic cold further develops, kidney yang will be impaired, leading to aversion to cold, weary lying, coldness in the limbs, diarrhea, clear and profuse urine, depression, and thin-faint pulse, etc.

2. *Cold is characterized by congealing*

Congealing means stagnation or coagulation. When pathogenic cold attacks the body, yang qi will be suppressed and impaired, and may become too weak to promote the smooth movements of qi, blood and body fluid, leading to pain due to obstruction.

3. *Cold is characterized by contracting*

Contracting means shrinkage or spasm. When cold invades the body, yang qi will be restrained, thus the interstices, meridians and tendons will be contracted. The blockage of interstices and obstruction of defense yang by the attack of cold pathogen often lead to the symptoms such as aversion to cold (due to insufficient defensive yang failing to warm the superficies), fever (due to accumulation of defensive yang), and absence of sweating. When pathogenic cold invades the blood vessels, there will be contracture of blood vessel, generalized pain, headache, tight pulse and cold limbs; if cold invades the tendons and vessels, there will be contraction of the tendons and vessels, spasm with pain, or disability of normal bending and stretching, etc.

Summer-heat

Summer-heat is predominant in summer, and often causes disease in summer. Its association with a particular season (summer) is the closest among the six climatic factors.

There are three characteristics of pathogenic summer-heat.

1. Summer-heat, a yang pathogen, is characterized by hotness. Summer-heat is transformed from the qi of fire-heat, so it is a yang pathogen.

Diseases due to summer-heat are often marked by hotness, redness, restlessness and agitation, e.g., high fever (steaming heat scorching the skin), vexation, reddened complexion, surging large pulse and so on.

2. Marked by ascending and dispersing, summer-heat can damage body fluid and consume qi. Summer-heat pertains to yang and tends to ascend, so it often disturbs and disperses yang qi or body fluid; besides, it can also consume body fluid, manifested as profuse sweating, thirst, frequent drinking, and red and scanty urine; if excessive yang qi is consumed, there will be insufficiency of qi, shortness of qi and lassitude, or even floating of yang qi, coma and insensibility, etc.

3. Summer-heat is often accompanied by dampness. Summer is hot, rainy and humid, so summer-heat often attacks the body in combination with dampness, which is a yin pathogen and characterized by heaviness, stickiness and turbidity. The percentage of summer-heat or dampness in a combined attack is decisive in the ensuing symptoms. So besides the common symptoms caused by summer-heat, there are other symptoms characteristic to dampness such as heaviness of head, dizziness, weary limbs, oppression in the chest, nausea with vomiting, sloppy stool and prolonged duration, etc.

Dampness

Dampness is predominant in the long summer, which refers to June in the lunar calendar. During the rainy season in the Yellow River Valley, people are prone to develop damp diseases with the accumulation of humidity. Our country covers an enormously vast area, so rainy seasons may vary from region to region, and even in the same region, humidity may vary due to different living or working environments. For this reason, it should be noted that damp diseases are not particular to long summer.

There are mainly four characteristics of pathogenic dampness.

1. Dampness is heavy and turbid. This is similar to the phenomenon that some objects, after being exposed to humidity for a long time, may become heavy, damp and turbid. Dampness is a yin pathogen and when it invades the body, yang qi will be stagnated, leading to different symptoms. For example, when it invades the skin and muscles, there will be a feeling of heavy-headedness; if it invades the meridians and joints, there will be prolonged aching of the joints, called damp

bi-syndrome or fixed bi-syndrome. There are also other symptoms due to invasion by dampness such as dirty complexion, excessive secretion in the eyes, sticky and greasy fur, diarrhea, turbid urine, leukorrhagia, and eczema, etc.

2. Dampness, a yin pathogen, is liable to obstruct qi movement. Dampness pathogen is heavy and turbid, so it is prone to inhibit qi activity, leading to disordered movements of qi marked by oppression in the chest and abdomen, heavy-headedness, unsmooth urination and defecation, etc. The spleen, pertaining to earth, likes dryness and dislikes dampness, so it is susceptible to pathogenic dampness. As a result, the qi movement and digestive function of the spleen may be impeded, characterized by gastric stuffiness, abdominal distention, torpid intake, loose stools or diarrhea, scanty urine, edema and ascites, etc.

3. Dampness is sticky and stagnant. This feature of dampness pathogen can be discussed from two aspects. One is the sticky nature of the secreta and excreta. The other one is the prolonged course of disease, which is marked by long duration and repetitive occurrence, such as damp bi-syndrome in arthritis, eczema in skin diseases, and damp-warm disorder in exogenous febrile diseases.

4. Dampness tends to go downward and attack the lower part of the body. Dampness pathogen is heavy and turbid, so it has the tendency to go downward, and often leads to edema and skin diseases of the lower limbs, as well as stranguria with turbid discharge, leucorrhea and diarrhea in the lower parts of the body.

Daily Exercises

1. What are the characteristics of pathogenic cold?
2. What are the characteristics of pathogenic summer-heat?
3. What are the characteristics of pathogenic dampness?

The Six Abnormal Climatic Factors

Dryness

Dryness is predominant in autumn. Similar to summer-heat, it is closely associated with a certain season, namely, late autumn.

There are two main characteristic of pathogenic dryness.

1. Dryness, marked by drying and astringing, is prone to impair the body fluid, leading to symptoms such as dry mouth and nose, dry throat, thirst, dry or unsmooth skin.

2. Dryness tends to impair the lung. The lung is a delicate organ preferring dampness to dryness. Among the five zang-organs, only the lung communicates with nature directly; besides, the lung pertains to metal, which is associated with autumn and dryness, so dryness often attacks the lung and tends to impair lung fluid, affecting the diffusion and purification function of the lung. Unlike pathogenic cold and wind, it invades the lung only in autumn, and is often marked by dry cough with scanty phlegm, sticky phlegm, and bloody phlegm (caused by incessant dry coughing), etc.

Fire (heat)

Unlike wind, cold, summer-heat, dampness and dryness, fire (heat) is not particular to a certain season. It is common in all the seasons. Once upon a time fire was classified into summer-heat and is correlated with the heart; this is probably due to its prevalence in every season. It frequently occurs in many seasons, not merely in summer, so gradually it becomes one of the six abnormal climatic factors. Different from wind, cold, summer-heat, dampness and dryness, fire is mainly transformed from them, or developed when weather turns warm or hot.

There are five characteristics of pathogenic fire.

1. Fire is a yang pathogen and tends to flame upwards. Fire is characterized by hotness, agitation, redness and dryness, such as fever, aversion to heat, reddened complexion and eyes, extreme thirst, vexation and rapid pulse, etc.

2. Fire tends to damage fluid and consume qi. Fire damages body fluid from two approaches: compelling fluid out or drying fluid up. Hence the diseases caused by pathogenic fire are often marked by profuse sweating (compelling fluid out), extreme thirst, dry tongue and throat, red and scanty urine, and constipation, etc.

3. Fire tends to engender wind and disturb blood. In nature, fire often disturbs air around it and produces wind. This is similar to fire invading

the body. In extreme cases, wind will be produced, called "excessive heat engendering wind." For example, after a high fever, there are often tic of the limbs, upward turning of the eyeballs, stiff neck, and opisthotonos, etc. besides, when fire scorches blood vessels and compels blood out, there will be bleeding symptoms such as vomiting of blood, coughing up blood, non-traumatic bleeding, bloody stool, bloody urine, skin macule, profuse menses or incessant vaginal bleeding, etc.

4. Fire tends to cause sores and ulcers. When fire invades blood phase and accumulates in local parts, it will causticize blood and muscles, leading to abscesses, sores and ulcers, which is characterized by redness, swelling, hotness and pain.

5. Fire tends to disturb the mind. Fire is connected with the heart, so the mind will be affected when fire invades the heart, leading to vexation and insomnia due to disquieted heart spirit. In more severe cases, the manifestations are manic psychosis, loss of consciousness or delirious speech.

Pestilence

Pestilence refers to the external pathogens which are highly epidemic and infectious. In ancient times, it has many other names such as "perverse qi," "usual qi," "alien qi" or "toxic qi," etc.

The Characteristics of Pathogenic Pestilence

It is marked by sudden onset, similar symptom, severe pathological state and strong infection. In ancient medical records, smallpox, cholera and plague, as we know today, are classified into this category.

Its outbreak is closely associated with abnormal climate, dense population, dirty environment and contaminated food, etc.

The Differences and Similarities Between Pestilence and the Six Excesses

Both are exogenous factors. The prevalence of pestilence is related to climatic abnormality, so there is a necessity to distinguish them.

In the long history of TCM, both co-existed from ancient times to the present. The difference between them is primarily based on their pathogenic characteristics. Those marked by sudden onset, similar symptom, severe pathological state and strong infection are called pestilence; otherwise, they are called six excesses.

However, with the in-depth observation of diseases by ancient doctors, it was found that some disease, though not prevalent in large areas, have similar characteristics of onset and turnover. They are also marked by sudden onset, similar symptoms and severe pathological state. Hence, as early as the Ming Dynasty, physician Wu Youxing has put forth the theory of pestilent qi, which holds that different diseases are caused by different pathogens (pestilent qi), and "one disease is attributable to one pestilent qi." This theory, a hundred years older than a similar theory of lemology in western world, is a major improvement in TCM on the recognition of infectious diseases. By comparing the characteristics, symptoms and descriptions of six excesses, pestilence and pestilent qi, we find that they are both related and differentiated, which should be noted during clinical treatment.

The theory of six excesses, with a complete system of principle, method, prescription and medication, plays a dominant role in the syndrome differentiation and treatment of exogenous febrile diseases. It is both effective and easy to learn during clinical practice. The pestilent qi theory, with an unique system of principle, method, prescription and medication, reveals the general pattern of the occurrence and development of infectious diseases. So it is very valuable and of great significance to clinical treatment.

And then, how can we grasp the differences and similarities between the six excesses and the pestilence?

The answer lies in their pathogenic characteristics instead of western lemology. This will help one when understanding the theory of six excesses, reading ancient classics and treating diseases.

Daily Exercises

1. What are the characteristics of pathogenic dryness?
2. What are the characteristics of pathogenic fire (heat)?
3. What is pestilence, and what are the pathogenic characteristics of pestilence?

Internal Impairment Due to Seven Emotions

The seven emotions refer to joy, anger, anxiety, contemplation, grief, fear and fright. Ancient physicians believed that the seven emotions are physiological responses of visceral qi. For example, in *Huang Di Nei Jing* (*The Yellow Emperor's Canon of Medicine*, 黄帝内经), the seven emotions are matched with the five viscera: the heart governs joy, the liver governs anger, the lung governs grief, the spleen governs contemplation and the kidney governs fear. Under normal circumstances, the seven emotions transformed from the five visceral qi are normal psychological responses of the body to the environmental stimuli. However, sudden, violent or prolonged emotional stimuli beyond the range of physiological activities will cause disorder of qi activity and disharmony of visceral yin, yang, qi and blood that consequently lead to diseases. Because the seven emotions originate from the five visceral qi, when the visceral qi is abnormal, the emotions will be in disorder; just as what is said in *Ling Shu* (*Miraculous Pivot*, 灵枢), "excess of liver-qi causes anger while deficiency of liver-qi brings out fear; excess of heat-qi brings out joy while deficiency of heart-qi leads to grief." Since the seven emotions are endogenous and directly affect visceral qi and blood, the internal disorder caused is called "internal impairment due to seven emotions." This is different from the six excesses and pestilence which invade the body exogenously.

The Pathogenic Characteristics of Internal Damage Due to Seven Emotions

1. *Directly impairing the internal organs.* It is clearly summarized in *Huang Di Nei Jing* (*The Yellow Emperor's Canon of Medicine*, 黄帝内经) that excessive anger impairs the liver, excessive joy impairs the heart, excessive contemplation impairs the spleen, excessive grief impairs the lung and excessive fear impairs the kidney, etc.

There are three points that should be noted: First, the heart houses spirit and serves as the monarch organ, so damage to other zang-organs may inevitably involve the heart. Whenever there are abnormal emotional changes, the heart will be the first to be influenced, marked by palpitation, forgetfulness, vexation, insomnia or constant laughter. Second, clinically the heart, the liver and the spleen are the most susceptible ones to abnormal emotional changes; for example, excessive thinking will weaken the heart and spleen, leading to palpitation, forgetfulness, night sweat, lassitude, anorexia and insomnia, etc. And depressed rage may obstruct the liver qi, leading to distending pain in the costal regions, irascibility, frequent sighing, irregular menstruation, difficult menstruation and suppression of menses. Third, when there are emotional disorders, different viscera may be involved directly or in succession. For example, depression and rage may impair the liver, and the adverse flow of liver-qi can also attack the spleen and the stomach, or the lung, leading to liver-fire scorching the metal (lung), imbalance between the liver and spleen as well as disharmony between the liver and stomach, etc.

2. *Affecting qi movement of zang-fu organs.* Unlike the six abnormal climatic factors, the emotional disorders often directly affect the qi movement, just like what is said in *Su Wen*, "Excessive anger drives qi to move upwards; excessive joy relaxes the activity of qi; excessive contemplation stagnates qi; excessive grief exhausts qi; excessive fear drives qi to move downwards; excessive fright disturbs qi; and excessive anxiety depresses qi." This is discussed in detail as follows:

Excessive anger drives qi to move upwards: Great anger or rage makes the liver qi surge upward, even driving up the blood with it, marked by distending pain in the head and eyes, reddened complexion and eyes, vomiting of blood, syncope, panting, wheezing, or even coughing with blood.

What should be noted is that anger may also drive liver qi to move transversely instead of upwardly, thus affecting the spleen and stomach, with the symptoms of reduced appetite, discomfort or distending pain in the stomach or abdomen, and diarrhea, etc.

Excessive joy relaxes the activity of qi: This covers two meanings. One refers to the healthy, normal state of qi movement that is smooth and ordered; the other refers to the unhealthy, abnormal state of qi movement that is unsmooth and disorganized. Normally joy can harmonize qi and blood, and ease the mind. But sudden, intense and excessive ecstasy may slack heart-qi and derange the mind, leading to inability to concentrate, absent-mindedness, and even mania.

3. *Excessive grief exhausts qi.* Excessive grief exhausts and depresses lung-qi, leading to sorrow, lassitude, dispiritedness and shortness of qi, etc.

Excessive fear drives qi to move downwards. Sudden terror impairs the kidney and drives renal or general qi to move downwards, leading to pale complexion, distending sensation in the lower abdomen, or even incontinence of urine and feces, or seminal emission.

Excessive fright disturbs qi. Fear and fright are different in the responses of visceral qi activity. Fright, dominated by the kidney, drives qi to move downwards; fear, originated from the heart, disturbs the activity of qi. So when frightened, the main responses are disorder of heart-qi, derangement of the mind, hesitation and bewilderment.

Excessive anxiety depresses qi. Excessive contemplation will cause stagnation of spleen-qi, leading to reduced digestive capacity, gastric and abdominal distension and fullness, anorexia and even diarrhea, etc.

Contemplation is attributed to the spleen, but as early as the period of *Nei Jing*, it has already been noticed that contemplation is closely associated with the heart. Prolonged indulgence in contemplation may disturb heart qi, often bringing on palpitation, amnesia, insomnia and dreaminess, etc.

4. *Emotional disorders may worsen or even deteriorate the conditions of a disease.*

Improper Diet, Overstrain and Indulgence in Leisure

Food, work and rest constitute the daily life of people. But if they are overdone or inadequate, discomforts and diseases may be induced.

1. Improper diet includes three aspects: irregular diet, unsanitary diet, and unbalanced diet, which are discussed below.

(1) Irregular diet. Irregular diet will not only damage the stomach directly, but also affect the transformation and production of qi and blood, the circulation and metabolism of body fluid, as well as other visceral functions, thus leading to various diseases.

Insufficient intake of food. This will lead to malnutrition, blood deficiency, insufficient visceral qi and essence, and weak healthy qi. As a result, many diseases can be induced and the body will also become susceptible to attacks of six excesses and pestilence. The weakness of healthy qi is the fundamental reason why most diseases due to inadequate food intake are complicated in pathogenesis, tough in treatment and unfavorable in prognosis.

Excessive food intake. This covers two aspects: First, it may impair the spleen and stomach and affect their functions; second, the production of excessive qi and blood accumulate internally and then transform into heat, which in turn damages the spleen and stomach, marked in adults by gastric and abdominal distension and fullness, fetid eructation, belching, anorexia or even vomiting and diarrhea; there are also complicated cases in which heat, phlegm or dampness are endangered, characterized additionally by reddened complexion, thirst, yellow fur, and rapid pulse, or shortness of qi, fatness, greasy fur and slippery pulse; in children, there may be stagnation syndromes due to malnutrition, marked by gastric and abdominal distension and fullness, yellow complexion and emaciated muscles, withered hair, irascibility, aptness to cry, and hot sensation in the centers of feet and hands, etc. The production of internal heat is similar to the complications manifested in diabetes in which superficial infection appears at the same time with polyphagia and polyorexia. This was recorded in *Huang Di Nei Jing* (*The Yellow Emperor's Canon of Medicine*, 黄帝内经) as early as 2000 years ago.

(2) Unsanitary diet. This refers to the contamination of food and drink by parasites, pathogens, toxins and harmful chemical substances, resulting in different parasitic diseases and gastroenteritis due to bacteria infection (featured by damp-heat and pestilence), or even intoxication.

(3) Unbalanced diet. This refers to the frequent, constant, or prolonged preference for a certain food and the decrease of or even abstinence from other food. The manifestations are various, being either imbalanced yin and yang or malnutrition.

Preference for cold or hot food. Preference for raw and cold food may damage yang qi of the spleen and stomach, leading to the syndrome of stomach cold marked by cold pain in the stomach and vomiting clear water; the syndrome of deficient cold in the stomach is characterized by slight pain in the stomach and abdomen, fear of cold and diarrhea; damp-cold encumbering the spleen is marked by reduced appetite, white-greasy fur, discomfort in the abdomen and stomach, and diarrhea, etc. Preference for spicy food can lead to thirst, foul breath, gastric and abdominal distension and pain, constipation and diarrhea, while preference for hot food may directly burn the mouth or gullet, or even lead to death in the long run.

Preference for a particular flavor: According to long-term clinical observation and the theory of five elements, the five flavors are attributed to the five zang-organs, respectively. The sour flavor is attributed to the liver, bitter to the heart, sweet to the spleen, pungent to the lung and salty to the kidney. Hence, partiality to a certain flavor may lead to unbalanced coordination among the five zang-organs, or even damage to other viscera as well as the organ to which this flavor is attributed. Take sweetness as an example, in *Su Wen*, it was recorded that sweetness is attributed to the spleen, but addiction to it may lead to obstruction of heart qi with dyspnea and imbalance of kidney qi, or bone pain and hair loss.

2. Overwork or addiction to leisure refers to frequent, excessive and prolonged work or rest, which may become the causative factor for many diseases.

(1) Overwork. This covers three aspects: excessive physical work, excessive mental work or sexual indulgence. In *Huang Di Nei Jing* (*The Yellow Emperor's Canon of Medicine*, 黄帝内经), it was said that overwork consumes qi, prolonged standing impairs the bone and protracted walking injures the tendon. This is marked by lassitude, shortness of qi and long-term fatigue, or sourness, distension and weakness in the laboring regions involved, such as the hands and feet. Excessive mental work refers to over thinking, which may impair the heart and spleen because the former houses the spirit while the latter stores ideation, characterized by palpitation, insomnia, anemia, indigestion, anorexia and loose stool, etc. Sexual indulgence refers to excessive sexual activities, marked by weak knees and loins, dizziness and tinnitus, and reduced sexual function, etc.

(2) Excessive rest. It refers to the lack of exercises and the indulgence in leisure. Constant lying in the bed due to idleness or unaccustomed

environment may lead to qi deficiency, qi stagnancy, depression, weak limbs, anorexia, lassitude, and panting on exertion, etc. Therefore it was said in *Nei Jing* that excessive lying impairs qi.

Daily Exercises

1. What is internal impairment due to seven emotions
2. How many aspects does improper diet include?
3. How many aspects does impairment due to overwork and excessive rest include?

Weekly Review

On Monday, we continued to study organs and orifices.

1. Mouth, tooth and tongue. The mouth, tooth and tongue are connected with the viscera through the meridians, particularly the spleen, stomach, heart and kidney. They are also closely related to the stomach meridian, large intestine meridian, kidney meridian, spleen meridian, liver meridian, conception vessel and thoroughfare vessel.

The lips are referred to as "Fei Men (flying porta)," and the tooth is called "Hu Men (the first entrance for passing food)."

The relationship between the viscera and the mouth, tooth and tongue. a. The spleen opens into the mouth. Pathologically, the disorders of the spleen and stomach often involve the mouth. b. The kidney governs the bone, and the tooth is the surplus of the bone. The physiological functions and pathological changes of the tooth are closely associated with the excess and deficiency of the kidney essence. c. The tongue is the sprout-organ of the heart. Pathologically, heart diseases may involve the tongue or be reflected in the tongue.

2. The throat is closely associated with the viscera such as the lung, stomach, spleen, kidney and liver as well as the meridians.

The main functions of the throat. a. Assisting respiration and vocalization. b. Assisting reception of water and food.

The relationships between the throat and the viscera are mainly manifested as "a solid bell (metal) cannot ring" and "a broken bell (metal) cannot ring." Besides, If the kidney yin is insufficient, the deficient fire will rise along the meridian, marked by dry and painful throat; and if the liver fails to govern the free flow of qi, phlegm and qi will be mixed and cause obstruction in the throat, leading to "globus hysteritis."

3. The external genitalia include male and female external genitals and urethral orifices.

The external genitalia is closely associated with the kidney, urinary bladder, liver and spleen. It is also related to the liver meridian and the conception vessel.

The kidney opens into the external genitalia, which has a certain effect on reproduction and urination. If the kidney essence is deficient, there will be symptoms such as weakened productive ability, impotence, bed-wetting, profuse urination and urinary incontinence. The liver promotes free flow of qi and stores blood, both exert a certain influence on the reproduction in male or female. The liver and the kidney must be coordinated in promoting free flow of qi and storing essence so as to ensure the normal reproductive activities of the external genitalia. The spleen is in charge of transporting and transforming water and fluid. So if the spleen fails to transport and transform properly, there will be profuse leucorrhea and metroptosis in women or scrotal edema and hernia in men.

4. The anus is also called the "doorway of corporeal soul," the last one in the seven important openings. The anus is closely associated with the large intestine, lung, kidney and spleen. It is also connected with the bladder meridian of foot taiyang.

From the second week in this month, we began to introduce the etiology.

It is important to memorize the characteristics and symptoms of different pathogenic factors. At the beginning, do not identify them with similar diseases in western medicine. When you are familiar with them, find some opportunities to learn in the clinic or hospital. Try to discern the pathogenic factors, invading either alone or in combination. Then you may take reference from western medical diagnosis. More practice and analysis will enable you to find their differences and understand the essence of Chinese etiology. So it is inadvisable to equate them to some similar diseases in western medicine.

Although pathogenic factors are many, we only discussed the six abnormal climatic factors, seven emotions, diet, or work and rest styles.

At the beginning, we outlined the etiological classification in different dynasties, such as the triple categories in the Eastern Han dynasty by Zhang Zhongjing, the triple categories in the South and North dynasty by Tao Hongjing, and the triple categories in the Song dynasty by Chen Wuze. These classifications, varying in some degree, have their own pros and cons. From the perspective of clinical practice, however, Chen Wuze's classification is more practical and hence is valued by many later physicians.

Discerning causes by syndrome differentiation is a distinct characteristic in TCM etiology, which seeks to determine the causative factors by syndrome differentiation rather than from the patient's main complaints or from laboratory tests. This is a concrete testimony to our ancestor's great intelligence. Moreover, Chinese etiology is closely intertwined with clinical medication and treatment, forming a fixed set of practice that is both simple and practical through millennia of tests and trials. Its profundity can only be comprehended through great amount of clinical practice.

As for the exogenous pathogenic factors, we discussed about the six abnormal climatic factors and pestilence. The six abnormal climatic factors are the general designation of pathogenic wind, cold, summer-heat, dampness, dryness and fire. They are different from the six normal climatic factors.

There are five common characteristics of the six abnormal climatic factors: (1) The diseases caused by six abnormal climatic factors have an obvious relationship with season and locality. (2) The six abnormal climatic factors are featured by sudden invasion, new contraction and short course of diseases. (3) The six abnormal climatic factors are characterized by invading the body from the superficies to the internal organs through the skin and muscle or mouth and nose. (4) Moreover, the six abnormal climatic factors can invade people either alone or in a combination of two or more. (5) From the perspective of discerning causes by syndrome differentiation, the six abnormal climatic factors may change their nature after invading the body according to the strength of the pathogenic factors, the constitution of the patients, or the intervention of the treatments.

In the early stage of TCM, the six abnormal climatic factors were not clearly differentiated from the endogenous five pathogenic factors (internal wind, internal heat (fire), internal dampness, internal dryness and internal cold). There were no detailed explanation about them theoretically and no clear difference in medication between them. That is because that at that time TCM is still immature, and the manifestations of the six endogenous pathogenic factors are very close to these of the six abnormal climatic factors; moreover, their treatment and medication are very similar. The difference between them is mainly demonstrated in the pathogenesis of stroke. In the Jin and Yuan dynasties, some scholars put forward that the cause of stroke is not exogenous pathogenic wind, both endogenous one due to disordered visceral qi and blood. The treatment, as a result, should be differentiated accordingly. This conforms to the clinical practice and is thus approved by most of the doctors, gradually forming a complete theory of five endogenous pathogenic factors. Again, it is absolutely necessary to accurately make a difference between them.

In the following, we will review the pathogenic characteristics of the six abnormal climatic factors.

Wind. There are four pathogenic characteristics of wind: 1. Wind, a yang pathogen, is characterized by ventilating and dispersing; it is also prone to invade the yang sites of the body. 2. Wind is swift and changeable. 3. Wind is the leading pathogen responsible for almost all diseases. 4. Wind tends to move.

Cold. There are three pathogenic characteristics of cold: 1. Cold, a yin pathogen, is prone to damage yang qi. 2. Cold is characterized by congealing. 3. Cold is characterized by contracting.

Summer-heat. There are three pathogenic characteristics of summer-heat: 1. Summer-heat, a yang pathogen, is characterized by hotness 2. With the nature of ascending and dispersing, summer-heat can damage body fluid and consume qi 3. Summer-heat is often accompanied by dampness.

Dampness. There are four pathogenic characteristics of dampness: 1. Dampness is heavy and turbid. 2. Dampness, a yin pathogen, is liable to obstruct qi movement. 3. Dampness is sticky and stagnant (This feature of dampness pathogen can be discussed from two aspects. One is the nature of stickiness of the secretion and excreta. The other one is the prolonged course of disease, which is marked by long duration and repetitive occurrence). 4. Dampness, prone to go downward, tends to attack the lower part of the body.

Dryness. There are two pathogenic characteristics of dryness: 1. Dryness, with the nature of drying, is prone to impair the body fluid. 2. Dryness tends to impair the lung.

Fire (heat). There are five pathogenic characteristics of fire: 1. Fire pertains to yang pathogen and tends to flame upwards. 2. Fire tends to damage fluid and consume qi. 3. Fire tends to engender wind and disturb blood. 4. Fire tends to cause sore and ulcer. 5. Fire tends to disturb the mind.

Another exogenous factor is pestilence. Pestilence refers to the external pathogens with severe epidemic and infectious nature. In ancient times, it has many other names such as "perverse qi," "usual qi," "alien qi" or "toxic qi," etc.

It is marked by sudden onset, similar symptom, severe pathological state and strong infection.

As for the internal damage, the impairment due to seven emotions is introduced.

The seven emotions refer to joy, anger, anxiety, contemplation, grief, fear and fright.

The seven emotions are matched with the five viscera: the heart governs joy, the liver governs anger, the lung governs grief, the spleen governs contemplation and the kidney governs fear. Sudden, violent or prolonged emotional stimuli beyond the range of physiological activities will cause disorder of qi activity and disharmony of visceral yin, yang, qi and blood that consequently lead to diseases.

There are mainly three pathogenic characteristics of internal damage due to seven emotions:

1. Directly impairing the internal organs: excessive anger impairs the liver, excessive joy impairs the heart, excessive contemplation impairs the spleen, excessive grief impairs the lung and excessive fear impairs the kidney.

2. Affecting qi movement of zang-fu organs: It is said in *Su Wen*, "Excessive anger drives qi to move upwards; excessive joy relaxes the activity of qi; excessive contemplation stagnates qi; excessive grief exhausts qi; excessive fear drives qi to move downwards; excessive fright disturbs qi; and excessive anxiety depresses qi."

The above-mentioned two points constitute the main manifestation and characteristics of impairment due to the seven emotions.

3. Affecting disease conditions. Emotional disorder may worsen or deteriorate the disease conditions.

As for the non-internal-external causes, improper diet, overstrain and indulgence in leisure were introduced.

Improper diet includes three aspects: irregular diet, unsanitary diet, and unbalanced diet, which are discussed as follows:

1. Irregular diet. Irregular diet, including insufficient intake of food and excessive intake of food, may not only damage the stomach directly, but also affect the transformation and production of qi and blood, the circulation and metabolism of body fluid, as well as other visceral functions, thus leading to various diseases.

2. Unsanitary diet. This refers to the contamination of food and drink by parasites, pathogens, toxins and harmful chemical substances, resulting in different parasitic diseases and gastroenteritis due to bacteria infection (featured by damp-heat and pestilence), or even intoxication.

3. Unbalanced diet. This refers to the frequent, constant, or prolonged preference for a certain food and the decrease of or even abstinence from other food. The manifestations are various, being either imbalanced yin and yang or malnutrition. Unbalanced diet includes preference for cold or hot food and reference for a particular flavor.

Injury due to work and rest includes overwork or idleness.

1. Overwork. This covers three aspects: excessive physical work, excessive mental work or sexual indulgence. This is marked by impairment of qi and direct damage to the involved organs and tissues, and is manifested as lassitude, shortness of qi and long-term fatigue, or sourness, distension and weakness in the laboring regions. Excessive mental work refers to over thinking, which may impair the heart and spleen, characterized by palpitation, insomnia, anemia, indigestion, anorexia and loose stool, etc. Sexual indulgence refers to excessive sexual activities, marked by weak knees and loins, dizziness and tinnitus, and reduced sexual function, etc.

2. Excessive rest. This refers to the lack of exercises and the indulgence in leisure, marked by depression, weak limbs, anorexia, lassitude, and panting on exertion, etc.

Daily Exercises

1. What is discerning causes by syndrome differentiation?
2. What are the concept of six abnormal climatic factors and their common pathogenic characteristics?
3. What are seven emotions and what are their pathogenic characteristics?
4. Closely observe people around you and see if they are overworked or excessively rested, and find out the relative manifestations.

THE TENTH WEEK

External Injury

External injury refers to injury from fall and knock, bullet wounds, metallic weapon wounds, injury from overload, frost bite, burns and scalds, and injury by insects or animals, etc.

Injury From Fall and Knock, Bullet Wounds, Metallic Weapon Wounds, and Injury from Overload

All the above-mentioned injuries can a damage the body, leading to swelling pain of the skin or muscles, bleeding, injury of soft tissues, bone fracture, dislocation, or even massive bleeding in the viscera and skull, coma, or death.

Frost bite

Frost bite is a local or general injury due to hypothermia or failure of yang qi to warm the body. For example, long-term exposure to low temperature without warm-keeping measures, cold injury may be ensued. General frost bite is marked by decreased temperature, chills, pale complexion, numbness, or even coma and death; local frost bite is characterized by pale skin, cold feeling, and numb sensation at first, and swelling, cyanosis, itching or scorching pain later in the local regions, such as the hands, feet, ears or cheeks, etc.

Burns or scalds

Burns or scalds refer to the damage to the skin and muscles of the body due to flame, boiling water or oil, and other high-temperature objects. In mild cases, only the skin is injured, marked by red skin, swelling, hot sensation, pain and blisters, etc. In severe cases, bones and muscles may be badly injured, leading to pale-white or sallow wound surface, or even coma due to visceral disorders.

Injury Due to Insects or Animals

Injury due to insects or animals refer to the lesions due to poisonous snakes, scorpions, centipedes, bees, loins, tigers, wolves or dogs, etc. Poisonous snakes cause diseases by injecting venom into the body. The damage to the body depends on the types of venom, marked by dizziness, headache, chest distress, palpitation, sweating and lassitude in mild cases, or even coma and death in severe cases. Insects wound the body with their venomous stings or hairs, marked by red skin, swelling and pain in mild cases, or high fever and chills in severe cases, etc. Wild beasts, such as lions, tigers and wolves, may pose lethal threat to humanity; moreover, rabid dog is responsible for rabies.

Parasites

In *Hou Han Shu*, there is a story about Hua Tuo who treated parasitic diseases with herbal decoctions, indicating that the ancient Chinese people have long recognized the role played by parasites in etiology. The types of parasites inside the body are various, so are the ensuing diseases and syndromes. For instance, diseases caused by roundworms are marked by pain around the umbilicus, yellow-withered complexion, teeth-grinding while dreaming, roundworms in the feces or even in the gallbladder, etc. Diseases caused by hook worms are marked by extreme itching around the anus worsening in the evening, poor sleep and presence of tiny, white worms around the anus at night; diseases caused by tapeworms are marked by abdominal pain and diarrhea, bulimia, yellow complexion, emaciation, and presence of white, flat worms in the feces, and even other deteriorated cases.

Phlegm, Retained-Fluid and Blood Stasis

Phlegm, retained-fluid and blood stasis, which are pathological substances produced by disturbance of water metabolism of the human body, can directly or indirectly act on the human body and lead to the occurrence of new diseases or syndromes; so they are also regarded as pathogenic factors.

Phlegm and Retained-Fluid

Phlegm and retained-fluid are pathological substances produced by disturbance of water metabolism of the human body. Generally speaking, the thick part is called phlegm while the thin part is called retained-fluid.

Phlegm may be divided into tangible phlegm and intangible phlegm. The former refers to visible expectorated sputum such as frothy sputum in chronic pulmonary diseases, while the latter means invisible sputum retained in the viscera or meridians with specific pathological manifestations, such as local spreading swelling in patients with superficial nodules, etc. These particular manifestations or signs can be indicative of a certain disease or syndrome. Retained-fluid may linger in the lung, the stomach, the urinary bladder or the skin and muscles. In *Jin Gui Yao Lue*, the fluid retained under the costal region is called "suspending fluid" and the fluid accumulated in the four limbs is called "overflowing fluid."

The phlegm and retained-fluid are often caused by external contraction of six abnormal climatic factors, abnormal changes of seven emotions, dietary irregularities, dysfunction of the lung, spleen, kidney and triple energizers, and disturbance of water metabolism, etc. The lung is in charge of dispersing and descending as well as regulating waterways and distributing body fluid; the spleen is in charge of transporting and transforming water and fluid; the kidney is in charge of steaming and transforming water and fluid; the triple energizer serves as the passage of water and fluid; and the urinary bladder is in charge of storing and discharging urine. So if the above-mentioned organs function abnormally, there will be production of phlegm and retained-fluid, which may trigger off other diseases or syndromes.

Pathogenic characteristics of phlegm and retained-fluid: Phlegm and retained-fluid may cause various clinical manifestations due to their difference in location. They often impede the ascent and descent of qi, obstruct qi and blood circulation and affect visceral functions.

Summary for diseases and syndromes caused by phlegm: Phlegm usually result in asthmatic cough with expectoration if it is retained in the lung; obstruction of heart blood, chest oppression, palpitation and chest pain if it is stagnated in the heart; unconsciousness and dementia if it confuses the mind; mania if it transforms into fire and disturbs the heart; nauseas, vomiting and stomach fullness if it is retained in the stomach; dizziness or vertigo if it attacks the head and clouds the upper orifices; obstructive sensation in the throat if it stagnates in the throat; and scrofula, superficial nodules, numbness of limbs or paralysis, and dorsal furuncles with pus if it is retained in the meridians, tendons and bones.

Summary for diseases and syndromes caused by retained-fluid: Retained fluid often leads to chest and hypochondriac distension and fullness as well as pain during cough if it is retained in the chest and hypochondria; chest oppression, cough, dyspnea and inability to lie flat and edema if it is retained in the chest and diaphragm; subcutaneous edema and body pain or heaviness if it is retained in the skin; intestinal gurgling if it is retained in the intestines.

Blood Stasis

Blood stasis, called accumulated blood in ancient times, is a pathological product due to blood stagnation, including extravasated blood and blood congested in the vessels or zang-fu organs due to the unsmooth blood circulation. So it is both a pathological product and a causative factor.

Blood stasis is caused by unsmooth blood circulation due to external contraction of six abnormal climatic factors, abnormal changes of seven emotions, dietary irregularities, overwork, excessive rest and external injuries, etc. For example, pathogenic cold will lead to contraction of vessels and sluggish circulation of blood; pathogenic heat will result in accumulation of heat in the blood and unsmooth flow of blood; deficiency of qi or stagnation of qi will fail to propel the circulation of blood; injuries due to falls, knocks, sprains and contusions will cause blood to flow out of the vessel and stay inside the body. Hence pathogenic blood stasis, as a pathological product, is characterized by affecting the local or general blood circulation with inability to nourish and moisten the body properly.

The manifestations caused by blood stasis may be roughly summarized as follows: a. Pain. This is marked by stabbing sensation and tenderness with fixed location, especially at night. b. Lump. This is marked by cyanosis and swelling around the fixed region and masses inside the body with a fixed location. c. Bleeding. This is marked by dark-purple blood with clots, cyanosis, cyanotic complexion, lips and nails, or dark-black complexion, scaly skin, and dark-purple tongue with petechia or ecchymosis, etc. Moreover, there are also manifestations such as thin-unsmooth or knotted-intermittent pulses.

Summary of diseases and syndromes caused by blood stasis. Static blood frequently causes palpitation, chest oppression, heartache and cyanotic nails and lips if it is retained in the heart; chest pain, cough and hematemesis if it is retained in the lung; mania if it attacks the heart; hemoptysis and black feces if it is retained in the intestines and stomach; lower abdominal pain, irregular menstruation, dysmenorrhea, amenorrhea, purplish color of menses with blood clots or profuse vaginal bleeding if it is retained in the uterus; local swelling, pain and cyanosis if it is retained in the limbs and muscles.

Daily Exercises

1. What are the common types of diseases due to external injury?
2. How can one differentiate phlegm and retained-fluid?
3. What are the viscera involved in the formation of phlegm and retained-fluid?
4. What are the pathogenic characteristics of blood stasis?

SECTION 2 NOSOGENESIS

Nosogenesis refers to the regular patterns of the occurrence, development and transmutation of a disease, called "disease mechanism" in TCM. Disease, in contrast to health, is a collective term for disorders and syndromes. Normal functions of the viscera, meridians, qi and blood, yin and yang are signs of health, and the dysfunction of which will lead to imbalance between yin and yang, causing diseases and presenting clinical manifestations.

The occurrence and changes of a disease, though complicated, can be discussed in terms of two aspects: healthy qi and pathogenic factors. In the following pages, we will discuss the occurrence of disease in relation to the struggle between healthy qi and pathogenic factors, and to the internal and external environments.

The Relationship Between the Occurrence of Disease and the Struggle of Healthy Qi and Pathogenic Factors

The Relationship Between the Occurrence of a Disease and the Struggle of Healthy Qi and Pathogenic Factors is Very Close

The healthy qi refers to the functional activities of the body (such as the functions of the viscera, meridians, qi and blood, yin and yang, etc.), as well as its abilities to resist and recover from diseases; the pathogenic factors refer to various pathogenic factors. The occurrence and development of disease is actually the reflection of the struggle between the healthy qi and pathogenic factors under certain circumstances, so the outcome of conflict between healthy qi and pathogenic factors dominates the occurrence and development of diseases.

Insufficient Healthy Qi is the Intrinsic Factor Responsible for the Occurrence of Diseases

TCM lays considerable emphasis on the healthy qi and holds that as long as the viscera and meridians are normal in functions, qi and blood are exuberant, yin and yang are in a balanced state, and the defensive qi is powerful, pathogenic factors will find no way to invade and by no means will diseases occur. Otherwise, diseases will appear. In other words, the insufficiency of healthy qi is the intrinsic factor responsible for the occurrence of diseases.

Pathogenic Factors are Indispensable to the Occurrence of Diseases

Besides healthy qi, TCM also stresses that pathogenic factors play an important or even decisive role in the occurrence of diseases. Some etiological factors, such as injury from fall and knock, bullet wounds, metallic weapon wounds, frost bite, burns and scalds, and injury by insects or animals, may cause damage to the body even if the healthy qi is abundant. Take virulent epidemic disease as another example. In ancient Chinese medical classics, it is believed to be caused by pestilent qi which may impose instant affliction on people indiscriminately, no matter how strong or weak, and how old or young they are. This emphasizes the importance of pathogenic factors in the occurrence of diseases, indicating that pathogenic factors may cause diseases even if the body is strong and the healthy qi is exuberant.

The Struggle Between Healthy Qi and Pathogenic Factors Dominates the Occurrence and Development of Diseases

TCM holds that insufficient healthy qi is the intrinsic factor responsible for the occurrence of diseases, and pathogenic factors also play an important role in the occurrence of diseases. Therefore, the struggle between them will determine the occurrence and development of diseases. The main manifestations can be divided into the following aspects.

1. When pathogenic factors invade the body, if the healthy qi is powerful and can effectively resist the pathogenic factors, disease will not occur. In other words, pathogenic factors will not impose affliction on everyone, especially those with powerful healthy qi. That is why someone escapes certain epidemic invasion while others cannot even if they are in the same area.

2. When powerful pathogenic factors invade the body, if the healthy qi is weak and cannot effectively resist the pathogenic factors, disease will occur due to imbalance of the viscera, yin and yang, as well as qi and blood.

After the occurrence of disease, the combat between healthy qi and pathogenic factors will dominate the development of the disease. If pathogenic factors triumph over the healthy qi, the prognosis will be unfavorable and the treatment will be long and arduous. On the contrary, if healthy qi beats the weaker pathogenic factors without serious damage, the disease will be quickly cured. So if the healthy qi is exuberant, it can often lead to favorable prognosis and swift recovery.

The Relationship Between the Occurrence of Disease and the Internal or External Environment

The occurrence of disease is closely associated with the internal and external environments of the human body. External environment refers to the living and working surroundings, including climate, locality and hygiene, etc. Internal environment refers to the constitution, emotions and healthy qi of the human body, and so on.

External Environment and Occurrence of Disease

TCM holds that man and nature are closely related. Nature provides essential living conditions for man, and environmental changes, particularly when it comes to such factors as climate, locality or environmental hygiene, can influence the human beings directly or indirectly, leading to corresponding variations and reactions, or even diseases.

1. Climatic factors, such as wind, cold, summer-heat, dampness, dryness and fire, are normal environmental changes under common conditions. When climate takes an unusual turn, they will become pathogenic factors. For example, wind-warm diseases are predominant in windy spring; febrile diseases and sunstroke are prevalent in extremely hot summer; dry-natured diseases are common in dry and solemn autumn; and cold-induced diseases are frequently seen in cold winter. Moreover, when climatic factors do not occur at due time, disease will also be incurred. Many epidemic diseases are particular to certain seasons. For example, measles and epidemic cerebrospinal meningitis are prevalent in winter or spring, while epidemic encephalitis type B is often seen in summer and autumn.

2. Different locality and environment may foster various diseases, and this is especially true when it comes to endemic diseases; for example, simple goiter is often seen in iodine-deficient hinterland, and rheumatic arthritis is common in southern areas featuring humid climate.

3. Long-term exposure to hazardous substances in working or living areas, such as industrial waste gas or particles and acute-toxic pesticides, can lead to chronic intoxication and occupation diseases. For example, excessive intake of powder dust will cause grinder's disease, and poor environmental sanitation may breed mosquitoes or flies which contaminate air or water, giving rise to diseases.

Internal Environment and Disease Occurrence

Internal environment refers to factors such as body constitution, emotions and health qi.

TCM lays great emphasis on the relationship between body constitution and disease occurrence. In *Ling Shu* (*Miraculous Pivot*, 灵枢), the human body is divided into five types: taiyin, shaoyin, taiyang, shaoyang and moderate yin-yang; besides, different disposition, constitution, shape and physiological trait as well as their relationships with treatment are depicted in this book. It is also shown that people with different disposition or constitution are susceptible to different pathogenic factors. This is because they have different physique and healthy qi. For example, people with qi deficiency may be susceptible to common cold, while fat people are apt to contract phlegm-damp diseases or stroke, etc.

Emotional factors are also closely associated with the occurrence of diseases. Under normal circumstances, the seven emotions correspond physiological responses to the external environmental stimuli. In other cases, however, when sudden, violent or prolonged emotional stimuli go beyond the range of the body's regulative capacity, the physiological functions of the body will be hampered, and consequently diseases will be incurred. In this sense, the seven emotions are also regarded as key etiological factors, just as what is said in *Su Wen*, "Excessive anger drives qi to move upwards; excessive joy relaxes the activity of qi; excessive grief exhausts qi; excessive fear drives qi to move downwards; excessive fright disturbs qi; and excessive contemplation stagnates qi." Since the seven emotions may lead to dysfunction of the viscera, imbalance of yin-yang and qi-blood, and deficiency of healthy qi, we should pay attention to metal cultivation and always take an optimistic attitude towards life so as to contain the healthy qi, spirit and essence inside the body.

Daily Exercises

1. Describe the roles of healthy qi and pathogenic factors in the occurrence of diseases.
2. Why the internal and external environments are closely associated with the occurrence of diseases.

CHAPTER 10

Pathogenesis

Pathogenesis refers to the mechanism of the occurrence, development and variation of diseases. In other words, when pathogenic factors invade the body, the affected viscera or meridians will be impaired, leading to functional disorders and pathological manifestations. TCM lays considerable emphasis on identifying disease causes by syndrome differentiation, while pathogenesis is the intrinsic foundation for clinical manifestation, development, variation, diagnosis and medication of diseases. In *Su Wen* (*Plain Conversation*, 素问), it is stressed that the pathogenesis should always be followed, and also created 19 principles of pathogenesis, in which different symptoms or syndromes are attributed to a certain cause or a certain zang-organ. These principles of pathogenesis simplify the complicated clinical manifestations; therefore, by discussing pathogenesis, we can get a clear view about the mechanism of diseases, syndromes and symptoms, or about the occurrence, development and change of diseases. Generally it can be discussed from the perspectives of exuberance and debilitation of healthy qi and pathogenic factors, imbalance between yin and yang, disorder of qi and blood, abnormality of fluid metabolism and malfunction of the viscera and meridians.

SECTION 1 COMMON TYPES OF PATHOGENESIS

Exuberance and Debilitation of Healthy Qi and Pathogenic Factors

Exuberance and debilitation of healthy qi and pathogenic factors refer to the waxing and waning between healthy qi and pathogenic factors during their struggle in the occurrence and development of diseases. Such a struggle is influential and decisive in the onset, progress and turnover of diseases. The strength contrast between healthy qi and pathogenic factors determines the prognosis of disease. In this sense, many diseases are, in essence, a process of combat between healthy qi and pathogenic factors, as well as their waxing and waning.

Exuberance and Debilitation of Healthy Qi and Pathogenic Factors and Interchange Between Deficiency and Excess

In the occurrence and development of a disease, the strength contrast between healthy qi and pathogenic factors are not fixed, but in constant change. In other words, the process is marked by the waxing of one side and at the same time, the waning of the other. If the healthy qi is powerful, the pathogenic factors will retreat, and if the pathogenic factors are fierce, the healthy qi will withdraw. With the ongoing struggle between the two sides, the disease will develop towards either deficiency or excess.

1. *Develop towards excess*

In *Su Wen*, it is said that the abundance of pathogenic qi leads to excess while the consumption of essential qi results in deficiency. So an excess syndrome is characterized by predominant pathogenic factors. This is due to that both the pathogenic factors and the healthy qi are strong, or due to that the pathogenic factors are powerful and the healthy qi is not weak, leading to intense combat between the two sides, clinically marked by a series of dramatic pathological manifestations, or the so-called excess syndrome. Excess syndrome is commonly manifested in the initial and middle stages of diseases due to exogenous pathogenic invasion. At first, it is marked by fever, aversion to cold, headache, sore throat, cough, presence of sweating or absence of sweating, and floating pulse, etc. If the disease develops into the interior, it may be characterized by high fever, profuse sweating, extreme thirst, and surging large pulse, or impalpable pain and fullness in the abdomen, high fever, delirium, and sinking, excessive and powerful pulse, etc. Moreover, diseases due to retention of phlegm, food, water and blood are also deemed as excess syndromes, marked by internal accumulation of phlegm and saliva, undigested food, overflowing of water and dampness, and internal obstruction of blood stasis, etc.

2. Develop towards deficiency

This means that in the struggle between healthy qi and pathogenic factors, the deficiency of the former is the primary aspect. When the viscera, meridians, qi and blood, body fluid, defensive qi and nutritional qi are in deficiency, the healthy qi will be too weak to launch a fierce combat against the invading pathogens, leading to a series of clinical manifestations marked by debilitation, decline and deficiency. This is the so-called deficiency syndrome, which is commonly seen in people with weak constitution or inadequate innate endowment, or in advanced stage of diseases and chronic diseases, etc. Clinically insufficiency of healthy qi is often caused by severe or chronic diseases, excessive vomiting or diarrhea with fluid loss, and profuse bleeding with qi and blood deficiency, characterized by spiritual or physical lassitude, lusterless complexion, low and weak voice, spontaneous sweating, night sweating, feverish sensation over the five centers (the palms, the soles, and the heart), chilly, cold limbs, and feeble pulse, etc.

3. Mixed deficiency and excess

This refers to the pathological state of simultaneous existence of exuberant pathogenic factors and insufficient healthy qi. It is caused by the following conditions: (a) Pathogenic factors linger inside the body with impaired healthy qi; (b) Exogenous pathogenic factors invade the body when the healthy qi is weak, leading to clinical manifestations marked by both deficiency and excess; (c) Unaddressed or improperly treated disease leads to prolonged retention of pathogenic factors inside the body with impairment of healthy qi; (d) Insufficient healthy qi results in endogenous retention of water, dampness, phlegm, fluid and blood, etc.

Mixed deficiency and excess can be further divided into excess within deficiency and deficiency within excess according to their difference in proportion. The former is mainly the deficiency of healthy qi with complication of pathogenic factors, such as deficiency of spleen yang and kidney yang with complication of edema. The latter is mainly the excess of pathogenic factors with complication of insufficient healthy qi, such as exogenous diseases with the main syndrome of excess-heat accumulation and the complication of fluid consumption.

Besides, there are also genuine or false conditions of excess and deficiency; in other words, under unusual circumstances the clinical manifestations of a disease are not in accordance with its essence or nature. The false manifestations are the reverse reflection of the essence. For this reason, sometimes when the body is extremely weak, there will be false symptoms of excess; and when the body is in extreme excess, there will be false symptoms of deficiency.

With the ongoing struggle between healthy qi and pathogenic factors, the deficiency and excess of a syndrome may interchange. Therefore, deficiency and excess are relative rather than absolute. Clinically we should take a dynamic, relative approach instead of a static, absolute one to make a difference between excess and deficiency.

Exuberance and Debilitation of Pathogenic Factors and Healthy Qi and Turnover of Disease

During the occurrence and development of a disease, the struggle between pathogenic factors and healthy qi determines its turnover. If the healthy qi is not weak, it can resist the pathogenic factors overtime and make a favorable turn of the disease or has it completely cured; otherwise, if the healthy qi is originally weak, or becomes weak due to powerful pathogenic invasion, the disease may be exacerbated and even become lethal. In this sense, it is considered that the turnover of disease is determined by the exuberance and debilitation of pathogenic factors and healthy qi.

1. *Healthy qi triumphing over pathogenic factors*

This refers to the process in which the powerful healthy qi beats the relatively weak pathogenic factors and makes a favorable turn of the disease. This is due to that the healthy qi is abundant with effective resistance against the pathogens, or that timely and proper treatment is implemented to control, debilitate and even eliminate the pathogens. In this way the impaired the viscera and meridians are repaired and their functions are restored. For example, pathogenic wind-cold may cause common cold; however, if the healthy qi is not weak and is capable of launching an effective resistance against the pathogens, the disease will be relieved with some sweat-promoting herbs pungent and warm in flavor.

2. *Pathogenic factors retreats, leaving healthy qi weak and deficient*

This is a condition that the pathogenic factors are basically eliminated, while the healthy qi is also impaired due to the struggle between them. This case is commonly seen in the recovery phase of some severe diseases.

3. *Pathogenic factors triumphing over healthy qi*

This refers to the condition that healthy qi fails to resist the powerful pathogenic factors, leading to an unfavorable turn of the disease. This is because the healthy qi is too weak to effectively control the hyperactive pathogens which, consequently, become increasingly hazardous to the body, thus prolonging and exacerbating the disease. If the healthy qi becomes further debilitated and the pathogenic factors become rampant, the functions of the viscera and meridians will be severely damaged, leading to dissociation of yin and yang, or even death. For example, exogenous pathogenic cold may weaken the healthy qi and consume large amount of yang qi, leading to severe debilitation of the body, depletion of yang with profuse sweating, or even termination of life.

4. *Pathogenic factors and healthy qi in a deadlock*

This refers to the condition that pathogenic factors and healthy qi are well matched, resulting in an impasse in their long-term struggle. This can be seen in exogenous febrile diseases, such as shaoyang disease mentioned in *Shang Han Lun*, which is marked by alternated chills and fever due to the struggle between healthy qi and pathogenic factors; besides, it can also be seen in miscellaneous diseases due to internal impairment, such as chronic diarrhea marked by co-existence of spleen deficiency and pathogen retention.

Furthermore, there are also other conditions such as deficiency of healthy qi leading to retention of pathogens; in other words, when healthy qi is extremely weak and the pathogens are not completely eliminated, the disease course will be prolonged because either side is incapable of launching an effective battle to wipe out the other. This is common at the late stage of diseases or in chronic diseases. It is responsible for the lingering effects of some diseases or the transition of a disease from acuteness to chronicity.

Daily Exercises

1. Describe the relationship between the exuberance and debilitation of pathogenic factors and healthy qi and the interchange of pathogenic factors and healthy qi.
2. Describe the relationship between the exuberance and debilitation of pathogenic factors and healthy qi and the turnover of diseases.

Imbalance Between Yin and Yang

Imbalance between yin and yang refers to the relative exuberance or debilitation of yin and yang, failure of yin to control yang or yang to control yin, mutual consumption of yin and yang, and depletion of yin and yang, due to various pathogenic factors in the occurrence and development of diseases. Besides, it is also a generalization of the dysfunction of the viscera, meridians, qi and blood, nutrient qi and defensive qi as well as the disorder of qi movements.

The inter-restriction, inter-transformation and interdependence between yin and yang are both opposite and unified, existing in a dynamic balance. Yin and yang are the main factors responsible for regulating the metabolism and functional activities of the human body, and also the essential foundation for normal life activities. Under normal circumstances, yin and yang exist in a balance, ensuring the normal physiological activities; however, if such a balance is broken, diseases will occur. The six climatic factors, seven emotional variations, improper diet and lifestyle can all exert a pernicious influence on the body, leading to imbalance between yin and yang, and diseases.

The pathological changes of imbalance between yin and yang are very complicated. Clinically it includes relative exuberance, relative debilitation, mutual consumption, mutual repulsion and depletion of yin and yang.

Relative Exuberance of Yin and Yang

The relative exuberance of yin or yang is an excess syndrome due to invasion of abundant pathogenic factors. When pathogenic factors invade the body, corresponding responses will be triggered in different forms according to the nature of the pathogens; for example, when yang pathogen invades the body, there will be relative exuberance of yang, and when yin pathogen invades the body, there will be relative exuberance of yin.

Yin and yang are mutually restrained, and exuberance of either side will lead to debilitation of the other side. The interaction between yin and yang is revealed in *Su Wen*, which stated that exuberance of yang leads to yin disease, and exuberance of yin results in yang disease.

1. *Exuberance of yang*

This refers to the pathological state marked by hyperactive function, reinforced reaction and redundant heat energy. It is an excess-heat syndrome with exuberant yang and unimpaired yin. Exuberance of yang is mainly caused by invasion of pathogenic warm-heat, transformation of yin pathogen into yang-heat, transformation into fire due to hyperactivity of the seven emotions, or transformation into heat due to qi stagnancy, blood stasis, and improper diet and lifestyles, etc.

Yang is characterized by hotness, agitation and dryness, the exuberance of which is marked by a series of heat manifestations such as high fever, flushed complexion, reddened eyes, reddish urine, thirst, yellow fur and rapid pulse, etc. When pathogenic factors invade the superficies, the defensive qi will cover all over the body to resist them, leading to external manifestations of heat or fever. Exuberance of yang may result in insufficiency of yin fluid, which may fall into two categories: if yang is abundant and yin is relatively insufficient, there will be manifestations of excess-heat syndrome; and if hyperactive yang further develops and consumes yin fluid or even yin essence, the syndrome will transit from the previous one to a syndrome of excess-heat with yin depletion or a syndrome of deficiency-heat.

2. *Relative exuberance of yin*

This refers to the pathological state marked by exuberant yin qi, debilitated functional activities, reduced reaction, and insufficient production of heat, and accumulation of metabolic products. It is a excess-cold syndrome characterized by exuberant yin and unimpaired yang, mainly caused by contraction of pathogenic damp-cold or overtake of raw and cold food, leading to retention of cold in the middle energizer, obstruction of yang qi, and exuberance of yin-cold.

Yin is cold, quiet and damp by nature, and the exuberance of which may lead to cold sensation of the body, cold limbs, pale complexion, clear and profuse urine, loose stool and pale tongue, etc. If it is accompanied by retention of phlegm-dampness or water-fluid, there will be edema, clear and clod phlegm and slow pulse, etc. When pathogenic yin-cold attacks the interior, yang qi will be impaired, leading to debilitation of yang and exuberance of yin, intolerance of cold and internal abundance of yin, etc.

Exuberance of yin may lead to debilitation of yang, so excess-cold syndrome of yin exuberance is often accompanied by relative insufficiency of yang qi. Besides, further damage of yang qi will incur internal abundance of yin-cold with insufficiency of yang qi.

Relative Debilitation of Yin and Yang

The relative debilitation of yin or yang refers to the pathological changes due to deficiency of yin or yang of the body, or due to insufficiency of essence, qi, blood and body fluid and debilitation of their physiological functions as well as hypofunction or imbalance of the viscera and meridians. This is because essence, qi, blood, body fluid, viscera and meridians as well as their physiological functions are either yin or yang in nature. They are physiologically interdependent and inter-restricted, sustaining the life activities in a coordinated way. If certain pathogenic factors invade the body, however, there will substantial or functional impairment of one side, leading to relative hyperactivity of the other side. Such pathological manifestations are generally called "deficiency of yang leading to exuberance of yin," "deficiency of yang leading to cold manifestations," "deficiency of yin causing hyperactivity of yang" and "deficiency of yin resulting in heat manifestations."

1. *Relative debilitation of yang, or yang deficiency*

This refers to the pathological state of deficient yang qi, hypofunction or debilitation of the body, reduced metabolism and inadequate heat energy, etc. Its pathogenesis is marked by insufficient yang failing to restrain the relatively hyperactive yin. It is a deficiency-cold syndrome. The disorders of the spleen and kidney are primarily responsible for this phenomenon because the spleen is the acquired foundation while the kidney is the root of all kinds of yang. Therefore the insufficiency of yang qi is mainly attributed to the spleen and kidney, particularly the latter. Relative debilitation of yang is mainly characterized by hypofunction of yang qi in warming, propelling and stimulating, malfunction of the viscera and meridians, as well as coagulation of blood and retention of water due to sluggish circulation of blood and fluid. Besides, there are also manifestations such as intolerance of cold, cold limbs and depression due to failure of yang qi to warm and stimulate the body.

"Deficiency of yang leading to cold manifestations" means that debilitation of yang qi in warming the body causes clinical manifestations marked by cold sensation of the body, cold limbs, preference for warmth, pale complexion, pale tongue, slow pulse, spiritual or physical lassitude, clear and profuse urine, and diarrhea, etc. Besides, if the qi-transforming function of yang qi debilitates, there will be retention of water-dampness and edema. Hence, "deficiency of yang leading to cold manifestations" and "exuberance of yin leading to cold manifestations" are different both in pathogenesis and clinical manifestations; the former is marked primarily by deficiency while the latter by cold.

2. *Relative debilitation of yin, or yin deficiency*

This refers to the depleted essence, blood and body fluid fail to restrain yang-heat, leading to yang exuberance and false hyperactivity. Its pathogenesis is characterized by insufficient yin-fluid failing to restrain yang and moisten the body, resulting in relative hyperactivity of yang and the syndrome of deficiency-heat. This is due to pathogenic yang impairing yin, or hyperactivity of the five emotions transforming into fire and damaging yin, or chronic disease consuming yin.

The kidney is the root of all kinds of yin, and the kidney and liver share the same origin; so yin insufficiency is mainly manifested as yin deficiency of the liver and kidney, particularly the latter. Relative debilitation of yin is mainly marked by insufficient essence, blood and body fluid as well as weakened functions in moistening, nourishing and tranquilizing, with such signs as feverish sensation over the five centers (the palms, the soles and the heart), bone-steaming sensation with hectic fever, flushing complexion, emaciation, night sweating, dry throat and mouth, reddish tongue with scanty fur, and thin-rapid-feeble pulse, etc. Essence, blood and body fluid have their own distinct clinical manifestations when they are insufficient, and even different visceral fluids, when in short supply, have their own manifestations that are individually different. These manifestations, both connected and differentiated, come in different forms such as internal heat due to yin deficiency, fire hyperactivity due to yin deficiency, and yang hyperactivity due to yin deficiency.

Heat manifestations due to yin deficiency and yang abundance are different. The former is marked by insufficient yin-fluid failing to moisten the body and restrain yang, leading to a series of heat manifestations; while the latter is characterized by feverish sensation over the five centers (the palms, the soles and the heart), dry mouth, reddish tongue and thin-rapid pulse, etc. It is thus evident that they differ in both pathogenesis and clinical manifestations. In a nutshell, heat manifestations due to yin deficiency are marked by both deficiency and heat, particularly the former, while heat manifestations due to yang abundance are marked by hotness instead of deficiency.

Daily Exercises

1. What are the connotations of imbalance between yin and yang?
2. What are the pathogenetic characteristics of relative exuberance of yin and yang?
3. What are the pathogenetic characteristics of relative debilitation of yin and yang?

Imbalance Between Yin and Yang

Mutual Consumption Between Yin and Yang

Mutual consumption between yin and yang means that during the development of disease, the deficiency of yin or yang to a certain extent will inevitably involve the other side, resulting in simultaneous deficiency of yin and yang. Yang deficiency developed on the basis of yin insufficiency is called "yin impairment involving yang," whereas yin deficiency evolved on the basis of yang insufficiency is called "yang impairment involving yin." The interdependence between yin and yang is the underlying reason for simultaneous consumption between yin and yang. The kidney stores essence which is the material foundation for kidney yin and yang as well as the root of yang qi and yin fluid. So if yin or yang debilitates to a certain extent, no matter what viscus it may pertain to, the kidney yin or yang will be involved. Moreover, the deficiency of kidney yin to a certain extent will inevitably involve the kidney yang and *vice versa*. Therefore, imbalance between yin and yang is marked by two pathological states: yin impairment involving yang and yang impairment involving yin.

1. *Yin impairment involving yang*

This means that the deficiency of yin to a certain extent will inevitably involve yang, resulting in simultaneous deficiency of yin and yang, with yin deficiency as the dominant one. For example, hyperactivity of the liver yang is caused by yin failing to restrain yang, or insufficient kidney-water failing to nourish the liver-wood; further development may involve the kidney essence and lead to deficiency of kidney yang, marked by intolerance of cold, cold limbs, pale complexion, and clear, profuse urine. In the end, both yin and yang will be deficient.

2. *Yang impairment involving yin*

This means that the deficiency of yang to a certain extent will inevitably involve yin, leading to simultaneous deficiency of yin and yang, with yang deficiency as the dominant one. For example, edema due to kidney yang deficiency is mainly caused by malfunction of qi transformation and overflowing of water, and further development will affect the production of yin-fluid, marked by emaciation, irascibility and even spasm. In the end, both yin and yang will be deficient.

Relative Repulsion Between Yin and Yang

Relative repulsion between yin and yang is a special form of imbalance between yin and yang. When yin or yang becomes extremely exuberant or debilitated, the powerful aspect will push the weak aspect outside, leading to disassociation between yin and yang marked by false cold with genuine heat or genuine cold with false heat.

1. *Exuberant yin rejecting yang*

This refers to exuberant yin stagnates inside and blocks debilitated yang outside, leading to mutual repulsion and disassociation of yin and yang. Its essence is internal exuberance of yin marked by cold manifestations and false heat symptoms due to rejection of yang. For this reason, it is called syndrome of genuine cold with false heat. At first, this syndrome is manifested as cold limbs, diarrhea, pale complexion, depression, intolerance of cold, weariness, and extremely thin and feeble pulse, and then, with the aggravation of the disease, there will be symptoms such as flushed complexion, no aversion to cold, and irascibility due to predominant yin driving yang upward and outward. This is a critical condition and may bring on dissociation of yin and yang.

2. *Exuberant yang rejecting yin*

This refers to a pathological state that abundant yang-heat is stagnated inside the body, failing to reach the four limbs and rejecting yin outside. Its essence is internal exuberance of yang marked by heat manifestations and false cold symptoms due to rejection of yin; so clinically it is called syndrome of genuine heat with false cold. For example, in exogenous febrile diseases, abundant pathogenic yang-heat often lead to high fever, flushed complexion, irascibility, reddish tongue, and large-powerful pulse; with the development of the disease, however, there may also be cold manifestations such as cold limbs and sinking-hiding pulse. This is called in *Shang Han Lun* that the more exuberant the pathogenic yang, the colder the four limbs.

Inter-transformation Between Yin and Yang

Inter-transformation between yin and yang, a pathological state of imbalance between yin and yang, means that either yin or yang can transform into its opposite side, such as yin transforming into yang or yang into yin.

1. *Yang transforming into yin*

This means that the nature of a disease changes from yang to yin due to certain reasons. For example, in exogenous febrile diseases, there may be high fever, profuse sweating, extreme thirst, and surging-large pulse due to exuberance of pathogenic heat. When the disease further develops, however, yin fluid can be consumed, which may subsequently involve yang and lead to manifestations of yang depletion such as cold limbs, pale complexion or profuse cold sweat, etc. This is a pathological process characterized by yang converting into yin, excess into deficiency, or heat into cold. The primary reason for it is that abundant pathogenic heat impairs yin fluid and yang qi.

2. *Yin transforming into yang*

This means that the nature of disease changes from yin to yang due to certain reasons. For example, diarrhea with deficiency-cold may be manifested as abdominal pain, rugitus, loose stool or even watery diarrhea, intolerance of cold, pale tongue and soggy pulse. However, if it is mistreated or over-warmed, the nature of this disease will turn from deficiency cold into excess heat, bringing on manifestations such as constipation, abdominal fullness and pain, fever, red tongue and rapid pulse. This is a pathological process characterized by deficiency converting into excess and cold into heat, which can be explained primarily by the transformation of pathogenic factors and disease nature from deficiency-cold to excess-heat.

Depletion of Both Yin and Yang

Depletion of both yin and yang refers to a life-threatening pathological state characterized by massive loss of yin fluid or yang qi of the body. It can be mainly discussed in terms of loss of yin and loss of yang.

1. *Loss of yang*

This refers to a life-threatening pathological state characterized by massive deprivation of yang qi and severe prostration of yang functions. Yang qi is capable of warming, promoting, consolidating and defending, so if it is lost considerable, there will critical conditions due to functional prostration. Loss of yang is primarily caused by exuberance of pathogens, weakness of healthy qi, innate deficiency of yang qi, overstrain, excessive sweating, vomiting and purging, massive loss of qi, blood and body fluid, and chronic diseases.

Because loss of yang is a pathological state marked by extreme depletion and functional prostration of yang qi, it is manifested as deficiency cold symptoms such as cold limbs, depression, pale complexion, profuse sweating, intolerance of cold with curled body, and a thin, extremely feeble pulse, etc.

2. *Loss of yin*

This refers to a life-threatening pathological state characterized by massive deprivation of yin fluid and severe prostration of yin functions. Yin qi is capable of moistening, inner-preserving, and nourishing, so if it is lost excessively, there will be critical conditions due to functional prostration of yin fluid. Loss of yin is primarily due to that exuberant pathogenic heat severely damages yin fluid, or chronic diseases continuously consume yin fluid.

Because loss of yang is a pathological state marked by extreme depletion and functional prostration of yin qi, it is primarily manifested as symptoms such as thirst with preference for drinking, restlessness, panting, warm extremities with profuse sweating, and rapid pulse, etc.

Loss of yin and loss of yang, though different in pathogenesis and clinical manifestation, are intrinsically interrelated because yin and yang are physiologically interdependent and pathologically interchanged. For example, loss of yang may lead to exhaustion of source for production of yin whereas loss of yin may result in scattered yang due to deprivation of its attachment. In other words, loss of yang can cause immediate loss of yin and *vice versa*, ultimately resulting in loss of both.

From the above, we can learn that loss of yin, as a matter of fact, is attributable to severe depletion of yin fluid, and loss of yang to depletion of yang qi. With the continuous depletion of yin fluid or yang qi, their functions may debilitate, too. Despite their difference in clinical presentations, they are intrinsically interrelated because yin and yang are physiologically interdependent and pathologically interchanged. For this reason, clinically both yang and yang are often involved, giving rise to yin-yang dissociation.

Daily Exercises

1. What are the pathogenetic characteristics of mutual consumption between yin and yang?
2. What are the pathogenetic characteristics of mutual repulsion between yin and yang?
3. What are the pathogenetic characteristics of mutual transformation between yin and yang?
4. Explain why loss of yin and loss of yang are intrinsically interrelated?

Weekly Review

This week, we studied etiology, occurrence of disease (external injury, phlegm, fluid retention, blood stasis, the relationship between the occurrence of disease and the conflict between pathogens and healthy qi, and the relationship between the occurrence of disease and the internal and external environments), and pathogenesis (the exuberance and debilitation of pathogenic factors and healthy qi, and the imbalance between yin and yang). Now let us review about all these as follows.

External injury refers to injury from falls and knocks, bullet wounds, metallic weapon wounds, injury from overload, frost bite, burns and scalds, and injury by insects or animals, etc. These injuries can all damage the body, leading to painful swelling of the skin or muscles, bleeding, injury of soft tissues, or even death. So these factors cannot be neglected.

Parasites can also lead to various diseases, and the common parasites are roundworm, hookworm, pinworm, tapeworm, or blood fluke, etc. The pathogenic characteristics of parasites should be fully understood so as to reduce the hazards posed by parasites to the human body.

Phlegm and retained-fluid are pathological substances produced by disturbance of water metabolism of the human body. Generally speaking, the thick part is called phlegm while the thin part is called retained-fluid. Phlegm may be divided into tangible phlegm or intangible phlegm. The former refers to visible expectorated sputum, while the latter means invisible sputum retained in the viscera or meridians with specific pathological manifestations, such as local spreading swelling in patients with superficial nodules, etc. Retained-fluid may linger in the lung, the stomach, the urinary bladder or the skin and muscles. The phlegm and retained-fluid are often caused by external contraction of six abnormal climatic factors, abnormal changes of seven emotions, dietary irregularities, lifestyle abnormalities, dysfunction of the lung, spleen, kidney and triple energizers, and disturbance of water distribution and excretion, etc.

Blood stasis, called accumulated blood in ancient times, is a pathological product due to blood stagnation, including extravasated blood and blood congested in the vessels or zang-fu organs due to the unsmooth blood circulation. So it is both a pathological product and a causative factor. Blood stasis is caused by unsmooth blood circulation due to external contraction of six abnormal climatic factors, abnormal changes of seven emotions, dietary irregularities, overwork, excessive rest or external injuries, etc.

The occurrence and changes of a disease, though complicated, can be discussed from two aspects: healthy qi and pathogenic factors. The former refers to the functional activities of the body (such as the functions of the viscera, meridians, qi and blood, yin and yang, etc.) as well as its abilities to resist and recover from diseases; the latter refers to various pathogenic factors. The occurrence and development of disease is actually the reflection of the struggle between the healthy qi and pathogenic factors under certain circumstances, so insufficient healthy qi is the intrinsic factor responsible for the occurrence of diseases, while pathogenic factors are important conditions indispensable to the occurrence of diseases. The outcome of conflict between healthy qi and pathogenic factors dominates the occurrence and development of diseases. When pathogenic factors invade the body, if the healthy qi is powerful and can effectively resist the pathogenic factors, disease will not occur; nevertheless, when powerful pathogenic factors invade the body, if the healthy qi is weak and cannot effectively resist the pathogenic factors, disease will occur. After its occurrence, if pathogenic factors are strong and the conditions are severe, the prognosis will be unfavorable and the treatment will be long and arduous. On the contrary, if pathogenic factors are weak and the conditions are mild, the disease will be quickly cured.

The occurrence of disease is closely associated with the internal and external environments of the human body. External environment refers to the living and working surroundings, including climate, locality and hygiene, etc. TCM holds that man and nature are closely related and corresponded, so these external environmental factors have a lot to do with the health of the body. Internal environment refers to the constitution, emotions and healthy qi of the human body, which also exert certain influence on the health of the human body.

Pathogenesis refers to the mechanisms of the occurrence, development and transmutation of a disease. Each syndrome or symptom has its own mechanisms, so the timely recognition of the pathogenesis of disease is essential to every TCM doctors.

Exuberance and debilitation of healthy qi and pathogenic factors refer to the waxing and waning between healthy qi and pathogenic factors during their struggle in the occurrence and development of disease. The outcome determines the development of disease. If pathogen is abundant and predominant in the conflict, whereas the healthy qi is not weak and can fight fiercely against the intrusion, there will be violent and intense pathological manifestations called excess syndrome. If the healthy qi is weak and fails to resist the pathogens, there will be pathological manifestations marked by weakness, debilitation and inadequateness, called deficiency syndrome. If there is simultaneous existence of exuberant pathogens and debilitated healthy qi, a more complicated morbid state marked by mixed deficiency and excess will be present. Such a condition can be divided into excess within deficiency (if deficiency is dominant) and deficiency within excess (if excess is dominant).

During the occurrence and development of a disease, the struggle between pathogenic factors and healthy qi also determines its turnover. If the healthy qi is strong while the pathogens are relatively weak, the disease will take a favorable turn, called healthy qi triumphing over pathogenic factors. In some cases pathogenic factors are basically eliminated, but the healthy qi is also impaired due to the struggle between them; this is called withdrawal of pathogenic factors leaving healthy qi weak and fragile. There are other conditions in which pathogenic factors and healthy qi are well matched, resulting in a deadlock in their long-term struggle.

Imbalance between yin and yang refers to unbalanced and uncoordinated state between yin and yang. Its pathological changes are very complicated, including relative exuberance, relative debilitation, mutual consumption, mutual repulsion and depletion of yin and yang.

The relative exuberance of yin or yang is a pathological state due to invasion of abundant pathogenic yin or yang. Exuberance of yang refers to the pathological state marked by hyperactive functions, reinforced reaction and redundant heat energy. It is an excess-heat syndrome with exuberant yang and unimpaired yin. Relative exuberance of yin refers to the pathological state marked by exuberant yin, debilitated functional activities, and insufficient production of heat and accumulation of metabolic products. It is an excess-cold syndrome characterized by exuberant yin and unimpaired yang.

The relative debilitation of yin or yang refers to the pathological changes due to deficiency of yin or yang, or due to insufficiency of essence. Relative debilitation of yang, or yang deficiency, refers to the pathological state marked by deficient yang qi, functional debilitation, reduced metabolism and inadequate heat energy, etc. It is a deficiency-cold syndrome. Relative debilitation of yin, or yin deficiency, refers to the condition that the depleted essence, blood and body fluid fail to restrain yang-heat, leading to yang exuberance and false hyperactivity. It is a deficiency heat syndrome.

Mutual consumption between yin and yang means that during the development of disease, the deficiency of yin or yang to a certain extent will inevitably involve the other side, resulting in simultaneous deficiency of yin and yang. Yin impairment involving yang means that the deficiency of yin to a certain extent will inevitably involve yang, resulting in simultaneous deficiency of yin and yang, with yin deficiency as the dominant one. Yang impairment involving yin means that the deficiency of yang to a certain extent will inevitably involve yin, resulting in simultaneous deficiency of yin and yang, with yang deficiency as the dominant one.

Relative repulsion between yin and yang is a relatively special form of imbalance between yin and yang. When yin or yang becomes extremely exuberant or debilitated, the powerful aspect will push the weak aspect outside, leading to disassociation between yin and yang. Exuberant yin rejecting yang refers to that exuberant yin stagnates inside and blocks debilitated yang outside. It is a syndrome of true cold with false heat. Exuberant yang rejecting yin refers to a pathological state that abundant yang-heat is stagnated inside the body, failing to reach the four limbs and rejecting yin outside. It is a syndrome of true heat and false cold.

Inter-transformation between yin and yang, a pathological state of imbalance between yin and yang, means that either yin or yang can transform into its opposite side under certain circumstances. Yang transforming into yin means that the nature of disease changes from yang to yin due to certain reasons. Yin transforming into yang means that the nature of disease changes from yin to yang due to certain reasons.

Depletion of yin and yang refers to a life-threatening pathological state characterized by massive loss of yin fluid or yang qi of the body. Loss of yang refers to a critical condition characterized by massive deprivation of yang qi and severe prostration of yang functions. Loss of yin refers to a critical condition characterized by massive deprivation of yin fluid and severe prostration of yin functions. Loss of yin and loss of yang, though different in pathogenesis and clinical manifestations, are intrinsically interrelated because yin and yang are physiologically interdependent and pathologically interchanged.

Daily Exercises

1. Understand the characteristics of external injury, pathogenic phlegm, fluid-retention, and blood stasis in causing diseases.
2. Comprehend and grasp the concept of disease occurrence in TCM.
3. Comprehend and grasp the different variations of exuberance and debilitation between pathogenic factors and healthy qi.
4. Comprehend and grasp the different pathological states of imbalance between yin and yang.

THE ELEVENTH WEEK

Disorders of Qi and Blood

Disorder of qi and blood refers to the pathological state due to insufficient qi and blood, abnormal physiological functions of qi and blood, and failure of qi and blood to promote each other.

Qi and blood is the material basis for physiological functions of the viscera, meridians and tissues. Under normal circumstances, the energy required by the viscera, meridians and tissues comes from qi and blood (or body fluid). So if qi and blood are exuberant with normal functions, the viscera and meridians can work properly to sustain the life activities of the body. Otherwise, the viscera and meridians will be in disorder and diseases may be incurred. On the other hand, qi and blood are also products of visceral activities, so malfunction of the viscera may lead to local or general disorders of qi and blood, involving not only the viscera per se but also the whole body.

In conclusion, the pathogenesis of disorders of qi and blood, similar to that of exuberance and debilitation between pathogenic factors and healthy qi and imbalance between yin and yang, is not only the underlying reason for various disorders of the viscera and meridians, but also the foundation for analyzing the pathogenesis of various diseases.

Disorders of Qi

The disorders of qi refer to the insufficient production or excessive consumption of qi, debilitation of some physiological functions of qi, as well as the abnormal movements of qi characterized by qi deficiency, qi stagnancy, qi adverseness, qi sinking, qi blockage and qi collapse, etc.

1. Qi deficiency

This refers to the morbid conditions characterized by debilitated visceral functions and weakened disease-resistance due to insufficiency and functional disorders of primordial qi. The common causes of qi deficiency are innate deficiency due to lack of congenital essence, postnatal malnutrition due to functional disorders of the lung, spleen and kidney, or excessive consumption due to overstrain and chronic diseases. Both insufficient production and excessive consumption can contribute to the deficiency of qi.

Qi deficiency is seen in all aspects of the body with various manifestations characterized by depression, lassitude, weak limbs, dizziness, spontaneous perspiration and feeble pulse. As for qi deficiency of the viscera, it is marked by debilitated or declined visceral functions.

Qi is closely associated with blood and body fluid. Qi deficiency can directly affect the production, circulation and storage of blood and body fluid, leading to blood deficiency, abnormal blood circulation or bleeding, insufficiency of body fluid, and unsmooth circulation and excretion of body fluid.

2. *Disorders of qi movement*

This refers to the morbid conditions of qi stagnancy, qi adverseness, qi sinking, qi blockage and qi collapse due to abnormal ascending, descending, exiting and entering of qi.

Ascending, descending, exiting and entering, the basic forms of qi movement, are responsible for the maintenance of balanced functional activities of the viscera, meridians, qi, blood, and body fluid, such as respiration, dispersion, purification and descent by the lung, the ascent of the lucid by the spleen and the descent of the turbid by the stomach, the ascending of liver qi and the descending of lung qi, the descending of heart-fire and the ascending of kidney water, etc. These are all specific manifestations of qi movement. If it is abnormal, the physiological functions of the viscera, meridians, qi and blood, as well as yin and yang will be involved, leading to various disorders of the viscera and meridians, such as qi deficiency, qi stagnancy, qi adverseness, qi sinking, qi blockage and qi collapse, etc. Now we will discuss them one by one as follows.

(1) Qi stagnancy refers to unsmooth flow of qi caused by emotional depression, or by tangible pathogens such as phlegm, dampness, retained food and blood stasis, or by inhibition of qi activities by exogenous pathogenic factors, leading to local or general unsmooth circulation of qi and functional disorders of the viscera and meridians.

The clinical manifestations of qi stagnancy are multi-faceted, e.g., sensation of distension, fullness and pain, or retention of blood, water, fluid and phlegm in the affected regions if qi is stagnated in a local area; or visceral disorders of the liver, lung, spleen and stomach if qi is stagnated in them because these organs play an important role in regulating general qi activities.

(2) Qi adverseness refers to the morbid state of abnormal ascent and descent of qi and reversal flow of visceral qi due to emotional impairment, irregular diet, retention of phlegm, and contraction of pathogens or physical weakness. It commonly occurs in the lung, stomach and liver, and is often manifested as cough with dyspnea in cases of lung qi counterflow; headache, distension in the head, reddened complexion, blood-shot eyes and testiness in cases of liver qi counterflow; and nausea, vomiting, belching and hiccup in cases of stomach qi counterflow; Qi adverseness is mostly caused by excess; however, there are conditions in which deficiency may lead to adverse rising of qi, such as adverse rising of stomach qi due to deficiency of stomach qi, and adverse rise of lung qi due to deficiency of lung qi or kidney qi.

(3) Qi sinking refers to the pathological state marked by failure of qi in lifting-up and ascending the lucid on the basis of qi deficiency. Most cases are developed on syndrome of qi deficiency; for example, fragile constitution or chronic diseases may weaken the lifting ability of the spleen qi, or descend the middle qi, leading to qi sinking in the end.

The normal physiological functions of the viscera and the sustaining of their normal positions are both maintained by the normal movements of the ascending, descending, entering and exiting of qi. If qi is too weak to lift the viscera, there will be manifestations such as gastroptosis, nephroptosis, or uterine prolapse. If the spleen qi is too weak to ascend the cereal nutrients to the head and eyes, there will be symptoms such as dizziness, blurred vision, tinnitus and lassitude, etc.

(4) Qi blockage refers to the pathologic state of impeded qi movements due to emotional depression or turbid pathogens blocking the chest and clouding the upper orifices, leading to severe syncope or coma due to excessive heat, contraction of turbid qi, violent pain or physic trauma, etc.

(5) Qi collapse refers to the pathologic state marked by severe prostration of healthy qi and sudden failure of body functions due to excessive loss of qi. Sudden damage to the healthy qi and prolonged consumption by chronic diseases may both contribute to the deprivation of qi. It is usually seen in the cases of massive bleeding, profuse sweating, or excessive vomiting and over-purging, leading to deprivation of qi with depletion of blood or fluid. This is commonly manifested as incessant perspiration, pale complexion, involuntarily opened mouth with closed eyes, general weakness, relinquished hands, incontinence of urination and defecation, and extremely weak pulse, etc.

Disorders of Blood

The disorders of blood refers to pathological conditions of blood deficiency due to inadequate production or excessive loss of blood or weakened functions of blood in nourishment, accelerated blood flow driven by blood heat, and blood stasis caused by sluggish blood circulation. Now we will discuss them one by one as follows.

1. *Blood deficiency*

This refers to the morbid state marked by insufficient production of blood and reduced capacity in nourishment. It is often caused by insufficient production of blood by the spleen and stomach, excessive loss of blood without replenishment, or insidious consumption of blood due to chronic consumptive diseases.

One of the main functions of blood is to nourish the viscera and meridians as well as other organs and tissues of the whole body. So when the blood is deficient, there will be malnourishment of the related viscera or certain regions. It is often manifested as deficiency syndromes marked by pale complexion, dizziness, palpation, spiritual or physical lassitude, numb hands and feet, pale nails, dry eyes and thin pulse, etc.

2. *Blood heat*

This refers to the pathological state marked by heat in the blood, accelerated blood circulation, and even bleeding. When pathogenic heat invades the blood phase, or when the five emotions transform into fire, the blood will be heated-up.

Under normal conditions, blood circulates inside the vessels and nourishes the whole body. If the blood is heated-up, however, the circulation of blood will be speeded-up, manifested as flushed complexion and reddened eyes, reddish or dark-reddish tongue, upset, restlessness and rapid pulse; and if the blood is stirred and disturbed, there will be macules, non-traumatic bleeding, or presence of blood in the urine, etc.

3. *Blood stagnancy*

This refers to the morbid state marked by sluggish and unsmooth blood circulation due to deficiency of qi, obstruction of qi, retention of turbid phlegm, and accumulation of pathogenic cold or heat. Further development of blood stagnancy may lead to blood stasis. Blood stasis and blood stagnancy are mutually affected; the former is both the pathological product of the latter and the cause of the latter once it obstructs the vessels. Blood stagnancy is characterized by unsmooth circulation, general or local fixed pain in the affected regions, and masses. It may also be accompanied by dark complexion, scaly skin, and dark purple tongue and lips with ecchymoses, etc.

Once blood stagnancy is formed, it may worsen the obstruction of qi movements, resulting in a vicious cycle marked by mutual affection of qi obstruction and blood stagnancy.

4. *Blood cold*

This refers to the morbid state of cold in the blood phase marked by sluggish and impeded circulation of blood due to attack of pathogenic cold or debilitation of yang with exuberant yin. Cold in the blood is responsible for the sluggish or impeded circulation of blood, manifested as cold pain in the hands, feet and lower abdomen, aversion to cold with preference for warmth, alleviation upon warming, or cold extremities with cyanosis, delayed menstruation in women, dark purple menses with blood clots, dark purple tongue with white fur, and sinking, slow and unsmooth pulse, etc.

Daily Exercises

1. What are the common types of qi disorder?
2. Describe the pathogenetic characteristics of qi deficiency, qi stagnancy, qi adverseness, qi sinking, qi blockage and qi collapse.
3. What are the common types of blood disorder?
4. Describe the pathogenetic characteristics of blood deficiency, blood heat, blood stagnancy and blood cold.

Disharmony Between Qi and Blood

Qi and blood are closely related, the coordination between which sustains the normal physiological activities. Qi can promote, warm, transform and control blood, whereas blood can moisten, nourish and carry qi. Pathologically they are mutually affected. Disorder or deficiency of qi may involve blood and *vice versa*; for example, qi deficiency may lead to blood deficiency, while blood stasis can impede qi movement. Clinically the disharmony between qi and blood is mainly manifested as blood stasis due to qi stagnancy, blood stasis due to qi deficiency, failure of qi to control blood, qi collapse with blood depletion, and simultaneous deficiency of qi and blood, etc.

Blood Stasis Due to Qi Stagnancy

This refers to the pathological state marked by simultaneous existence of qi stagnancy and blood stasis due to emotional depression or injuries from tumbling down. It is closely related to the liver because the liver stores blood and promotes free flow of qi. If liver qi is stagnated and fails to disperse and dredge, blood circulation will be hampered, leading to simultaneous existence of qi stagnancy and blood stasis. Besides, it is also related to the heart because the heart governs blood and vessels and is in charge of blood circulation. So if the heart is in disorder, it will lead firstly to blood stasis, secondly to qi stagnancy, and finally to simultaneous existence of qi stagnancy and blood stasis. Qi stagnancy with blood stasis is clinically manifested as distension, fullness and pain, or ecchymosis, lumps and masses.

Blood Stasis Due to Qi Deficiency

This refers to a pathological state of blood stasis due to qi deficiency. Generally qi deficiency appears at first, and then blood stasis occurs because the deficient qi fails to promote blood circulation. The manifestations are marked by sluggish blood circulation in mild cases, or flaccidity and even atrophy in severe ones, such as hemiparalysis resulting from malnutrition of vessels and tendons, which is caused by blood stasis due to sudden prostration of healthy qi.

Failure of Qi to Control Blood

This refers to various pathological conditions marked by vomiting of blood, non-traumatic bleeding, bloody stool, and incessant extra-menstrual vaginal bleeding due to insufficient qi failing to contain blood within the vessels. If it is accompanied by insufficiency of middle qi or sinking of qi due to qi deficiency, there will be manifestations such as incessant extra-menstrual vaginal bleeding, bloody stool and bloody urine, etc. The root lies in the deficiency of qi.

Qi Collapse with Blood Depletion

This refers to the exhaustion of qi with massive loss of blood, resulting in the pathological state of simultaneous depletion or deficiency of qi and blood. It is often seen in profuse bleeding due to external injury, postnatal incessant bleeding, and acute vaginal bleeding, etc. This is because blood can carry qi, and if blood is exhausted, qi will have no place to stay in and may subsequently become depleted.

Simultaneous Deficiency of Qi and Blood

This refers to the pathological state of simultaneous existence of qi deficiency and blood deficiency. The causes are various. Qi deficiency may cause insufficient production of blood, and then lead to deficiency of both; blood loss may deprive the body of qi, leading to deficiency of both; and chronic diseases can impair qi and blood, leading to deficiency of both.

It is mainly manifested as pale complexion, spiritual or physical lassitude, shortness of qi, reluctance to speak, palpitation, insomnia, and thin-void pulse, etc. If simultaneous existence of qi deficiency and blood deficiency leads to malnutrition of tendons, there will be manifestations such as numb limbs with inhibited movements, as well as scaly and dry skin, etc.

Abnormal Metabolism of Body Fluid

Body fluid metabolism refers to the production, distribution and excretion of body fluid. Therefore, normal metabolism of body fluid is indispensable to the successful production, distribution and excretion of body fluid and the proper maintenance of the physiological functions of the body. The ascending, descending, entering and exiting of qi, as well as the transformation of qi play an important role in the regulation of general metabolism of body fluid. If qi moves and transforms normally, the metabolism of body fluid will be balanced. Besides, fluid metabolism is also closely related to the physiological functions of the related viscera. For example, the production of body fluid relies on the transportation and transformation of the spleen and stomach; the distribution and excretion of body fluid depend on the essence-dispersing function of the spleen, the diffusing, purifying and descending function of the lung, the ventilating and dredging function of the liver, the steaming and qi-transforming function of the kidney and urinary bladder, and the unblocking and regulating function of the triple energizer. In this sense, we can say that the aforementioned viscera play a very important role in the sustaining of normal metabolism of body fluid. If qi movement and qi transformation are abnormal, or visceral functions are in disorder, fluid metabolism will be disturbed, leading to inadequate body fluid inside the body due to insufficient production or excessive consumption and excretion of body fluid; or accumulation of water and body fluid or even edema due to obstructed distribution and excretion, as well as sluggish circulation of body fluid.

Insufficiency of Body Fluid

This refers to the pathological state marked by dryness due to inadequate body fluid failing to moisten and nourish the viscera, meridians, body constituents, orifices, skin and hair, etc. Insufficient body fluid is commonly caused by exuberant heat in exogenous febrile diseases, abundant heat in endogenous febrile diseases, and scorching heat in yin-deficiency disorders; or by excessive sweating, vomiting and purging, large-area burning, and chronic consumptive diseases, etc.

According to the difference in property, function and distribution, body fluid is subdivided into jin (fluid) and ye (liquid). Generally speaking, the thin fluid, jin, is dilute, more fluidic, and mainly distributed in the body' surface so as to fill up the vessels and to moisten and nourish the muscles, orifices, skin and hair; fluid is apt to be consumed and supplemented. Excessive vomiting, sweating and purging can all contribute to the loss of fluid, manifested as dry mouth, scanty urine, diminished elasticity of the skin, sunken eyes, wailing without tears, or flat and dry nails, etc. Besides, high fever with profuse sweating can also lead to severely damaged fluid marked by dry mouth with desire for drinking, scanty urine and constipation, etc.

The thick fluid, ye, is dense, less fluidic, and generally distributed in the viscera, bone marrow, brain marrow, spinal cord and joints to perform its nourishing and moistening functions. Liquid cannot be easily consumed, but once it is impaired, the recovery will be slow and tough. Liquid depletion is often caused by severe febrile diseases or chronic consumptive diseases. For example, at the late stage of febrile diseases, there are often manifestations such as dry and reddish tongue with scanty or no fur, dry lips, emaciation, lusterless skin and hair, or even squirming feet and hands, etc.

Fluid impairment and liquid depletion are different in pathogenesis and clinical manifestations; fluid and liquid, however, share the same origin and are of no difference in nature. Physiologically they are inter-complemented and inter-transformed; while pathologically they are mutually affected. Commonly fluid impairment is not necessarily accompanied by liquid depletion while liquid depletion is definitely accompanied by fluid impairment.

Distribution and Excretion Disturbance of Body Fluid

The distribution and excretion of body fluid are two important aspects of fluid metabolism. Normal distribution ensures the successful transportation, dispersion and circulation of body fluid; while normal excretion guarantees the proper discharge of metabolized fluid in the forms of urine and sweat. If distribution and excretion are abnormal, body fluid will accumulate and stay inside the body, leading to internal retention of water-dampness, phlegmatic fluid, and even edema, etc.

1. *Distribution disturbance of body fluid*

This refers to the abnormal transportation and distribution of body fluid, leading to sluggish circulation or retention of body fluid manifested as endogenous water-dampness and phlegmatic fluid, etc. The causes may be various; the lung, spleen, liver and triple energizer play a key role in the process. If the lung fails to diffuse and descend qi, the phlegmatic fluid will accumulate in the lung; if the spleen fails to transport and transform food properly, there will be phlegmatic retention due to accumulation of body fluid and dampness; if the liver fails to maintain the normal flow of qi, there will be fluid retention; and if the triple energizer fails to dredge and regulate the waterways, there will internal retention of fluid and water. Among the aforementioned organs, the spleens play a dominant role.

2. *Excretion disturbance*

This refers to the functional disorder of transforming body fluid into urine and sweat, leading to retention of water and edema. The lung is responsible for turning fluid into sweat while the kidney is in charge of transforming fluid into urine. If the lung and kidney are in disorder, excretion disturbance marked by retention of water and edema will be inevitable. The kidney plays a more important role than the lung. If the lung fails to turn the fluid into sweat, it can still be transformed into urine by the kidney; if the kidney fails to transform the fluid into urine, there will inevitably be overflowing of water-dampness and edema.

Despite their differences, distribution disturbance and excretion disturbance are mutually affected, playing a synergic role in causing fluid retention and edema.

Daily Exercises

1. What are the common types of imbalance between qi and blood?
2. What are the pathogenetic characteristics of blood stasis due to qi stagnancy, blood stasis due to qi deficiency, failure of qi to control blood, qi collapse with blood depletion, and simultaneous deficiency of qi and blood?
3. What are the common factors responsible for abnormal metabolism of body fluid?
4. How can one differentiate the characteristics of jin deficiency and ye deficiency in terms of pathogenesis?
5. What are the frequently involved viscera in the distribution disturbance and excretion disturbance of body fluid?

Functional Disorders of Body Fluid, Qi and Blood

The production, distribution and excretion of body fluid are closely related to the functions of qi and blood. If qi and blood are normal in function, body fluid will be sufficiently supplied so as to fill up the blood vessels and circulate smoothly throughout the body to perform its physiological functions. If any of them is in disorder, however, there will be corresponding pathological manifestations such as stagnancy of qi due to fluid retention, collapse of qi due to fluid depletion, dryness of blood due to fluid exhaustion, and stagnancy of blood due to fluid consumption, etc.

Stagnancy of Qi Due to Fluid Retention

This refers to the pathological state marked by stagnancy of qi due to abnormal fluid metabolism and retention of water, dampness, and phlegm, etc. For example, when water attacks the heart, the heart qi and heart yang may be obstructed, leading to palpation and heartache, etc.; when phlegmatic fluid accumulates in the lung, the lung qi will be stagnated, leading to cough, panting, and chest fullness with inability to lie down calmly; when fluid retains in the middle energizer, qi movements will be inhibited, marked by abnormal ascending and descending, marked by gastric and abdominal distension and fullness, anorexia, dizziness and drowsiness, etc.

Collapse of Qi Due to Fluid Depletion

This refers to the collapse of qi due to massive loss of fluid because qi is attached to fluid. For example, in exogenous febrile diseases, abundant interior heat often drives fluid out of the body, manifested at first as high fever, profuse sweating, and unquenchable extreme thirst, and then as cold limbs, intolerance of cold and faint pulse, etc. Besides, excessive vomiting and purging can also consume a large amount of fluid, and finally leads to collapse of qi with the depletion of fluid.

Dryness of Blood Due to Fluid Exhaustion

This refers to the endogenous production of wind due to lack of blood and depletion of body fluid. Fluid shares the same origin with blood and is also an important constituting part of blood, so if fluid is excessively lost due to high fever, burning, chronic consumptive diseases, blood will inevitably become inadequate and condensed, marked by vexation, dry mouth and throat, feverish sensation over the five centers (the palms, soles, and heart), emaciation, and dry or scaly skin with itching, etc.

Stagnancy of Blood Due to Fluid Consumption

This refers to the pathological state marked by sluggish and unsmooth blood circulation due to excessive consumption of body fluid. For example, high fever, severe burning, profuse sweating, and excessive vomiting or purging can consume the body fluid, which may further involve the blood and lead to unsmooth circulation of blood or even blood stasis. Besides the symptoms of fluid depletion, it is also manifested as dark purple tongue, macular eruption or ecchymosis, etc.

Endogenous Production of "Five Pathogenic Factors"

The five endogenous pathogenic factors, caused by imbalance of visceral functions and disorders of qi, blood and body fluid in the occurrence and development of disease, are similar in manifestations to the exogenous pathogenic factors, namely wind, cold, dampness, dryness and fire. Since the pathogens are derived from the interior rather than the exterior, they are collectively called the "five endogenous pathogenic factors," namely internal wind, internal cold, internal dampness, internal dryness and internal fire.

Internal Stirring of Liver-Wind

Internal stirring of liver-wind is closely associated with the liver. It refers to the morbid conditions marked by dizziness, spasm and tremor due to hyperactivity of yang or failure of debilitated yin to suppress the overabundant yang. Generally speaking, it is caused by internal disturbance of yang qi inside the body. According to the specific causes, it can be divided into liver-yang transforming into wind, extreme heat engendering wind, deficient yin stirring wind, and blood deficiency producing wind, etc.

1. *Liver-yang transforming into wind*

This is usually caused by emotional depression, hyperactivity of five emotions, or overstrain, leading to yin deficiency of the liver and kidney which fails to restrain the hyperactive yang and finally produces wind. It is commonly manifested as dizziness with tendency to fall, numbness and tremor of limbs, muscular twitching and cramp, deviated eyes and mouth, or even hemiparalysis, sudden fall, excess-syncope (syncope due to blockage) or deficiency-syncope (syncope due to prostration).

2. *Extreme heat engendering wind*

This is also called exuberant heat stirring wind, and is mainly seen in the high-fever stage of exogenous febrile diseases when exuberant heat scorches the body fluid and blazes the nutrient blood, leading to malnutrition of the tendons and generation of wind. It is mainly manifested as convulsion, spasm, superduction, or even loss of consciousness and delirious speech.

3. *Deficient yin stirring wind*

This is usually occurs in the late phase of febrile diseases or in chronic cases, in which deficient body fluid fails to moisten and nourish the muscles and tendons, resulting in yang hyperactivity. It is commonly manifested as wind-stirring symptoms marked by muscular twitching, spasm, and involuntary movements of limbs. It is different from the syndromes of liver-yang transforming into wind and extreme heat producing wind.

4. *Blood deficiency producing wind*

This refers to the endogenous production of deficient wind due to malnourished muscles and tendons resulting from poor production or excessive loss of blood, or chronic consumptive illnesses. Clinically it is marked by both blood deficiency symptoms and wind stirring symptoms such as pale complexion, white nails, numbness of the body, twitching of the muscles, or even tremor of the feet and hands.

5. *Blood dryness generating wind*

This is caused by chronic consumptive diseases, senility, or malnutrition, leading to depletion of fluid and blood which fail to moisten and nourish the muscles and skin. It is commonly manifested as dry or scaly skin, itching or falling-off of tiny skin tissues, etc.

Endogenous Production of Cold

Endogenous production of cold, or internal cold, refers to the morbid state marked by overabundance of deficiency cold or yin cold originating from the interior due to debilitation of yang qi with weakened functions of warming and transforming.

Yang deficiency will lead firstly to yin exuberance and secondly to internal cold, characterized by insufficient yang-heat and endogenous deficiency-cold, or contraction of blood vessels with sluggish blood circulation due to internal cold, marked by cold body, pale complexion, painful limbs with cold sensation, and contracture of tendons. It is mainly caused by insufficient yang of the spleen and kidney because the kidney yang is the root of all kinds of yang qi while the spleen is the source for the production of qi and blood. So if the spleen yang and kidney yang are insufficient, there will be inadequate production of yang qi, and endogenous generation of cold.

Insufficient yang may lead to malfunction of qi transformation and steaming function with inability to warm and transport water and dampness, leading to retention of water, phlegm and fluid. Clinically it is manifested as prolonged urination, or clear, thin and cold saliva and snivel, loose stool, and even edema, etc. Internal cold and external cold are connected to as well as different from each other. The former is marked by both cold and deficiency, with deficiency as the dominant one, while the latter is characterized mainly by cold with mild deficiency occasionally. They are both caused by invasion of pathogenic cold damaging yang qi, leading to yang deficiency which makes the body even more vulnerable to cold attack.

Endogenous Production of Turbid Dampness

Endogenous production of turbid dampness, or "internal dampness," refers to the morbid state marked by retention of water, dampness, phlegm and turbidity inside the body due to malfunction of the spleen in transportation, transformation and distribution of body fluid. Since internal dampness is closely associated with the spleen, it is also called production of dampness due to spleen deficiency.

Internal dampness is usually seen in fat people with overabundance of phlegmatic dampness inside the body, and is primarily caused by excessive intake of sweet and greasy or row and cold food which may impair the functions of spleen and stomach in transportation and transformation.

So it can be seen that the spleen plays a key role in the production and accumulation of fluid, phlegm, dampness and water. The transportation and transformation of the spleen rely on the warming, steaming and transforming functions of the kidney because the kidney yang is the root of all kinds of yang qi and is in charge of water. So if kidney yang is insufficient, the spleen will be involved, leading to endogenous production of water dampness. Since dampness is a yin pathogen which tends to impair yang qi, the symptoms of yang debilitation can also be seen.

Dampness is a yin pathogen characterized by heaviness, stickiness, and turbidity. So it tends to impair qi movements. Its clinical manifestations vary with the focuses at which dampness accumulates. For example, oppression in the chest or cough may appear if dampness invades the upper energizer; stomach and abdomen stuffiness, poor appetite, greasy taste in the mouth, or thick and slimy fur may manifest if dampness obstructs the middle energizer; sloppy stool and inhibited urination may occur if dampness stagnates in the lower energizer; edema may be seen if dampness permeates all over the skin and muscles; and swollen head or inflexible movements may be present if dampness lingers in the meridians.

Internal dampness and external dampness, although formed in different ways, are mutually affected once they come into existence. For instance, exogenous invasion of pathogenic dampness into the spleen will affect the spleen and produces internal dampness by impairing its function of transformation; and people with overabundant dampness may be vulnerable to external attack of pathogenic dampness.

Daily Exercises

1. What are the common types of imbalance between body fluid and qi- blood?
2. What are the pathogenetic characteristics of stagnancy of qi due to fluid retention, collapse of qi due to fluid depletion, dryness of blood due to fluid exhaustion, and stagnancy of blood due to fluid consumption?
3. What does endogenous production of five pathogenic factors refer to?
4. What are the common types and the pathogenetic characteristics of internal stirring of liver-wind?
5. What are the pathogenetic characteristics of endogenous production of pathogenic cold and endogenous production of pathogenic turbid dampness?

Endogenous Production of "Five Pathogenic Factors"

Impaired Fluid Transforming into Dryness

Impaired fluid transforming into dryness, also called internal dryness, refers to the morbid conditions marked by dryness and malnutrition of the related organs, orifices and tissues due to lack of body fluid. Insufficient body fluid is commonly caused by impairment of exuberant heat in exogenous febrile diseases, or excessive sweating, vomiting and purging, or massive bleeding because blood and fluid share the same origin, or insidious consumption by chronic consumptive diseases, etc.

Insufficient body fluid failing to moisten and nourish the viscera and orifices is characterized by dryness and hotness such as dry and lusterless skin with scurf or chap, dry throat and mouth, reddened tongue with little or no fur, absence of fluid, dry and painful eyes, dry nasal cavity, dry stool and scanty urine, etc.

Pathogenic dryness invading the stomach is marked by deficient stomach yin with dry mouth, preference for drinking, reddened tongue, and absence of fur; pathogenic dryness attacking the lung is characterized by dry cough with no sputum, or constipation if the large intestine lacks fluid.

Internal dryness, caused by consumption of yin fluid inside the body, is predominant in autumn and is often complicated by exogenous manifestations. So it is not difficult to be identified.

Endogenous Production of Fire-Heat

Endogenous production of fire-heat, commonly called internal heat or internal fire, refers to the hyperactive conditions marked by generation of fire-heat from the interior due to predominance of yang, debilitation of yin, obstruction of qi and blood, or stagnation of pathogenic factors transforming into heat, etc. Both fire and heat pertain to yang, and there is a saying indicating the connection between them, "fire is the extreme form of heat, whereas heat is the initial form of fire." Despite their similarity in pathogenesis and clinical manifestations, fire and heat differ in degree and may be divided into two types: deficiency and excess.

1. *Predominant yang transforming into fire*

Innate excess of yang in the body often becomes hyperactive and produces fire which scorches the body fluid. So it is called "vigorous fire" due to "excess of qi."

2. *Stagnation of pathogens transforming into fire*

Accumulation of pathogenic wind, cold, dryness or dampness may transform into fire if they are not expelled timely; and pathological products such as retention of fluid, phlegm and blood, if not removed immediately, may also produce fire.

3. *Hyperactivity of fire due to yin deficiency*

Depletion of yin-essence will lead to yang hyperactivity and endogenous production of deficient fire, marked by general manifestations of deficiency-heat such as reddened complexion in the afternoon, high fever, dry mouth and lips, or toothache and dry throat due to up-flaming of deficient fire.

4. *Hyperactivity of five emotions*

Hyperactivity of five emotions, or five emotional fires, is marked by overabundance of fire, heat and yang and malfunction of the viscera, yin and yang due to prolonged emotional depression transforming into fire. Since the five emotional fires are all related to the stagnation of liver qi, they are also regarded as a kind of liver fire.

SECTION 2 PATHOGENESIS OF THE MERIDIANS

Meridians, the passages connecting the human viscera, superficies, four limbs, five sensory organs and nine orifices, can circulate qi and blood of the whole body, connect the viscera with the limbs, link the interior with the exterior, and regulate the physiological functions of the internal organs and tissues. Pathogenesis of the meridians, the pathological changes due to invasion of pathogens into the meridians, is classified as relative exuberance or debilitation of qi and blood, circulatory disturbance of qi and blood, rebellious flow of qi and blood and depletion of qi and blood, and so on.

Relative Exuberance or Debilitation of Qi and Blood within the Meridians

Meridians can circulate qi and blood of the whole body, connect the viscera, tissues and organs, and regulate the physiological functions of qi, blood and the internal organs. So if qi and blood inside the meridians are relatively exuberant or debilitated, the physiological functions and the balanced state of the body will be affected. If the qi and blood within the meridians are exuberant, the pertaining viscera will be hyperactive in function; on the contrary, if qi and blood within the meridians are deficient, the pertaining viscera will be weak in function. For example, in *Ling Shu*, it is recorded that if the qi inside the stomach meridian of foot yangming is vigorous, there will be symptoms such as fever, polyorexia, and yellowish urine. If the meridian qi is insufficient, there will be chilly sensation, and stomach coldness and fullness, etc. From the above, it can be seen that the exuberance and debilitation of qi and blood inside the meridians can be influential on the functions of the related viscera.

Circulatory Disturbance of Qi and Blood within the Meridians

Circulatory disturbance of qi and blood within the meridians refers to the inhibited circulation of meridian qi which affects the flow of qi and blood and leads to pathological conditions of the related meridians or viscera. For example, in *Shang Han Lun*, it is stated that in taiyang disease, pathogenic wind-cold invade the taiyang meridian, leading to unsmooth flow of the meridian qi and pathological manifestations such as painful and stiff sensation in the head and neck, aversion to cold, and other symptoms related to the meridian; another point to note is that when pathogens invade the shaoyang meridian, there will be inhibited flow of meridian qi, presenting symptoms such as fullness of the chest and hypochondria, bitterness of the mouth, dryness of the throat, and dizziness, and so on.

Rebellious Flow of Qi and Blood within the Meridians

Rebellious flow of qi and blood within the meridians refers to the morbid conditions marked by abnormal uprising or sinking of qi and blood due to the vicious interaction between dysfunction of meridian qi and malfunction of qi and blood.

Rebellious flow of qi and blood can result in acute thoracic pain by disconnecting yin qi and yang qi of the body. Upward flowing of qi of the taiyang meridian may lead to upper excess symptoms marked by heaviness and distension of the head and lower deficiency symptoms marked by inability to walk, dizziness and tumbling down.

Rebellious flow of qi and blood can give rise to functional disorders of the related viscera. For example, the dysfunction of qi of the spleen meridian of foot taiyin may cause disorders of the stomach and intestines, marked by cholera with the symptoms of simultaneous vomiting and diarrhea.

Rebellious flow of qi and blood is also responsible for various bleeding symptoms. For example, liver fire invading the lung, marked by emptysis, is due to rebellious flow of qi of the liver meridian into the lung, which scorches the lung collaterals. Moreover, non-traumatic bleeding may be present when rebellious qi of the stomach meridian of foot yangming, combined with exuberant heat, attacks the upper energizer.

Depletion of Qi and Blood within the Meridians

Depletion of qi and blood within the meridians refers to the critical conditions of yin-yang separation and life termination due to depletion of meridian qi and the ensuing exhaustion of qi and blood. The clinical manifestations may be various due to the different functions of the meridians and related viscera.

Daily Exercises

1.　What are the pathogenetic characteristics of impaired fluid transforming into dryness and endogenous production of fire-heat?
2.　In which aspects is the pathogenesis of meridians reflected and what are their characteristics?

SECTION 3 PATHOGENESIS OF THE VISCERA

Visceral pathogenesis refers to the mechanisms of physiological dysfunction of the viscera in the occurrence and development of disease. The causes responsible for visceral dysfunction and diseases are various. In TCM, these causative factors are identified by analyzing the syndromes. So visceral pathogenesis plays a very important role in syndrome differentiation and treatment, and serves as the primary foundation for it.

TCM lays a particular stress on visceral pathogenesis; for example, in *Su Wen*, it was recorded, "All wind disorders and dizziness are attributed to the liver; all cold manifestations and contracture are attributed to the kidney; all stagnations of qi are attributed to the lung; all symptoms of dampness, edema, and fullness are attributed to spleen; and all pains, itching and ulcers are attributed to the heart." It was further developed by *Shang Han Za Bing Lun* and *Zhu Bing Yuan Hou Lun*, thus laying a firm foundation for the TCM visceral pathogenesis.

Visceral pathogenesis is reflected by the excess and deficiency of, or imbalance between, the physiological functions of zang-fu organs. Besides, the imbalance between yin and yang or qi and blood of the viscera per se are also important aspects of visceral pathogenesis. The yin, yang, qi and blood of the viscera pertain to, as well as correlate with, the yin, yang, qi and blood of the whole body. To master the visceral pathogenesis, the physiological functions of all the viscera may be well comprehended. Every TCM doctor should pay special attention to it, so as to build a firm foundation for syndrome differentiation.

Visceral pathogenesis is mainly classified into three categories: disorders of qi, blood, yin and yang of the five zang-organs, functional disorders of the six fu-organs, and functional disorders of the extraordinary fu-organs.

Disorders of Qi, Blood, Yin and Yang of the Five Zang-Organs

The disorders of qi, blood, yin and yang of the five zang-organs refer to the pathological state of functional abnormality of the five zang-organs due to dysfunction of their qi, blood, yin and yang. Since their functions are different, the disorders of qi, blood, yin and yang of the five zang-organs are also complicated.

Disorders of Qi, Blood, Yin and Yang of the Heart

(1) The heart is the monarch organ which governs all the viscera and life activities. Its main functions are to control blood and vessels as well as govern the spirit. The former propels blood circulation inside the vessels all around the body; while the latter is in charge of the mind, consciousness and thinking activities. This is due to the synthetic efforts of the cardiac yin, yang, qi and blood, the imbalance of which is mainly reflected in the aforementioned two major aspects of the cardiac functions.

The disorders of the heart yang and the heart qi are mainly manifested as relative exuberance or relative debilitation of heart yang qi.

(1) Relative exuberance of the heart yang qi is, in essence, the hyperactivity of the heart fire which is marked by either excess or deficiency. Pathogenic heat, phlegmatic fire or emotional depression may lead to excess fire; while mental overstrain may damage the heart yin and blood, leading to hyperactivity of deficiency fire. Clinically they are interchangeable, manifested in the following aspects.

Uneasiness of the heart spirit: yang qi is characterized by ascending and moving, so hyperactivity of the heart yang may disturb the spirit, leading to restlessness or hyperactivity of the heart sprit such as palpitation, vexation, insomnia, dreaminess, talkativeness, and even ravings.

Hastened blood flow driven by heat. Exuberance of heart yang produces heat while excess of heart qi generates fire, leading to accelerated circulation of blood inside the vessels with the symptoms of palpitation, fluster, rapid pulsation, reddened tongue with prickles, or even bleeding due to deviated flow of blood driven by heat.

Uprising of heart fire and downward moving of heart fire. The heart opens into the tongue and fire is characterized by flaming up, so uprising of the heart fire along the meridian is manifested as erosion of mucous membrane in the oral cavity, reddened tongue, and painful, eroded tongue tip with prickles. The heart and the small intestine are internally and externally related, so the downward migration of heart fire is marked by yellowish red urine with burning pain.

(2) The relative debilitation of heart yang, or deficiency of heart qi and heart yang, is a deficiency syndrome due to long-term consumption of healthy qi in chronic diseases. For example, insufficiency of pectoral qi will weaken its function of propelling qi and blood circulation inside the vessels; deficiency of the spleen qi will lead to internal obstruction of the heart vessels by turbid phlegm; and weakness of the kidney yang may result in insufficiency of heart yang due to water attacking the heart. Besides, severe debilitation of heart yang may also be seen in some acute diseases and is manifested in the following aspects.

Depression of heart spirit: Insufficiency of heart yang leads to weakened stimulation and enhanced depression of the spirit, consciousness, and mental activities, marked by spiritual lassitude, torpidity, somnolence and drowsy expression, etc.

Cold congealing the blood vessels. Deficiency of heart yang not only fails to effectively propel the blood, but also produces cold due to its weakened action of warming, leading to sluggish circulation or even stagnation of blood, marked by slow, knotted, intermittent, or unsmooth pulses, cold body, whitish complexion, palpitation, chest oppression with stabbing pain, spontaneous sweating, or even profuse sweating and depletion of yang, etc.

The relative debilitation of heart yang is related to other viscera such as the lung and kidney. Since both heart qi and lung qi are related to the pectoral qi, deficiency of heart qi may involve the lung qi by impairing the pectoral qi. Since deficiency of heart yang is developed on the insufficiency of heart qi, so deficiency of heart yang may involve the lung qi with the manifestations of weakened respiration, wheezing, palpitation and unsmooth blood flow, etc. Besides, if the deficiency of heart yang persists, the kidney yang may be involved, leading to deficiency of both with the manifestations of overflowing of water like edema, or panting with inability to lie flat and palpitation due to water qi attacking the heart.

2. Disorders of heart yin and heart blood are mainly manifested as insufficiency of heart yin, consumption of heart blood and stagnation of heart blood, etc.

(1) Insufficiency of heart yin, or deficiency of heart yin, is mostly due to mental overstrain, prolonged malnutrition and impairment of heart yin; or due to emotional depression transforming into fire which consumes the heart yin; or due to hyperactivity of liver fire or heart fire scorching the heart yin, and so on. Deficiency of heart yin is characterized by yin deficiency and yang hyperactivity with the manifestations of feverish sensation over the five centers, reddish complexion, night sweat, dry mouth and throat, reddened tongue, and thin-rapid pulse, etc. Another aspect of deficiency of heart yin is marked by uneasiness of heart spirit due to weakened action of tranquilization, manifested as restlessness, insomnia, and spiritual uneasiness, etc.

(2) Consumption of heart blood, or depletion of heart blood, is mostly due to excessive loss of blood or inadequate production of blood, or insidious consumption of heart blood by fires transformed from emotional depression, etc. Deficiency of blood is marked by insufficient blood inside

the vessels due to malnutrition with the manifestations of thin and feeble pulse, etc. Besides, it is also accompanied by general blood deficiency manifested as pale and lusterless complexion, mental and physical lassitude, and pale tongue and lips, etc. Another aspect of deficiency of heart blood is marked by mental derangement due to malnutrition of heart spirit, manifested as listlessness, distraction, absentmindedness, insomnia, dreaminess, palpitation or even fright and terror, etc.

(3) Stagnation of heart blood, or obstruction of heart vessels, refers to the morbid conditions marked by unsmooth or even obstructed circulation of blood. It is mostly due to deficiency of heart qi or heart yang, congealment of pathogenic cold, or accumulation of turbid phlegm inside the heart vessels, etc. It is often triggered or aggravated by overstrain or emotional factors. Stagnation of heart blood is marked by qi stagnancy and blood stasis due to unsmooth or obstructed blood circulation, with signs such as depressed or painful sensation in the pericardial region, terrified feelings, or even incessant ache, pale complexion, massive sweating, and even separation of yin and yang.

The following are the pathological conditions due to disorders of yin, yang, qi and blood of the heart. It is mainly classified into two types; dysfunction of the heart in controlling blood and vessels and malfunction of the heart in governing the spirit. So the common clinical manifestations of heart diseases are palpitation, vexation, insomnia, dreaminess, forgetfulness, constant laughter, or even delirium, mania and dementia, depressed or painful sensation in the pericardial region, coma, dark purplish complexion and nails, pale and lusterless complexion, knotted-intermittent pulse, thin-rapid pulse, scattered-large-rapid pulse, slow-unsmooth pulse, or deficient-large-feeble pulse, etc.

Daily Exercises

1. What is visceral pathogenesis?
2. What are the common types and pathogenetic characteristics of disorder of the heart yang and heart qi?
3. What are the common types and pathogenetic characteristics of disorder of the heart yin and heart blood?

Weekly Review

This week, we have studied the disorders of qi and blood, metabolism disturbance of body fluid, endogenous production of five pathogenic factors, pathogenesis of the meridians and disorders of qi, blood, yin and yang of the heart in visceral pathogenesis. Now we will have a review as follows.

Disorders of qi and blood refer to the pathological state due to insufficient qi and blood, abnormal physiological functions of qi and blood, and failure of qi and blood to promote each other.

The disorders of qi refer to the insufficient production or excessive consumption of qi, debilitation of some physiological functions of qi, as well as abnormal movements of qi.

The common forms are as follows.

Qi deficiency refers to the morbid conditions characterized by debilitated visceral functions and weakened disease-resistance ability due to insufficient primordial qi and functional disorder.

Qi stagnancy refers to dysfunction of some viscera and meridians due to unsmooth flow of qi movements.

Qi adverseness refers to the morbid state of abnormal ascent and descent of qi and reversal flow of visceral qi.

Qi sinking refers to the pathological state marked by failure of qi in ascending and lifting the lucid on the basis of qi deficiency.

Qi blockage refers to the pathologic state marked by impeded qi flow of entering and exiting.

Qi collapse refers to the pathologic state marked by severe prostration of healthy qi and sudden failure of body functions due to excessive loss of qi.

The disorders of blood refer to the pathological conditions of blood deficiency due to inadequate production or excessive loss of blood or weakened functions of blood in nourishment, accelerated blood flow driven by blood heat, blood stasis caused by sluggish blood circulation, and cold in the blood phase.

Clinically disharmony between qi and blood is mainly manifested as qi stagnancy with blood stasis, qi deficiency with blood stasis, failure of qi to control blood, qi collapse with blood depletion, and simultaneous deficiency of qi and blood, etc.

Abnormal metabolism of body fluid refers to the pathological conditions due to disordered production, distribution and excretion of body fluid. It is associated with qi movements and qi transformation, as well as the spleen, stomach, lung, liver, kidney and triple energizer, etc. It is mainly manifested as follows.

Insufficiency of body fluid refers to the pathological state marked by dryness due to inadequate body fluid failing to moisten and nourish the viscera, meridians, body constituents, orifices, skin and hair, etc. Jin and Ye are different to some degree.

Distribution disturbance of body fluid refers to the abnormal transportation and distribution of body fluid, leading to sluggish circulation or retention of body fluid marked by endogenous water-dampness and phlegmatic fluid, etc.

The excretion disturbance refers to the functional disorder of transforming body fluid into urine and sweat, leading to retention of water and edema.

Imbalance between qi-blood and body fluid is mainly manifested as stagnancy of qi due to fluid retention, collapse of qi due to fluid depletion, dryness of blood due to fluid exhaustion, and stagnancy of blood due to fluid consumption, etc.

The five endogenous pathogenic factors, caused by imbalance of visceral functions and disorders of qi, blood and body fluid in the occurrence and development of disease, are similar in manifestations to the exogenous pathogenic factors, namely wind, cold, dampness, dryness and fire.

Internal stirring of liver-wind refers to the morbid conditions marked by dizziness, spasm and tremor due to hyperactivity of yang or failure of debilitated yin to suppress the overabundant yang.

Liver-yang transforming into wind is usually caused by yin deficiency of the liver and kidney which fails to restrain the hyperactive yang and finally produces wind. It is commonly manifested as dizziness with tendency to fall, numbness and tremor of limbs, muscular twitching and cramp, deviated eyes and mouth, or even hemiparalysis, sudden fall, and excess-syncope or deficiency-syncope.

Extreme heat producing wind refers to the morbid state due to exuberant heat scorching body fluid and blazing nutrient blood, leading to malnutrition of the tendons and generation of wind. It is mainly manifested as convulsion, spasm, superduction, or even loss of consciousness and delirious speech.

Deficient yin stirring wind refers to the morbid state marked by muscular twitching, spasm, and involuntary movements of limbs due to deficient body fluid failing to moisten and nourish the muscles and tendons.

Blood deficiency engendering wind refers to the morbid state marked by co-existence of blood deficiency and wind disturbance due to malnutrition of the muscles and tendons.

Blood dryness generating wind refers to the morbid state marked by co-existence of blood-fluid deficiency and wind production due to malnutrition of the muscles and skin.

Endogenous production of cold, or internal cold, refers to the morbid state marked by overabundance of deficiency cold or yin cold originating from the interior due to debilitation of yang qi with weakened functions of warming and transforming.

Endogenous production of turbid dampness, or internal dampness, refers to the morbid state marked by retention of water, dampness, phlegm and turbidity inside the body due to malfunction of the spleen in transportation, transformation and distribution of body fluid.

Impaired fluid transforming into dryness, also called internal dryness, refers to the morbid conditions marked by dryness and malnutrition of the related organs, orifices and tissues due to lack of body fluid.

Endogenous production of fire-heat, commonly called internal heat or internal fire, refers to the hyperactive conditions marked by generation of fire-heat from the interior due to predominance of yang, debilitation of yin, obstruction of qi and blood, or stagnation of pathogenic factors transforming into heat, etc.

Pathogenesis of the meridians, the pathological changes due to invasion of pathogens into the meridians, includes relative exuberance or debilitation of qi and blood within the meridians, circulatory disturbance of qi and blood within the meridians, rebellious flow of qi and blood within the meridians and depletion of qi and blood within the meridians, and so on.

Relative exuberance or debilitation of qi and blood within the meridians can promote or inhibit the functions of the related viscera. Circulatory disturbance of qi and blood within the meridians can cause disorders of the related meridians and lead to qi stagnancy and blood stasis. Rebellious flow of qi and blood within the meridians can cause disorders of the related meridians. Depletion of qi and blood within the meridians can cause disorders of the related meridians or even lead to critical conditions of yin-yang separation and life termination.

Visceral pathogenesis refers to the mechanisms of physiological dysfunction of the viscera in the occurrence and development of disease. Visceral pathogenesis is marked by the excess and deficiency of the physiological functions of zang-fu organs as well as disorders of yin, yang, qi and blood of the viscera per se. It is an important aspect of TCM pathogenesis.

The pathogenesis of the heart is mainly disorders of qi, blood, yin and yang of the heart.

Relative exuberance of heart yang qi is, in essence, the hyperactivity of heart fire which may be divided into different morbid conditions such as uneasiness of the heart spirit, hastened blood flow driven by heat, uprising of heart fire and downward moving of heart fire, etc.

The relative debilitation of heart yang, or deficiency of heart qi and heart yang, is a deficiency syndrome marked by depression of heart spirit and cold congealing the blood vessels, etc.

Disorder of heart yin or heart blood is mainly manifested as insufficiency of heart yin, consumption of heart blood and stagnation of heart blood, etc.

Daily Exercises

1. Master the different morbid states of dysfunction of qi and blood.
2. Master the different morbid states of dysfunction of fluid metabolism.
3. Familiarize with the different morbid states of the five endogenous pathogenic factors.
4. Master the different morbid states of the disorders of yin, yang, qi and blood of the heart.

THE TWELFTH WEEK

Disorders of Qi, Blood, Yin and Yang of the Five Zang-Organs (Continued)

Disorders of Yin, Yang, Qi and Blood of the Lung

The lung, located above all the viscera like a canopy, is the place where exchange of qi takes place. The main functions of the lung is governing qi and in charge of respiration. It can also disperse and descend the nutrients and body fluid, regulate and dredge the waterways, and connect all the vessels to facilitate the heart in blood circulation. The disorders of yin, yang, qi and blood of the lung are mainly manifested as abnormal respiration, disordered production of qi and metabolism of body fluid, and failure to facilitate the heart to control blood circulation, etc.

The disorders of yin, yang, qi and blood of the lung are unique. Generally the insufficiency of yang qi of the lung is called deficiency of lung qi instead of deficiency of lung yang. And since all the blood vessels convene at the lung, blood deficiency of the lung is very rare. Hence, the pathological changes of the lung are mainly demonstrated in two aspects: the lung qi and lung yin.

1. *Disorders of lung qi*

The lung governs respiration and controls qi of the whole body. By dispersing and descending, it regulates qi movement and fluid metabolism of the whole body. So the disorders of lung qi are primarily manifested as abnormal dispersing and descending function of the lung and insufficiency of lung qi.

The dispersing function and descending function are two aspects of the ascending, descending, exiting and entering activities of lung qi. They are different from as well as closely associated with each other. The dysfunction of the lung in dispersing and descending is primarily due to invasion of exogenous pathogenic factors into the superficies and the lung, retention of phlegm and fluid in the air tube, attack of liver fire on the lung, and deficiency of lung qi or lung yin.

Failure of lung qi to disperse is a sign of respiratory malfunction of the lung marked by unsmooth respiration, nasal obstruction, unpleasant cough, wheezing, throat itching, frequent sneezing, or absence of sweat due to stagnation of defensive qi and failure of the lung to open the sweat pores, and liability to perspire due to weakness of defensive qi and failure of the lung to close the sweat pores.

Failure of lung qi to descend is also called dysfunction of lung qi in descending and purifying the respiratory tracts, marked by symptoms of adverse rising of lung qi such as cough, chest distress, panting, and wheezy phlegm, or symptoms of malfunction of the lung in regulating waterways such as scanty urine and edema, etc.

Deficiency of lung qi, or insufficiency of lung qi, is mostly caused by prolonged dysfunction of the lung in dispersing and descending, excessive overstrain impairing lung qi, or failure of the spleen to produce adequate qi. Deficiency of lung qi will debilitate the physiological functions of the lung, manifested as weakened respiratory function, reduced amount of gas exchange, and shortness of breath aggravated on exertion. Besides, it can also result in spontaneous sweating due to weakness of defensive qi unable to tighten the sweat pores; moreover, if fluid metabolism is involved, there will be retention of fluid, phlegm and water.

2. *Disorders of lung yin*

These are mainly due to pathogenic dryness or heat scorching the lung, turbid phlegmatic fire burning the lung, prolonged cough impairing the lung yin, or deficiency of the kidney yin involving the lung. Disorders of lung yin, or deficiency of lung yin, are marked by internal exuberance of fire due to attenuated moistening function of the lung fluid and deficiency of lung yin, with the symptoms such as dry cough, scanty and sticky sputum, dry mouth and throat, flushed cheeks, feverish sensation over the five centers (the palms, soles and heart), high fever, reddened tongue, scarce fur, thin-rapid pulse, or even bloody sputum.

The aforementioned are all about disorders of qi, blood, yin, and yang of the lung, which falls into two major aspects: disorders of lung qi and disorders of lung yin. So clinically lung diseases are generally manifested as cough, shortness of qi, wheezing, asthma, chest oppression and pain, coughing-up of sputum and blood or bloody sputum, spontaneous sweating and hoarse voice, etc.

Disorders of Yin, Yang, Qi and Blood of the Spleen

The main physiological functions of the spleen are to transform water and food into nutrients and transport them so as to nourish the whole body. So the spleen is called the postnatal foundation and the source for production of qi and blood. The spleen also controls blood and prevents it from deviation; besides, the spleen governs ascending of the lucid so as to disperse the water and food nutrients to the heart, lung, head and eyes, and to sustain the normal position of the internal organs. The pathological conditions of the spleen is marked by hypofunction of transporting and transforming water and food nutrients, inability to ascend, disorder of distributing and excreting body fluid and loss of control in blood circulation, etc.

1. *Disorders of spleen qi and spleen yang*

Deficiency of the spleen may be characterized by internal retention of water-dampness due to dysfunction of the spleen in transportation and transformation, bleeding due to failure of the spleen in controlling blood, and inability to ascend or sinking of middle qi due to weakness of spleen yang. Therefore, the disorder of spleen qi and spleen yang is mainly manifested as the deficiency of spleen qi and spleen yang.

Deficiency of spleen qi, or insufficiency of middle qi, is primarily caused by improper diet, emotional depression, excessive contemplation, overstrain, poor body constitution, or consumption by chronic diseases. Deficiency of spleen qi is marked by manifestations of reduced digestive functions such as anorexia, indigestion of food and abdominal distension; or by manifestations of insufficient production of qi and blood such as etiolate complexion, emaciation, speechlessness and lassitude; or by manifestations of sinking of middle qi such as dizziness, sinking sensation in the lower abdomen, diarrhea, anal prolapse or even visceroptosis; or by manifestations of qi failing to control blood such as bloody stool, excessive menses and muscular bleeding, etc.

Deficiency of spleen yang is mostly developed from deficiency of spleen qi, or caused by excessive intake of uncooked or cold food and insufficiency of kidney yang. Deficiency of spleen yang is characterized by hypofunction of warming and promoting, with signs such as cold and pain in the stomach and abdomen, watery diarrhea with indigested food in the stool, and diarrhea before dawn. If the spleen fails to effectively transport and transform the body fluid, there will be retention of fluid, water and phlegm. So spleen deficiency is closely associated with retention of water-dampness and edema.

2. Disorders of spleen yin

These are mainly manifested as deficiency of spleen yin. The spleen qi is the material foundation for spleen yin and since yin and yang are interdependent and inter-affected, deficiency of spleen yin may generally involve deficiency of spleen qi, leading to simultaneous deficiency of spleen qi and spleen yin. In other words, deficiency of spleen yin is mostly developed on the basis of deficiency of spleen qi. Besides, deficiency of spleen yin may also be caused by excessive contemplation, overstrain, impairment by deficient fire, insufficiency of kidney yin, and long-term overtake of spicy and dry food or herbs.

Deficiency of spleen yin is, as a matter of fact, the insufficiency of both spleen qi and spleen yin, so it is manifested on the one hand as symptoms of weakened digesting and absorbing functions due to deficiency of spleen qi marked by torpid intake, abdominal distension and loose stools, and on the other hand as symptoms of malnutrition and inadequate moistening due to deficiency of spleen yin marked by dry mouth and throat, reddish tongue with scanty fur, and emaciation, etc.

Deficiency of spleen qi, spleen yang and spleen yin are both different from and closely related to each other. Deficiency of spleen qi is the basis, marked by weakened food-transforming function, lucid-ascending function, and blood-controlling function. If there are no cold or dry manifestations, the syndrome of spleen-qi deficiency is simple. However, if it is accompanied by cold manifestation and debilitated warming function, this syndrome will transform into deficiency of spleen yang; and if deficiency of spleen qi is accompanied by dry manifestation due to malfunction of fluid distribution, it will turn into deficiency of spleen yin.

The above-mentioned are pathological conditions of disorders of qi, blood, yin and yang of the spleen, mainly manifested as the disorders of spleen qi, disorders of spleen yang and disorders of spleen yin. So clinically spleen diseases are generally manifested as poor intake of food, loose stools, pain, distension and fullness in the abdomen and lassitude, or jaundice, anal prolapse, metroptosis, hemafecia, metrorrhagia-metrostaxis, and peliosis, etc.

Daily Exercises

1. What are the common types of disorders of yin, yang, qi and blood of the lung?
2. What are the pathogenetic characteristics of failure of the lung to disperse and descend?
3. What are the pathological characteristics of deficiency of lung qi and lung yin?
4. What are the common types of disorders of yin, yang, qi and blood of the spleen?
5. What the pathological characteristics of deficiency of spleen qi and spleen yang?
6. What are the pathological characteristics of deficiency of spleen yin?

Disorders of Qi, Blood, Yin and Yang of the Five Zang-Organs (Continued)

Disorders of Yin, Yang, Qi and Blood of the Liver

The main physiological functions of the liver are controlling free flow of qi and storage of blood. The liver being in charge of free flow of qi ensures the smooth circulation of blood and body fluid, unrepressed fluctuation of emotions and normal movements of visceral qi. The liver stores enough amount of blood so as to restrict hyperactivity of liver and maintain free flow of qi. The liver is marked by firmness, activeness and ascent, so the liver qi and liver yang are constantly in excess while liver blood and liver yin are generally in deficiency. This is the pathological characteristic of disorders of liver yin, yang, qi and blood.

1. Disorders of liver qi and liver yang. The liver is marked by firmness, and liver qi and liver yang are constantly in excess, so disorders of liver qi and liver yang are generally manifested as the hyperactivity of liver qi and

liver yang whereas deficiency of liver qi and liver yang is seldom seen. The hyperactivity of liver yang and liver qi is marked by stagnation of liver qi and up-flaming of liver fire.

(1) Stagnation of liver qi, or liver stagnation for short, is mostly due to emotional depression, chronic consumption, or impairment by other viscera. Malfunction of the liver in promoting free flow of qi is responsible for stagnation of liver qi within the related meridians and viscera, marked by depression, hypochondriac or lower abdominal distension, frequent sighing, and belching, etc.

If qi stagnates in the chest and hypochondriac region, there will be distension, fullness and pain in the costal regions or the right hypochondriac region; if there is stagnation of qi and phlegm or stagnation of qi and blood, localized mass or accumulation, or gall and globus hysteritis will be present; if the liver attacks the stomach, there will be belching, acid regurgitation, or even gastric pain; if the liver qi invades the spleen, there will be rugitus and diarrhea with or without pain. Besides, prolonged stagnation of liver qi may transform into fire because excess of qi can generate fire, leading to up-flaming of liver fire.

(2) Up-flaming of liver fire is caused by stagnation of liver qi transforming into hyperactive fire. It is mostly due to emotional depression transforming into fire or sudden anger impairing the liver, leading to hyperactivity of liver fire. It is characterized by excessive ascending of yang qi accompanied by fire. Fire, a heat pathogen pertaining to yang, is active by nature. So up-flaming of liver fire is marked by ascending, hotness and activeness, clinically manifested as reddish complexion and eyes, headache and distension of head, irascibility, sudden tinnitus or deafness of the ear, reddened tongue, and rapid pulse, etc. Excessive ascending of liver yang or impairment of the collaterals by liver fire are manifested as bleeding symptoms such as coughing-up blood when the lung collaterals are impaired, and vomiting of blood when stomach collaterals are scorched. If the situation of up-flaming of liver fire persists, hyperactivity of fire with yin deficiency will eventually take place, thus further consuming the yin fluid.

2. Disorders of liver yin and liver blood. These are mainly marked by insufficiency of liver yin and live blood, leading to uncurbed ascending of

liver yang such as hyperactivity of liver yang and internal stirring of liver wind. Therefore the disorders of liver yin and liver blood are mainly manifested as deficiency of liver yin and liver blood, and the ensuing hyperactivity of liver yang and internal stirring of liver wind.

(1) Deficiency of liver yin, or insufficiency of liver yin, is marked by functional debilitation of tranquilizing, moistening, nourishing and restraining actions of yang heat. It is mostly due to stagnation of the liver transforming into fire and consumes yin, malnourishment of the liver by insufficiency of kidney yin, or impairment of liver yin by intruding pathogenic heat at the late stage of exogenous febrile diseases. Deficiency of liver yin is often manifested as hot or dry manifestations such as flushed complexion, feverish sensation over the five centers (the palms, the soles and the heart), dry mouth and throat, and reddened tongue, etc. Besides, there are also such symptoms as blurred vision, dry eyes, or even spasm, tremor and involuntary movements of the hands and feet, etc.

(2) Hyperactivity of liver yang is mainly transformed from deficiency of liver yin, or developed on the basis of deficiency of liver yin. It is a morbid state marked by uncurbed yang exuberance due to insufficiency of liver yin. Since liver and kidney share the same origin, deficiency of liver yin is often accompanied by insufficiency of kidney yin, and hyperactivity of liver yang is characterized by upper excess and low deficiency. The former refers to the excessive ascending of liver yang with signs such as head distension, dizziness, flushed complexion, red eyes, tinnitus, irascibility and vexation, etc. The latter refers to the deficiency of kidney yin or liver yin in the lower energizer with the manifestations of waist soreness, lumbago, or weak legs and knees, etc.

(3) Deficiency of liver blood is a reflection of general blood deficiency in the liver. The liver stores blood, so it is closely related to blood deficiency of the whole body. Deficiency of liver blood is mostly caused by excessive loss of blood, prolonged consumption of liver blood in chronic diseases, or inadequate production of blood due to deficiency of the spleen and stomach. It is mainly manifested as pathological changes of the eyes, tendons and nails due to malnutrition such as dry and painful eyes, blurred vision, inhibited extension and flexion of the limbs, spasms, muscular tremor, or pale nails, etc. Besides, it is also accompanied by general blood

deficiency such as lusterless complexion, dizziness, lassitude, and pale tongue and lips, etc.

(4)   Internal stirring of liver wind refers to the morbid conditions marked by uncurbed hyperactivity of liver yang and excessive ascending of yang qi. It is mainly caused by malnutrition of liver yang due to insufficient liver yin or liver blood, malnutrition of tendons due to prolonged consumption of yin blood by chronic diseases, or invasion of exuberant pathogenic heat. The most common one, however, is deficiency of liver yin or kidney yin failing to restrain the hyperactive liver yang. Internal stirring of liver wind is manifested in milder cases as dizziness, muscular tremor, and involuntary movements of the feet and hands and, in severer cases, as convulsion of the limbs, or even coma and partial paralysis. In some exogenous febrile diseases, when exuberant heat fails to restrain the hyperactive yang and generates wind, there will be manifestations such as high fever, spasm, convulsion, syncope, and even delirium and coma. This syndrome is also called exuberant heat produces wind.

The above-mentioned are pathological conditions of disorders of yin, yang, qi and blood of the liver, mainly manifested as disorders of liver qi and liver yang and disorders of liver yin and liver blood. The common symptoms of liver diseases are dizziness, parietal headache, bilateral hypochondriac pain, breast distension and pain, lower abdominal pain, cyst pain, inhibited movements of the joints, contraction of tendons, numbness and spasms of the four limbs, irascibility, emotional depression, and taut pulse, etc.

Disorders of Qi, Blood, Yin and Yang of the Kidney

The main function of the kidney is to store essence, which contains genuine yin and genuine yang and serves as the postnatal foundation. The kidney essence, constantly nourished and supplemented by cereal nutrients after birth, is the foundation for life and the root of yin and yang. Only when kidney essence is replenished and kept full can physiological functions of the kidney come into full play. The kidney also governs water and receives qi, which works to regulate the distribution and excretion of body fluid and assist the lung to inhale the lucid qi. The pathological manifestations of the kidney are mainly manifested as insufficient kidney essence qi and imbalance between kidney yin and yang.

1. Insufficiency of kidney essence qi. Kidney essence qi, including kidney essence and kidney qi, is a combination of kidney yin and yang and the material foundation for physiological functions of the kidney. Insufficiency of kidney essence qi is mainly manifested as deficiency of kidney essence and lack of kidney qi.

(1) Depletion of kidney essence refers to the inadequate storage of essence inside the kidney, marked by attenuated promoting effect on the growth, development and reproduction of the body, as well as on the nourishment of the bones, marrows, teeth and hair, etc. It is mostly caused by impairment of the kidney essence in chronic diseases, insufficient production of kidney essence due to senility, consumption of kidney essence by excessive sexual activities, and poor innate endowment of congenital essence. It is generally manifested in children as hypoevolutism, weak or deformed bones, inadequacy of kidney essence and brain marrow, underdevelopment of intelligence, and retarded growth of teeth; in young people as delayed arrival of tiangui, maldevelopment of sexual functions, presenility, loss of teeth, early whitening of hair, or poor sexual activities; and in old people as flaccidity of the lower limbs, difficulty in walking, lags in response, deafness, and fragile bones, etc.

(2) Lack of kidney qi refers to the pathological changes marked by insufficient kidney qi and debilitated functions in storage and reception. It is mostly caused by insufficient production of kidney essence due to prematurity, decline of kidney essence due to senility, indulgence in sexual activities and prolonged consumption by chronic diseases. Insufficiency of kidney qi is mainly manifested as attenuated function of storage such as premature ejaculation, nocturnal emission, involuntary emission, clear and thin leucorrhea, incessant extramenstral vaginal bleeding, habitual abortion, bed-wetting, urinary incontinence, and slipping diarrhea, etc. Moreover, it can also lead to inefficient reception of qi marked by shallow breath and panting on exertion, etc.

2. Imbalance between kidney yin and kidney yang. Kidney yin and kidney yang, an essential part of kidney essence, is the root of yin and yang

of the whole body. They represent the physiological functions of the kidney and are mutually restricted and coordinated, thus maintaining the normal physiological functions of the kidney. The imbalance between kidney yin and kidney yang are primarily manifested as deficiency of kidney yin and deficiency of kidney yang.

(1) Deficiency of kidney yin refers to lack of kidney yin with the pathological conditions marked by hypofunction of yang heat in nourishing, moistening, tranquilizing and restraining. It is mostly caused by innate deficiency of yin, emotional depression transforming into fire and scorching kidney yin, excessive sexual activities impairing kidney yin, severe and chronic diseases consuming kidney yin, or over intake of warm and dry herbs damaging yin, etc. Deficiency of kidney qi is manifested as emaciation, dry mouth and throat, insomnia, dreaminess, tinnitus, waist soreness and lower limb flaccidity. Besides, if deficiency of yin fails to restrain yang, there will be high fever, flushed cheeks, feverish sensation over the five centers (the palms, the soles and the heart), night sweat, thin-rapid pulse, and red tongue with scanty fur, etc.; if the kidney fails to restrict the hyperactive yang, there will be rampancy of kidney fire marked by nocturnal emission and premature ejaculation, etc.

(2) Deficiency of kidney yang, or insufficiency of kidney yang, is a morbid state marked by hypofunction in warming, promoting, activating and qi-transforming. It is mostly due to chronic diseases, senility, excessive sexual activities, or innate deficiency of yang. It is manifested as intolerance of cold, cold limbs, weary lying, pale and moistening tongue, thin-weak pulse, and pale complexion. If spleen yang and kidney yang are deficient, there will be diarrhea with undigested food or diarrhea before dawn. If there are disturbance of fluid metabolism, there will be phlegm retention, fluid retention, and edema. Besides, there are deficiency symptoms of the kidney such as weakness and soreness of the waist and knees, tinnitus, impotence, cold sperm, or sterility due to cold in the uterus, etc.

The above-mentioned are pathological conditions of yin, yang, qi and blood of the kidney, mainly manifested as insufficiency of kidney essence qi and imbalance between kidney yin and kidney yang. Clinically the common kidney diseases are marked by impotence, involuntary emission, premature ejaculation, soreness and weakness of the loins and knees, flaccidity of the lower limbs, panting, tinnitus, deafness, nocturnal emission, bone heat with high fever, forgetfulness, unsmooth urination, frequent urination, incontinent urination and edema, etc.

Daily Exercises

1. What are the common types of disorders of yin, yang, qi and blood of the liver?
2. What are the pathological characteristics of stagnation of liver qi and up-flaming of liver fire?
3. What are the pathological characteristics of deficiency of liver yin, hyperactivity of liver yang, deficiency of liver blood and internal stirring of liver wind?
4. What are the common types of disorders of yin, yang, qi and blood of the kidney?
5. What are the pathological characteristics of deficiency of kidney essence and insufficiency of kidney qi?
6. What are the pathological characteristics of deficiency of kidney yin and deficiency of kidney yang?

Functional Disorders of the Six Fu-Organs

Functional disorders of the six fu-organs refer to the morbid state marked by functional disorders of the six fu-organs caused by pathogenic factors.

Functional Disorders of the Gallbladder

The main physiological function of the gallbladder is to store and excrete bile, which is transformed from the surplus qi of the liver. The secretion and excretion of the bile, as a result, is regulated by the liver with the functions of governing free flow of qi. So the normal function of the gallbladder is closely determined by the function of the liver in governing free flow of qi.

The disorder of the gallbladder in secreting and excreting bile can be caused by emotional depression and failure of the liver to regulate free flow of qi, or due to accumulation of damp-heat in the middle energizer or the liver and gallbladder. Conversely, the disorder of the gallbladder in secreting and excreting bile can aggravate the malfunction of the liver in regulating free flow of qi, leading to manifestations of distension and pain in the chest and hypochondriac region, etc. If damp-heat drives the bile out of the gallbladder and flow all over the skin, there will be presence of jaundice. If stagnation of gallbladder qi transforms into heat, goes upward and disturbs the mind accompanied by phlegm, there will be distension in the chest and hypochondriac region, vexation, and insomnia, etc. If the gallbladder qi is insufficient, symptoms such as terror and panic will occur.

Functional Disorders of the Stomach

The stomach, a sea of water and cereal, is characterized by unobstructed and downward transportation and has the functions of receiving and digesting water and food. The functional disorders of the stomach is mainly about the malfunction of the stomach in receiving and digesting water and food as well as the adverse rising of stomach qi due to failure of the stomach to descend.

Functional disorders of the stomach are generally manifested as deficiency of the stomach qi, deficiency of the stomach yin, cold in the stomach, heat in the stomach, and food retention in the middle energizer, etc.

1. Deficiency of stomach qi

This refers to the morbid state marked by hypofunction of the stomach in receiving and digesting water and food. It is mainly caused by impairment of stomach qi due to improper diet, poor innate constitution, and chronic diseases, etc. Deficiency of stomach qi will lead to malfunction of reception and digestion and is manifested as poor appetite and food intake, or anorexia, etc. Failure of the stomach to descend is marked by gastric and abdominal distension, fullness and pain, etc. Adverse rising of stomach qi is characterized by nausea, vomiting, belching and hiccups, etc.

2. Deficiency of stomach yin

This refers to the morbid state marked by functional disorders due to insufficient yin fluid of the stomach. It is mostly caused by chronic diseases consuming stomach yin, or exuberant heat damaging yin and involving the stomach at the late stage of febrile diseases. Deficiency of stomach yin may weaken the ability of the stomach in reception and digestion of water and food, leading to manifestations such as poor appetite and food intake, red tongue with little or no fur, or even mirror-like tongue, belching, unproductive vomiting, and gastric and abdominal distension and fullness, etc.

3. *Stomach cold*

This refers to the morbid state marked by functional disorders of the stomach due to invasion of pathogenic cold. It is generally caused by impairment of stomach yang due to excessive intake of cold and uncooked food, or innate cold-deficiency in the middle energizer, etc. Pathogenic cold often invades the stomach and damages the stomach yang, leading to hypofunction of digestion, with signs such as distension after intake of food and indigestion, etc. Cold can also congeal and stagnate qi and blood, leading to severe pain in the stomach, pale complexion and cold limbs, etc.

4. *Stomach heat, or stomach fire*

This refers to the morbid state marked by hyperfunction of the stomach in digestion of water and food due to heat in the gastric region. It is generally caused by emotional depression transforming into fire, with signs such as polyorexia, bulimia, thirst with desire for cold drinks and constipation, etc. Besides, fire is characterized by flaming-up, so there are also manifestations of adverse rising of stomach qi marked by nausea and vomiting of sour and bitter juice; if the stomach fire flames upwards along the meridians, there will be manifestations such as red, swelling and painful gums; if stomach fire scorches the collaterals or vessels, symptoms of non-traumatic bleeding and vomiting of blood will be present.

5. *Retention of food in the middle energizer*

This refers to the morbid state marked by abnormal ascending and descending of qi due to accumulation of food in the stomach. It is mostly caused by overtake, accumulation and indigestion of food. Abnormal ascending and descending of qi due to accumulation of food in the stomach is manifested as distending pain in the stomach, frequent belching, increased breaking of wind, foul breath and stink vomitus and excreta.

Functional Disorders of the Small Intestine

The main physiological functions of the small intestine are to receive and transform foodstuff as well as separate the lucid from the turbid. Functional disorder of the small intestine is mostly due to improper diet and contraction of damp-heat or damp-cold, etc. Malfunction of reception is marked by abdominal pain, diarrhea or vomiting; dysfunction of transformation is characterized by abdominal distension after food intake and indigestion; failure of the small intestine to separate the lucid from the turbid is manifested as diarrhea and unsmooth urination; shifting of fire-heat from the small intestine to the urinary bladder is marked by frequent or painful urination with burning sensation and red color. Clinically most disorders of the small intestine are attributed to the spleen and stomach.

Functional Disorders of the Large Intestine

The main physiological functions of the large intestine are to transport and transform residues as well as govern fluid. Functional disorders of the large intestine are mostly caused by failure of the stomach qi or lung qi to descend, internal accumulation of dryness and heat, insufficient production of intestinal fluid, or contraction of damp-heat or damp-cold, etc. Clinically, depletion of intestinal fluid will lead to malfunction of transportation and transformation marked by dry stools or constipation; pathogenic damp-water in the intestine is marked by loose stools, diarrhea and tenesmus due to unsmooth flow of qi; and weakness of kidney qi or sinking of middle qi is marked by chronic diarrhea, slipping diarrhea, and anal prolapse, etc.

Functional Disorders of the Urinary Bladder

The main physiological functions of the urinary bladder are to store and discharge urine. The functional disorders of the urinary bladder are mostly caused by abnormal qi transformation due to invasion of pathogenic damp-heat, or malfunction of the urinary bladder due to kidney deficiency. Disorders of the urinary bladder are generally manifested as frequent urination, urgent urination, painful urination, turbid urine, dripping urination, scanty urine, suppression of urine, bed-wetting and incontinence of urination.

Functional Disorders of the Triple Energizer

The triple energizer, a collective term for the upper, middle and lower energizers, serves as the passage for the ascending, descending, entering and exiting activities of qi, as well as the distribution and excretion of body fluid. The disorders of triple energizer are mostly caused by dysfunction of the viscera, so the disorders of qi activities of the triple energizer are generally manifested as dysfunction of qi activities of the viscera. For example, disorder of qi activities of the upper energizer is marked by failure of the lung to disperse and descend, or insufficiency of heart qi; disorder of qi activities of the middle energizer is marked by abnormal ascending and descending actions of the spleen and stomach, or inability of the liver to regulate free flow of qi; disorder of qi activities of the lower energizer is marked by malfunction of the large intestine in transportation, or inhibited qi transformation of the kidney and urinary bladder, etc. The qi transformation of the triple energizer, together with other functions of the lung, spleen and kidney, can regulate the circulation of body fluid. So if the lung in the upper energizer fails to disperse and descend as well as regulate the waterways, or if the spleen in the middle energizer fails to transport and transform normally, and if the kidney in the lower energizer weakens in steaming ability and qi transformation, the triple energizer will be affected, resulting in malfunction of qi transformation marked by internal retention of water-dampness, water-fluid, and edema, etc.

Functional Disorders of the Extraordinary Fu-Organs

Functional Disorders of the Brain

The brain, an extremely important organ to the human body, dominates the spiritual, cognitive and mental activities of body as well as the seeing, hearing, smelling, tasting, speaking and moving abilities of different organs or constituents of the body. The disorders of the brain, is primarily manifested as dysfunction or malfunction of the aforementioned abilities. These are mostly caused by insufficient production of brain marrow, deficiency of yin, yang, qi and blood of the whole body, emotional depression or stimulation, and retard development of the brain or deteriorated brain functions due to senility, etc. Disorders of the brain are commonly manifested as dizziness, lags in response, poor memory, hearing and seeing inability, depression or abnormal spiritual and mental activities, etc.

Functional Disorders of the Bone and Marrow

Marrow, including bone marrow, brain marrow and spinal marrow, is located inside the bones and can nourish the bones and the brain to promote development of the body and maintain normal physiological cerebral functions. The bones, the framework of the human body, are capable of protecting the viscera and ensuring their physiological functions. Disorders of the marrow and bone are mostly caused by general insufficiency of qi, blood, yin and yang, deficiency of kidney essence due to poor innate constitution, consumption of essence-blood due to excessive sexual abilities, or impairment of essence-blood due to chronic diseases, etc. The pathological changes of the marrow are generally manifested as cerebral malfunctions due to insufficient brain marrow. These changes are primarily characterized by malnutrition of the bone, with signs such as poor development, flaccidity, deformation, or bone fracture, etc.

Functional Disorders of the Vessel

As the house of blood, the vessel can circulate qi and blood within itself. Its functional disorders are mostly caused by malnutrition of the vessel due to depletion of body fluid, unsmooth movements of qi due to internal accumulation of turbid phlegm, or obstruction of the vessel due to cold congealment, qi stagnation and blood stasis, etc. The pathological changes of the vessel are mainly manifested as unsmooth circulation of qi and blood, localized pain, distension, swelling and numbness, or bleeding symptoms due to failure of the spleen to control blood.

Functional Disorders of the Uterus

The uterus, or womb, is also called the palace of the fetus in TCM. Its main physiological functions are to govern menstruation and conceive the fetus. Its functional disorders, however, are mostly caused by the influence of other viscera, the malfunction of thoroughfare meridian and conception meridian, or the contraction of exogenous pathogenic factors. Its functional disorders are generally manifested as abnormalities in the menses, leucorrhea, pregnacy and delivery. If the liver fails to store blood, or the spleen fails to control blood, or heat exists in the blood, there will be excessive bleeding of the uterus with signs such as preceeded menorrhea, excessive menstrual blood volume, prolonged menstrual period, or incessant vaginal bleeding, etc. If qi and blood are insufficient, or qi and blood are obstructed, there will be menstrual colic, amenorrhea, and unsmooth or inhibited menstruation, etc. If the functions of the liver, heart, spleen and kidney debilitate, there will be abnormalities of the uterus in pregnancy and delivery. If damp-heat invades the uterus, there will be profuse leucorrhea. In other words, the disorders of the uterus are closely associated with the viscera and meridians of the whole body.

The human body is an organic whole, and the disorders of the viscera, meridians, yin and yang, qi and blood are mutually affected, leading to a complicated pathological state marked by simultaneous malfunction of different viscera such as deficiency of both the heart and spleen, invasion of the liver into the stomach, attack of the liver fire on the lung, and yang deficiency of both the spleen and the kidney. Given the limited length of writing, we will not discuss them here in detail.

Daily Exercises

1. What are the common types of functional disorders of the six fu-organs and what are their respective pathological characteristics?
2. What are the common types of functional disorders of the extraordinary fu-organs and what are their respective pathological characteristics?

CHAPTER 11

Life Cultivation, Therapeutic Principles and Methods

Life cultivation is also called life preservation or life protection. Life has its own cycle of birth, growth, maturity, aging, and death. Despite the limited life span, human beings can enjoy longevity if they have a strong body constitution with powerful disease-resistance capacity as well as mental and physical soundness. Life cultivation is exactly a way to strengthen the body constitution, improve the body's resistance against diseases and adaptability to natural environment. It can also reduce the incidence of diseases, minimize the impairment incurred by diseases, and delay the aging process so as to attain longevity. From the above, we can see that life cultivation is of great significance to the improvement of body constitution, prevention of diseases and promotion of longevity.

Therapeutic principle, the rule for disease treatment, is the essential constituent of syndrome differentiation and treatment in TCM with prevalent guiding significance for different branches of clinical Chinese medicine from establishment of the treating regimen to prescription and medication, etc.

Therapeutic method, also a constituting part of syndrome differentiation and treatment, is the specific curative method formulated under the direction of therapeutic principle.

SECTION 1   LIFE CULTIVATION

Life cultivation is a proactive method for the improvement of body constitution, prevention of diseases and promotion of longevity. It is created by the ancient people who recognized the intimate and delicate correspondence between man and nature and mastered the rules of the occurrence and development of diseases as well as the normal physiological activities of the human body. *Nei Jin* accords great importance to the prevention of diseases, and under such a therapeutic philosophy, a complete set of life cultivation regimen was created. It is of profound national characters and practical efficacy, contributing significantly to the prevention of diseases for the later generations.

The Basic Principles of Life Cultivation

To promote health, improve immunity, prevent diseases and enjoy longevity, the ancient people summarized a set of principles on the basis of practice, namely compliance with the seasonal changes, emphasis on physical exercises, cultivation of mentality and spirit, regulation of diet and lifestyle, and obviation of pathogens, etc.

Compliance with the Seasonal Changes

In *Ling Shu* (*Miraculous Pivot*, 灵枢), it is said that man should be in full compliance with nature. Seasonal alternation plays an important role in the birth, growth and death of all things on earth. Under the influence of seasonal changes, all living things in nature follow the cycle of birth, growth, harvest and storage. So the four seasons, together with yin and yang, are regarded in *Su Wen* (*Plain Conversation*, 素问) as the root and dominator of myriads of things on earth, incompliance of which will lead to occurrence of diseases and disasters, and submission to which will result in elimination of even the most refractory diseases. Hence, people should follow the rhythm of seasonal alternation in their daily lives to adapt themselves to the external environmental changes and ward off exogenous pathogenic factors. This is not only an important measure for disease prevention, but also a principle for life cultivation.

Emphasis on Physical Exercise

Physical exercise is a proactive approach for the prevention of diseases created by the ancient people. Life lies in motion, so the survival of the human race is closely related to exercise, just as the old saying goes,

"Running water is never stale and a door-hinge never gets worm-eaten." TCM believes that physical exercise can facilitate the flow of qi and blood, lubricate the joints, strengthen the tendons and muscles, and promote the functions of the viscera so as to ward off diseases and enjoy longevity. The amount of exercise, however, should be moderate. A well-balanced regimen between rest and exercise, if practiced with perseverance, can be efficacious.

Cultivation of Mentality and Spirit

One of the most important aspects of life cultivation is the cultivation of mentality and spirit because mental activities are closely associated with diseases. Long-term adverse emotional stimulation can cause the occurrence of diseases by impairing the normal physiological functions of the human body. In *Su Wen*, it was recorded, "excessive anger impairs the liver, excessive joy impairs the heart, excessive contemplation impairs the spleen, excessive grief impairs the lung and excessive fear impairs the kidney" and "excessive anger drives qi to move upwards; excessive joy relaxes the activity of qi; excessive contemplation stagnates qi; excessive grief exhausts qi; excessive fear drives qi to move downwards; excessive fright disturbs qi; and excessive anxiety depresses qi." Under normal circumstances, the seven emotions will not cause diseases; however, sudden, violent or prolonged emotional stimuli beyond certain limitations will cause visceral disorders and diseases. It is evident that the seven emotions are very important to the health of the human body. So we should be in full compliance with the external environment and avoid the adverse stimuli to the body. A quiet natural surrounding, a stable social environment, a happy family background, and a good interpersonal relationship are all indispensable to the normal maintenance of human emotions. Once the emotional stimulation goes to extremes, prompt self-regulation should be performed to stabilize the agitated emotions and maintain a good mood.

Regulation of Diet and Lifestyle

Proper diet and lifestyle are very important to the health of the body. Excessive drinking and eating, or indulgence in alcohol and sexual activities often leads to diseases.

In TCM, diet is regarded as an important factor responsible for the occurrence of disease. Nutrients from food are indispensable to the sustaining of life, excessive eating and drinking or intake of putrid or poisonous food, however, may lead to diseases. So food prohibition or preference should be taken notice of so as to keep a scientific, reasonable and well-balanced diet.

TCM holds that appropriate physical exercise is beneficial to the body. However, overstrain may consume the healthy qi and excessive rest may also be detrimental to the health of the body. So moderate exercise, or a balance of rest and work, should be implemented. Besides, excessive sexual activities are also harmful to the body, so the ancient doctors always stressed the importance of continence and essence-preservation.

Warding off Pathogenic Factors

Warding off pathogenic factors is also an important aspect of life cultivation. It is the first principle of disease prevention pointed out in *Su Wen*. Some diseases may be contagious, but a powerful healthy qi inside the body will ward off the infectious factors. So we should preserve the healthy qi to ward off pathogenic factors at the same time of evading the pestilent qi. Besides, some medicines can be taken as a way of warding off the pathogens. In conclusion, avoidance of pestilent qi, preservation of healthy qi and pre-comsumption of medicine are three effective approaches for the obviation of pathogens and the prevention of diseases.

Daily Exercises

1. What are the clinical significances of life cultivation?
2. What are the basic principles of life cultivation?

The Main Methods of Life Cultivation

Life cultivation is of great significance to the improvement of body constitution and the prevention of diseases. So the ancient people developed many effective methods for life cultivation during their long-term practice.

Life Cultivation by Following Climatic Changes

It is a method for life preservation by keeping in compliance with the rhythm of seasonal climatic changes. Human beings should follow the cycle of seasonal alternation and adjust their diet and lifestyle so as to strengthen the body constitution and get accustomed to the climatic variations. In spring and summer, when yang qi is predominant, everything flourishes, so it is time for people to preserve yang by sleeping late and rising early or going outside for exercises. In this way they keep a good mood, get rid of the stale, and take in the fresh. In autumn and winter, when yin becomes predominant and yang gets restrained, everything tends to contain their essence and luster inside. So it is time for people to astringe yang and preserve yin by resting early and rising early, or resting early and rising late, and taking measures to ward off cold. In this way they store yin essence inside and keep yang qi from dissipating. In other words, there are different regimens for different seasons, and only by keeping in compliance with the seasonal changes can one be safe and sound.

Regulation of Emotions

This is a method for life preservation by constantly regulating emotions to be in a good mood. It requires people to keep a peaceful and joyful mind, a good mood and a purified or lofty spirit. Moderate exercise, such as walking or jogging, are recommended to promote the circulation of qi and blood, facilitate the movements of the tendons, and coordinate the functional activities of the viscera. As a result, the body can be refreshed and the mind can be carefree. When something bad happens, it is advised to divert one's attention to other things and let out the depressed emotions so that the normal state of mind is recovered.

Abstinence from Excessive Coitus to Conserve Essence

Essence, qi and spirit are considered to be the three treasures of the body by the ancients. Among them, essence can transform into qi and generate spirit. So essence is the root of qi and spirit, or the foundation for life activities. Yin essence is apt to be used-up and takes a long time to recover, so excessive sexual activities will inevitably lead to yin depletion that threatens health. In this sense, the ancient people valued the practice of abstinence from excessive coitus so as to conserve essence and promote longevity.

Life Cultivation by Diet

This is an important aspect of life cultivation in TCM. Nutrients from water and food are the source for the production and transformation of qi and blood. In TCM, there is a saying that food and medicine share the same origin. So diet regulation is also an important way to prevent and treat diseases. Sun Simiao, a famous doctor in the Tang dynasty, said that food can expel pathogens and nourish the viscera, or refresh the mind and supplement qi and blood, so excellent doctors often use dietary therapy to regulate emotions and cure diseases.

To cultivate life by diet, it should be kept in mind that the amount of food should be moderate, the types of food should be well-balanced and the time of meals should be regular. While eating, one should chew and swallow the food slowly and carefully so as to fully absorb the nutrients instead of gluttonizing without discrimination. The diet should be light because over intake of any of the five flavors may impair the body. Oily or indigestible food should be prohibited. Food that is too cold or too hot is also prohibited because it may impair the spleen and stomach. Besides, medicinal diet is advisable to treat some diseases after analyzing the types of body constitution. For example, people with qi deficiency can take food with qi-replenishing herbs, whereas people with yin deficiency can take food with yin-nourishing herbs.

Life Cultivation by Exercise

This is an important aspect of life preservation in TCM with a rich collection of experience. TCM holds that the body is the house of life and the existence of life relies on the body, so by exercising, the body will become strong and powerful, the essence qi will flow smoothly, and the spleen and stomach will be vigorous in digestion so as to nourish the body with nutrients.

The ancients have developed many methods. For example, moderate physical work can adjust the mental activities, promote circulation of qi and blood, and strengthen the bones and tendons. Walking is also a good way for life cultivation, especially a brisk walk after meals, which is conducive to the promotion of digestion. There is a folk saying which goes, "a hundred steps after meals, a long-living person happier than immortals." Walking around inside the house before rest is also beneficial to sleeping. Besides, the ancient Chinese cultivated their life by dancing, which was initiated in the periods of Spring-Autumn and Warring states. They believed that dancing can promote the circulation of qi and blood and soothe or activate the tendons and collaterals. Daoyin is the most frequently used method for life cultivation, represented by Wu Qin Xi (five-animal frolic), Tai Ji Quan (traditional Chinese shadow boxing), and Ba Duan Jin (Eight-sectioned Exercise), etc.

Life Cultivation by Tuina, Acupuncture and Moxibustion

Tuina, or Chinese massage, is a method for regulating yin, yang, qi and blood so as to strengthen the body, as well as prevent and treat diseases by applying certain manipulations on some specific regions of the body surface. It can be self-applied or performed by specialists after careful selection of acupoints and manipulations on the basis of syndrome differentiation. The effects can be satisfactory.

Acupuncture and moxibustion include needling method and moxa-fumigating method. Acupuncture is used for the regulation of meridian qi, yin and yang or qi and blood so as to strengthen the body and treat diseases by stimulating certain acupoints with needling manipulations.

Moxibustion is used to promote the circulation of qi and blood, strengthen the healthy qi, improve the body's resistance ability, maintain health and treat diseases by fumigating certain acupoints with ignited moxa products. It should be carried out on the basis of syndrome differentiation according to the differences in constitution or illnesses.

Life Cultivation by Medication

It is unique to TCM because Chinese herbs can strengthen the body and prevent diseases as well as treat diseases. So these who are weak or old can enhance their health by using Chinese herbs. This method is also applicable to the normal people. According to the differences in body constitution, the herbs are grouped into qi-nourishing herbs, blood-replenishing herbs, yin-supplementing herbs and yang-invigorating herbs. The kidney and the spleen, being the prenatal foundation and postnatal foundation respectively, are often nourished to promote health by doctors after the differentiation of body constitutions. The preparing forms can be various, such as single-herb prescription, compound prescription, patent prescription, or ointment prescription, etc. All of them are efficacious.

Weekly Review

In this week, we studied the disorders of qi, blood, yin and yang of the lung, spleen, liver and kidney, the functional disorders of the six fu-organs and extraordinary fu-organs, and life cultivation. Now we will take a brief review as follows:

The disorders of qi, blood, yin and yang of the lung are mainly manifested in two aspects: lung qi and lung yin.

Disorders of the lung qi are mainly manifested as malfunction of the lung in dispersion and descent and the deficiency of lung qi.

Failure of lung qi to disperse is a sign of respiratory malfunction of the lung marked by unsmooth respiration, nasal obstruction, unpleasant cough, wheezing, throat itching, frequent sneezing, and absence of sweat or sweating.

Failure of lung qi to descend is also called dysfunction of lung qi in descending and purifying the respiratory tracts, marked by symptoms of adverse rising of lung qi such as cough, chest distress, panting, and wheezy phlegm, or symptoms of malfunction of the lung in regulating waterways such as scanty urine and edema, etc.

Deficiency of lung qi, or insufficiency of lung qi, is manifested as weakened respiratory function, reduced amount of gas exchange, and shortness of breath aggravated on exertion. Besides, it can also result in spontaneous sweating.

Disorders of lung yin, or deficiency of lung yin, are marked by internal exuberance of fire due to deficiency of lung yin failure of lung fluid to moisten the body, with signs such as dry cough, scanty, sticky or even bloody sputum, dry mouth and throat, feverish sensation over the five centers (the palms, soles, and heart), and reddened tongue with scarce fur, etc.

Disorders of yin, yang, qi and blood of the spleen are mainly manifested as deficiency of spleen qi, deficiency of spleen yang and dysfunction of spleen yin, etc.

Deficiency of spleen qi, or insufficiency of middle qi, is marked by manifestations of reduced digestive functions such as anorexia, indigestion of food and abdominal distension; or by manifestations of insufficient production of qi and blood such as etiolate complexion, emaciation, speechlessness and lassitude; or by manifestations of sinking of middle qi such as dizziness, sinking sensation in the lower abdomen, diarrhea, anal prolapse or even visceroptosis; or by manifestation of qi failing to control blood such as bloody stool, excessive menses and muscular bleeding, etc.

Deficiency of spleen yang, or insufficiency of spleen yang, is characterized by hypofunction of warming and promoting, with the manifestations of cold and pain in the stomach and abdomen, watery diarrhea with indigested food in the stool, and diarrhea before dawn, as well as fluid retention, phlegm retention and edema.

Dysfunction of spleen yin, or deficiency of spleen yin, is mainly developed from deficiency of spleen qi, so it is manifested on the one hand as symptoms of weakened digesting and absorbing functions due to deficiency of spleen qi such as torpid intake, abdominal distension and loose stools, and on the other hand as symptoms of deficiency of spleen yin such as dry mouth and throat, reddish tongue with scanty fur, and emaciation, etc.

Disorders of yin, yang, qi and blood of the liver are mainly manifested as stagnation of liver qi, up-flaming of liver fire, deficiency of liver yin, hyperactivity of liver yang, deficiency of liver blood, and internal stirring of liver wind, etc.

Stagnation of liver qi, or liver stagnation for short, is mostly due to malfunction of the liver in dredging and dispersing or unsmooth flow of qi. It is commonly manifested as depression, hypochondriac or lower abdominal distension, frequent sighing, and belching, etc. Besides, there are also clinical manifestations of liver depression leading to qi stagnation, liver qi invading the stomach, or liver qi invading the spleen, etc.

Up-flaming of liver fire is caused by stagnation of liver qi transforming into hyperactive fire. It is manifested as reddish complexion and eyes, headache and distension of head, irascibility, sudden tinnitus or deafness of the ear, reddened tongue, and rapid pulse, etc. Besides, there are bleeding symptoms due to impairment of the collaterals by liver fire.

Deficiency of liver yin, or insufficiency of liver yin, is marked by functional debilitation of yang heat in tranquilizing, moistening, nourishing and restraining. It is often manifested as hot or dry manifestations, marked by flushed complexion, feverish sensation over the five centers (the palms, soles, and heart), dry mouth and throat, and reddened tongue, etc. Besides, there are also symptoms such as blurred vision, dry eyes, or even spasm, tremor and involuntary movement of the hands and feet, etc.

Hyperactivity of liver yang is mainly developed from deficiency of liver yin, or on the basis of deficiency of liver yin. It is characterized by upper excess and low deficiency. The former refers to the excessive ascending of liver yang with the manifestations of head distension, dizziness, flushed complexion, red eyes, tinnitus, irascibility and vexation, etc. And the latter refers to the deficiency of kidney yin or liver yin in the lower energizer with the manifestations of waist soreness, lumbago, or weak legs and knees, etc.

Deficiency of liver blood is a reflection of general blood deficiency in the liver. It is mainly manifested as pathological changes of the eyes, tendons and nails due to malnutrition such as dry and painful eyes, blurred vision, inhibited extension and flexion of the limbs, spasm, muscular tremor, or pale nails, etc. Besides, it is also accompanied by symptoms of general blood deficiency.

Internal stirring of liver wind refers to the morbid conditions marked by uncurbed hyperactivity of liver yang and excessive ascending of yang qi. It is manifested as dizziness, muscular tremor, involuntary movement of the feet and hands, convulsion of the limbs, or even coma and partial paralysis.

Disorders of qi, blood, yin and yang of the kidney are mainly manifested as insufficiency of kidney essence, insufficiency of kidney qi and deficiency of kidney yin and deficiency of kidney yang.

Depletion of kidney essence refers to the inadequate storage of essence inside the kidney, marked by attenuated promoting effect on the growth, development and reproduction of the body as well as on the nourishment of the bones, marrows, teeth and hair, etc. It is generally manifested in children as hypoevolutism, weak or deformed bones, inadequacy of kidney essence and brain marrow, underdevelopment of intelligence, and retard development of teeth; in young people as delayed arrival of tiangui, maldevelopment of sexual functions, presenility, loss of teeth, early whitening of hair, or debilitated sexual activities; and in old people as flaccidity of the lower limbs, difficulty in walking, lags in response, deafness, and fragile bones, etc.

Lack of kidney qi refers to the pathological changes marked by insufficient kidney qi and debilitated functions of storage and reception. Insufficiency of kidney qi is mainly manifested as attenuated function of storage such as premature ejaculation, nocturnal emission, involuntary emission, clear and thin leucorrhea, incessant extramenstral vaginal bleeding, frequent abortion, bed-wetting, urinary incontinence, and slipping diarrhea, etc.

Deficiency of kidney yin refers to lack of kidney yin with the pathological conditions of weakened functions of yang heat in nourishing, moistening, tranquilizing and restraining. Deficiency of kidney yin is manifested as emaciation, insomnia, dreaminess, tinnitus, waist soreness and lower limb flaccidity, high fever, feverish sensation over the five centers (the palms, soles, and heart), night sweat, thin-rapid pulse, and red tongue with scanty fur, etc.

Deficiency of kidney yang, or insufficiency of kidney yang, is a morbid state marked by weakened actions of warming, promoting, activating and qi-transforming on the whole body. It is manifested as intolerance of cold, cold limbs, weary lying, pale and moistening tongue, thin-weak pulse, and pale complexion. If spleen yang and kidney yang are deficient, there will be diarrhea with undigested food or diarrhea before dawn. If there are disturbance of fluid metabolism, phlegmatic fluid, water fluid, and edema will be seen. Besides, there are deficiency symptoms of the kidney such as weak and sore waist and knees, tinnitus, impotence, cold sperm, or sterility due to cold in the uterus, etc.

Functional disorders of the six fu-organs refer to the morbid state due to malfunctions of the gallbladder, stomach, small intestine, large intestine, urinary bladder, and triple energizer, etc.

The disorders of the gallbladder are closely related to failure of the liver to regulate free flow of qi, and mainly manifested as disturbances in secretion and excretion, marked by distension and pain in the chest and hypochondriac region, presence of jaundice, and terror or panic.

Functional disorders of the stomach are generally manifested as deficiency of the stomach qi, deficiency of the stomach yin, cold in the stomach, heat in the stomach, and food retention in the middle energizer, etc.

Deficiency of stomach qi refers to the morbid state marked by hypofunction of the stomach in receiving and digesting water and food. It is manifested as poor appetite, anorexia, gastric and abdominal distension and pain, nausea, vomiting, belching and hiccups, etc.

Deficiency of stomach yin refers to the functional disorders due to insufficient yin fluid of the stomach. It is mainly manifested as poor appetite and food intake, red tongue with little or no fur, or even mirror-like tongue, belching, unproductive vomiting, and gastric and abdominal distension and fullness, etc.

Stomach cold refers to the functional disorders of the stomach due to invasion of pathogenic cold. It is manifested as gastric pain and distension after intake of food, pale complexion and cold limbs, etc.

Stomach heat, or stomach fire, refers to the hyperfunction of the stomach in digestion of water and food due to heat in the gastric region. It is generally manifested as polyorexia, bulimia, thirst with desire for cold drink and constipation, vomiting of sour and bitter juice, red, swelling and painful gums, and foul breath, etc.

Retention of food in the middle energizer refers to the abnormal ascending and descending of qi due to accumulation of food in the stomach. It is manifested as distending pain in the stomach, frequent belching, increased breaking of wind, foul breath and stink vomitus and excreta, etc.

Functional disorders of the small intestine refer to the abnormal reception, transformation and separation of the lucid from the turbid. It is marked by abdominal pain, diarrhea or vomiting, and unsmooth urination. Clinically most disorders of the small intestine are attributed to the spleen and stomach.

Functional disorders of the large intestine refer to the malfunctions of the large intestine in transportation and transformation of dregs as well as governance of fluid. It is commonly marked by dry stools and constipation, or chronic diarrhea, slipping diarrhea, or prolapse of the anus, etc.

Disorders of the triple energizer refer to the abnormal movement of qi within the triple energizer and malfunction of fluid in distribution and excretion. The common manifestations are about inhibited qi movements of the related viscera in the upper, middle or lower energizer such as unsmooth urination, retention of fluid, dampness and water, etc.

Functional disorders of the extraordinary fu-organs refer to the malfunction of the brain, marrow, bones, vessels and uterus. Each of them has its unique pathogenesis.

Disorders of the brain are commonly manifested as dizziness, lags in response, poor memory, hearing and seeing inability, abnormal spiritual or mental activities, etc.

Functional disorders of the bone and marrow are mainly manifested as cerebral malfunctions due to insufficient brain marrow. The pathological changes of the bone are primarily characterized by malnutrition of the bone, with signs such as poor development, flaccidity, deformation, or bone fracture, etc.

The pathological changes of the vessel are mainly manifested as unsmooth circulation of qi and blood, localized pain, distension, swelling and numbness, or bleeding symptoms.

Functional disorders of the uterus are generally manifested as abnormalities of the menses, leucorrhea, fetus and delivery.

The basic principles of life cultivation are compliance with the seasonal changes, emphasis on physical exercises, cultivation of mentality and spirit, regulation of diet and lifestyle, and prevention of diseases, etc.

The main methods of life cultivation are cultivation of life according to seasonal variations, regulation of emotions, abstinence from excessive sexual activities, adjustment of diet, emphasis on exercise, and application of tuina, acupuncture and moxibustion, or medication, etc.

Daily Exercises

1. Grasp the pathological conditions marked by disorders of qi, blood, yin and yang of the lung, spleen, liver and kidney.
2. Grasp the pathological conditions marked by functional disorders of the six fu-organs and extraordinary fu-organs.
3. Comprehend the basic principles and methods of life cultivation.

THE THIRTEENTH WEEK

SECTION 2   THERAPEUTIC PRINCIPLES

Therapeutic principle, the rule for treating diseases, is a constituent part of syndrome differentiation and treatment in TCM. It is made by generalizing the symptoms and signs collected through the four diagnostic methods into a certain syndrome or disease under the guidance of TCM theories. So syndrome differentiation is a prerequisite, or the basis, for therapeutic principles and the following medications. In other words, the establishment of therapeutic principles is of great significance to the treatment of diseases.

The commonly used basic therapeutic principles are treatment of disease before occurrence, treatment of disease in terms of root, regulation of yin and yang, regulation of qi and blood, regulation of the viscera, and treatment of disease in accordance with three factors (climate, individuality, and locality).

Treatment of Disease before Occurrence

Traditional Chinese medicine accords great importance to this principle, which can be discussed in terms of prevention of disease, early treatment of disease and preparation for transmission of disease.

Prevention before occurrence refers to the adoption of preventive measures before the occurrence of diseases. A doctor who excels at this practice is referred to as "the superior doctor." For the prevention of diseases, there is a rich collection of theories and practices in TCM such as the basic principles and methods of life cultivation introduced in the previous week.

Early treatment refers to the prompt diagnosis and treatment of a disease during its early stage so as to control the disease and prevent it from further developing. Hence there is an old saying that the superior doctor treats a disease during its infancy.

Early treatment requires a knee observation of the doctor who can discern the subtle signs of abnormality during the very beginning of a disease, and thus take timely measures to prevent it from deteriorating. Early diagnosis and treatment, however, require a full comprehension of the rules of the occurrence and development of diseases. For example, in

Shang Han Lun (*Treatise on Febrile Diseases*), it was pointed out that at the early stage of taiyang disease, the symptoms of aversion to cold and a floating pulse appear before the manifestation of fever, so as long as these main symptoms are noticed, the doctor can make a timely diagnosis. It also holds that once the disease occurs, it should be promptly addressed. As for the miscellaneous diseases due to internal damage, they also have their intrinsic patterns; for example, failure of the liver in governing free flow of qi may lead to stagnation of liver qi, and chronic stagnation of liver qi may cause hyperactivity of liver yang which may subsequently result in internal stirring of liver wind. Therefore, only if the doctors learn these intrinsic patterns, prompt diagnosis and treatment can be made to prevent the disease from further developing.

Preparation for transmission of disease means to prevent disease from further developing. Each disease has its own way of developing, and the responsibility of a doctor is to control the disease by either taking proactive measure or adopting preventive measures. An excellent doctor can control the disease by fully comprehending its developing patterns. For example, according to the theory of five elements, liver disease is apt to involve the spleen, so the doctor should take preventive measures to reinforce the spleen, making it insusceptible to invasion by the liver. In *Shan Han Lun* (*Treatise on Febrile Diseases*), it was also pointed out that in the treatment of taiyang disease, the meridian of foot yangming can be needled for consolidation and prevention of pathogens from transmitting. In another example, Ye Tianshi, a famous doctor in the Qing dynasty, pointed out in *Wen Ren Lun* (*Treatise on Warm-Heat Diseases*) that when pathogenic heat sinks into the nutrient phase with eruptions, it is prone to further invade the lower energizer which is deficient at the time, so the kidney yin should be reinforced with salty and cold herbs, apart from the sweet and cold ones, to prevent the disease from developing.

Treatment of Disease from the Root

In *Su Wen*, it was pointed out that a disease must be treated by focusing on its root. In other words, the essence of the disease must be found and treated, which is an indispensible basic principle for treatment in TCM. The root of a disease, or the essence of it, is the nature of this disease reflected by its etiology or pathogenesis. Hence the ancient doctors also put forth the idea of seeking causative factors by discerning the syndromes. There is a rich collection in this aspect, but we only discuss treatment of the primary aspect and treatment of the secondary aspect as well as routine treatment and contrary treatment.

Treatment of the Primary Aspect and Treatment of the Secondary Aspect

Primary aspect and secondary aspect are a pair of comparative concept. As far as the etiology and symptom are concerned, the former is the primary aspect and the latter is the secondary aspect; as far as the sequence of disorders is concerned, the initial disorder is the primary aspect and the following one is the secondary aspect. In this sense, treatment of the primary aspect and treatment of the secondary aspect refer to the prioritization of treatment procedures on the basis of analyzing the syndromes and diseases. Commonly the secondary aspect is firstly treated in acute diseases and the primary aspect, or both the primary aspect and secondary aspect, takes priority in chronic diseases.

Treating the Secondary Aspect in Acute Diseases

In the development of diseases, if some symptoms are extremely severe and life-threatening, or if some new acute disorders develop on the basis of old diseases, these symptoms and disorders should be addressed immediately even if they are the secondary aspects. For example, in shaoyang disease, the patient will have alternated chills and fever or bitterness and fullness sensation in the chest and hypochondria, which could be cured with Xiao Chai Hu Decoction. However, if acute abdominal pain deficient and cold in nature appears at the same time, the pain, being the secondary aspect, should be relieved by using Xiao Jian Zhong Decoction and subsequently Xiao Chai Hu Decoction, to treat the root of the disease. Besides, abdominal flatulence and unsmooth urination and defecation are also secondary aspects acute in nature, so they should be treated with priority. Treating the secondary aspect in acute diseases is also a way of targeting at the principal contradiction.

Treating the Primary Aspect in Chronic Diseases

In less severe or recovery period of a disease when healthy qi becomes deficient and pathogenic factors still remain, treatment of the primary aspect can be implemented if there are no acute symptoms or syndromes at this time. For instance, patients with indigestion due to spleen deficiency may be manifested as poor appetite and distension after intake, and may also be accompanied by lassitude, lack of speech and shortness of qi; since the secondary aspects are not urgent, the primary aspect shall be addressed by nourishing qi.

The two principles are actually the prioritization of treatment procedures on the basis of syndrome differentiation. They are comparative, not absolute. Under special circumstances, the primary aspect could also be treated at first. For example, sometimes patients are manifested with cold limbs, diarrhea with undigested food, and interior deficiency-cold of shaoyin, and meanwhile are accompanied by aversion to cold and fever. In this case, although the deficiency-cold of shaoyin is the primary aspect, it should be addressed with Hui Yang Jiu Ni Decoction to restore yang and then with Gui Zhi Decoction to relieve the exterior. For the above, we can see that the principles used clinically are very flexible.

Simultaneous Treatment of the Primary and Secondary Aspects

This refers to the treatment of the primary aspect and secondary aspect at the same time because the two are both severe, or closely related. For instance, exterior syndrome of taiyang, due to misuse of purgation, may be accompanied by deficiency-cold diarrhea; in this case, Guizhi Renshen Decoction should be used to simultaneously relieve the interior and the exterior. Renshen is used to treat deficiency-cold diarrhea and Guizhi is applied to relieve the exterior. Simultaneous treatment of the primary aspect and secondary aspect does not mean to put the essential aspect and the non-essential aspect on an equal footing, but emphasize on a certain aspect. Guizhi Renshen Decoction is just an example of simultaneous treatment of the primary aspect and secondary aspect with particular emphasis on addressing deficiency-cold diarrhea in the interior.

Daily Exercises

1. What are the meanings of therapeutic principles?
2. What are the meanings of treatment before occurrence?
3. How to understand treatment of the primary aspect and treatment of the secondary aspect?

Routine Treatment and Contrary Treatment

Routine treatment and contrary treatment are also referred to as regular treatment and paradoxical treatment. Clinical manifestations are generally the reflection of the disease, and under most circumstances they are not contradictory; for example, heat manifestations may be a reflection of heat syndrome, and excess manifestations are presented in excess syndromes. For some special or complicated disorders, however, their clinical manifestations may be contradictory to the essence, or even be false. The false manifestations reflect the essence of a disease from the contrary aspect. Hence, before giving corresponding treatment, the doctors should see through the false manifestations and seize the essence of the disease. Routine treatment and contrary treatment are exactly the therapeutic principles made according to the above-mentioned situations. Both of them are an embodiment of "treating disease in terms of the root."

Routine Treatment

Routine treatment refers to the treatment of diseases in contradiction to the manifestations. It is also called reverse treatment in which the actions of the herbs are contradictory to the manifestations of the disorder. For example, herbs cold in nature are used to treat heat syndromes, and herbs tonifying in nature are applied to treat deficiency syndromes. They are common therapeutic principles. Generally there are many principles of this kind such as treating cold syndrome with herbs hot in property, treating heat syndrome with herbs cold in property, treating deficiency syndrome with herbs tonifying in action and treating excess syndrome with herbs purging in action, etc.

1. *Treating cold syndrome with herbs hot in property*

This refers to a therapeutic principle of treating cold syndromes or disorders by using herbs warm or hot in nature. For example, exuberance of yin cold due to yang deficiency, marked by cold limbs, diarrhea with undigested food, thin and feeble pulse, aversion to cold and weary lying on bed, is treated with herbs or prescriptions pungent in flavor and warm in property to restore the depleted yang. In another example, external contraction of pathogenic wind-cold, marked by fever, aversion to cold, headache, or floating and tense pulse, is treated with herbs or prescriptions pungent in flavor and warm in property to relive the exterior.

2. *Treating heat syndromes with herbs cold in property*

This refers to the therapeutic principle of treating febrile syndromes or disorders with herbs or prescriptions cool and cold in nature. For example, invasion of pathogenic heat into the interior, manifested as high fever, profuse sweating, red tongue, yellow fur and rapid pulse, should be treated with herbs or prescriptions cool or cold in nature to clear away heat. In another example, invasion of pathogenic heat into the nutrient phase, manifested as fever, thirst with desire for drinking, unclear macular eruption, dark red tongue and rapid pulse, should be treated with herbs or prescriptions with the functions of clearing away heat in the nutrient phase and cooling blood.

3. *Treating deficiency syndromes with herbs tonifying in action*

This refers to the therapeutic principle of treating deficiency syndromes or disorders with herbs or prescriptions with the function of nourishment. For example, qi deficiency syndrome, marked by lassitude, lack of speech, shortness of qi, sweating on exertion, pale tongue, or thin and feeble pulse, should be treated with herbs or prescriptions with the function of supplementing qi; for another example, bloody deficiency syndrome, characterized by lusterless or etiolate complexion, pale lips and nails, dizziness, palpitation, insomnia, numbness in the feet and hands, pale and scanty menses, pale tongue, and thin and feeble pulse, should be treated with herbs or prescriptions with the function of replenishing blood.

4. Treating excess syndrome with herbs purging in action

This refers to the therapeutic principle of treating excess syndromes with herbs with the function of expelling pathogenic excess. For example, interior excess-heat syndrome, marked by high fever, delirium, abdominal stiffness and pain, constipation, and a sinking, excessive and forceful pulse, can be treated with herbs or prescriptions cool and cold in property for purgation. "Purging," however, cannot be simply interpreted as purgation. Rather, it should be regarded as elimination of pathogenic factors in a broader sense, such as treating exterior-cold excess syndrome with herbs pungent in flavor and warm in property to relieve the exterior, or treating syndrome of exuberant interior heat with herbs cool and cold in property to clear away heat.

Contrary Treatment

Contrary treatment, also called compliance treatment, refers to the therapeutic principle of treating disease in compliance with the false manifestations. The properties of the herbs or prescriptions conform to the false manifestations of the syndrome or disorder. Since the false manifestations still reflect the essence of a disease, but from the contrary aspect, this principle is, in essence, still a way of treating diseases by focusing on the root. There are many types of this principle, such as treating heat syndromes with herbs hot in property, treating cold syndromes with herbs cold in property, treating obstructive disorders with herbs nourishing in action and treating diarrhea with herbs unblocking in action, etc.

1. Treating heat syndromes with herbs hot in property

This refers to the therapeutic principle of using herbs or prescriptions hot in property to treat syndromes of genuine cold and false heat. For example, in *Shang Han Lun*, it was mentioned that predominant yin rejecting yang is marked by symptoms of exuberant yin-cold such as diarrhea with undigested food, cold limbs and extremely feeble pulse; at the same time, it is also accompanied by symptoms of false heat such as non-aversion to cold and red complexion. Since its essence is exuberance of cold in the interior with false heat in the exterior, Tongmai Sini Decoction, pungent in flavor and warm in property, can be used to restore yang. This is called treating heat syndromes with herbs hot in property.

2. *Treating cold syndromes with herbs cold in property*

This refers to the therapeutic principle of using herbs or prescriptions cold in nature to treat syndromes of genuine heat and false cold. For example, in S*hang Han Lun*, it was mentioned that syndrome of coldness in the extremities due to blockage of excessive heat in the interior is marked by high fever, thirst with preference for cold drink, red tongue, yellow fur and rapid pulse; at the same time it is also accompanied by peripheral coldness or cold limbs. Since its essence is exuberance of heat in the interior with false cold in the exterior, Bai Hu Decoction or Cheng Qi Decoction, pungent cold or bitter cold in nature, can be used to treat this disease. This is what is called treating cold syndromes with herbs cold in property.

3. *Treating obstructive disorders with herbs nourishing in action*

This is also called unblocking obstruction by nourishment, and refers to the therapeutic principle of using herbs or prescriptions with the functions of nourishment to treat blocked syndromes. For instance, deficiency of spleen qi is marked by anorexia, lassitude, pale tongue and void pulse; meanwhile, it is also accompanied by gastric and abdominal distension and fullness after food intake, or irregular abdominal distension, and unsmooth defecation, etc. These obstructive symptoms are caused by spleen deficiency, so they can be treated by herbs or prescriptions with the functions of replenishing qi and invigorating the spleen. This is called treating obstructive disorders with herbs nourishing in action.

4. *Treating diarrhea with herbs unblocking in action*

This refers to the therapeutic principle of using herbs or prescriptions dredging or unblocking in action to treat diarrhea due to stagnation of pathogenic excess. For example, in *Shang Han Lun*, diarrhea with retention is marked by both diarrhea and retention of dry stools due to abundance of interior heat; in this case, Cheng Qi Decoction can be used to clear away heat for promoting defection. This is called treating diarrhea with herbs unblocking in action. Besides, bleeding syndromes due to internal retention of blood stasis is often treated by activating blood to eliminate stasis so that bleeding is checked. It is also a specific application of this principle.

Reinforcing Healthy Qi and Expelling Pathogenic Factors

The occurrence and development of disease is actually a struggle between the pathogenic factors and healthy qi, the result of which determines the prognosis of the disease. Hence, reinforcing the healthy qi to expel pathogenic factors is a basic principle of treating diseases in TCM.

Reinforcing the healthy qi refers to the supplement of healthy qi, the strengthening of body constitution, and the improvement of body's resistance against diseases. To reinforce the healthy qi, herbs with the function of nourishment are often used; besides, there are other methods such as acupuncture and moxibustion, qi exercise, physical exercise, mental regulation, and diet adjustment, etc. This principle is applicable to syndromes with deficiency of healthy qi and non-exuberance of pathogenic factors.

The types of deficiency should be firstly clarified before applying this principle, such as supplementing qi in case of qi deficiency, warming yang in case of yang deficiency, nourishing yin in case of yin deficiency, and replenishing blood in case of blood deficiency. If there is simultaneous deficiency of qi and blood, both of them should be nourished in this case. Besides, the deficiency syndrome may be mild or severe, or be chronic or acute, so different approaches such as moderate nourishment, drastic nourishment, gradual nourishment and urgent nourishment can be adopted, respectively. Moreover, the location of deficiency, either in a certain zang-organ or fu-organ or a combination of both, must be discerned beforehand so as to effectively reinforce the healthy qi.

Expelling of pathogenic factors refers to the therapeutic principle of eliminating pathogens to ensure health with herbs purging in action. It is suitable for exuberance of pathogenic factors and non-deficiency of healthy qi, with the former as the primary aspect. Before using this method, the nature of pathogenic factors should be firstly clarified. The common ones are wind, cold, summer-heat, dampness, dryness, fire, blood stasis, phlegmatic fluid, and food retention. Different eliminating methods are used for different pathogenic factors. For example, pathogenic dampness, marked by stickiness and long-term duration, is removed gradually with herbs mild in action. Besides, pathogenic factors with varying degrees of severity or acuteness should be prioritized in treatment. For instance, with regard to acute and severe diseases, large dose of medicine is used, and for chronic and mild ones, small dose of medicine is applied. Moreover, the location of diseases, either in the exterior or interior and either in the zang-organs or the fu-organs, should be discerned before eliminating the pathogens.

Reinforcement of healthy qi and elimination of pathogenic factors, though different from each other, are mutually promoted. For example, reinforcement of healthy qi is beneficial to the elimination of pathogenic factors and *vice versa*. So clinically they are used synthetically. For example, in *Shang Han Lun*, Shaoyang disease, caused by invasion of pathogenic factors into shaoyang and struggle between healthy qi and pathogenic factors, is treated by Xiao Chai Hu Decoction with the function of both reinforcing the healthy qi and eliminating pathogenic factors. Clinically they are used either alone or synthetically, such as reinforcement of healthy qi supplemented with elimination of pathogenic factors, or elimination of pathogenic factors added by reinforcement of healthy qi, etc.

Daily Exercises

1. What are the therapeutic principles of routine treatment and contrary treatment?
2. How can one use the therapeutic principles of reinforcement of healthy qi and eliminate pathogenic factors?

Regulation of Yin and Yang

The occurrence and development of disease is actually a pathological manifestation of imbalance between yin and yang. Under the influence of pathological factors, yin and yang of the body begin to lose imbalance, leading to relative exuberance or debilitation of yin and yang, or yin failing to restrain yang and yang failing to restrain yin, and finally, resulting in diseases. In this sense, the imbalance of yin and yang is considered a pathological generalization of disease. In *Su Wen*, it was pointed out that yin and yang should be carefully resulting in regulated to ensure its balance. In *Shang Han Lun*, it was also said that disorders due to excessive sweating, vomiting, discharging, bleeding or loss of body fluid can be naturally cured if the balance of yin and yang are reestablished. For this reason, it can be understood in such a way that the occurrence of diseases is due to the imbalance of yin and yang, and the responsibility of the doctors is to restore their equilibrium. This principle is widely used clinically, but we will only introduce two aspects: subduing relative exuberance and supplementing relative debilitation.

Subduing Relative Exuberance

This refers to the subjugation of relative exuberance of either yin or yang, whereas none of the two sides is in deficiency. The common practice is subduing exuberance of yin or subduing exuberance of yang.

1. Subduing exuberance of yang

This refers to the treatment of disorders with relative exuberant yang and non-debilitated yin by purging heat or descending fire. Most diseases of this category are caused by contraction of pathogenic yang-heat, or due to relative hyperactivity of yang in the body, which ascends excessively. For example, yangming disorder in *Shang Han Lun* is manifested as interior heat syndrome of high fever, profuse sweating, extreme thirst, and surging-large pulse. It is treated with Bai Hu Decoction to clear away heat, following the principle of subduing exuberance of yang. For another example, up-flaming of liver fire is manifested as dizziness, head distension, tinnitus, red complexion with red, swelling and painful eyes, irascibility, vexation, insomnia, mouth bitterness and dryness, constipation, red urine, scorching hypochondriac pain, red tongue, yellow fur, and taut-rapid pulse. In this case, Long Dan Xie Gan Decoction is applied to purge the excess fire. This is also an example of subduing exuberance of yang.

2. Subduing exuberance of yin

This refers to the treatment of disorders with relative exuberant yin and non-debilitated yang by warming yang and dissipating cold. Most diseases of this category are caused by contraction of pathogenic yin cold, or due to cold excess syndrome marked by relative predominance of yin and non-debilitation of yang. For example, bi-syndrome due to wind, cold and dampness are manifested as sore and painful limbs and joints aggravated by exertion, or localized cold pain alleviated upon warmth, white-greasy fur, and tense or taut pulse, etc. So Zhuo Bi Decoction or Gancao Fuzi Decoction are applied to warm yang and dissipate cold, following the principle of subduing exuberance of yin. In another example, chest obstruction due to congealment of heart vessels by yin cold is manifested as palpitation, oppressed painful sensation in the thoracic region occurring intermittently and involving the inner region of the arms or even the back, or aversion to cold with cold limbs relived upon warmth, pale tongue with white fur, and sinking pulse, etc. It is treated with Gualou Xiebai Baijiu Decoction to activate yang, following the principle of subduing exuberance of yin.

Supplementing Relative Debilitation

This refers to the therapeutic principle of treating disorders of relative debilitation of yin or yang or simultaneous deficiency of both yin and yang by nourishment. The relative debilitation of yin or yang is very complicated. Since yin and yang are both inter-promoted and mutually restricted, the relative debilitation of one side will inevitably lead to comparative exuberance or debilitation of the other side, or simultaneous deficiency of both sides. Clinically this principle should be applied flexibly.

1. *Nourishing yin*

This refers to the treatment of disorders of yin deficiency or insufficiency of yin fluid with yin-supplementing herbs or prescriptions. Clinically the disorders of insufficiency of yin fluid are common in many areas, particularly the insufficiency of yin fluid in the viscera and the whole body. Visceral insufficiency of yin fluid is manifested as deficiency of kidney yin, liver yin, heart yin, lung yin and stomach yin, etc. Generally deficiency of yin fluid is commonly a pathological manifestation of visceral insufficiency of yin fluid. They can be treated by nourishing the kidney yin, liver yin, heart yin, lung yin, stomach yin and general yin, respectively. The kidney is the root of yin and yang of the whole body, and the kidney and liver share the same origin, so the kidney and liver yin are closely associated with the general yin. Insufficiency of yin fluid often leads to hyperactivity of yang, internal abundance of heat, or exuberance of fire. Therefore, simultaneous application of nourishing yin and subduing yang should be carried out. The ancient doctors once suggested strengthening kidney yin to inhibit predominant yang. According to the inter-dependence and inter-promotion of yin and yang, when using yin-nourishing herbs, yang-invigorating herbs should be combined to replenish yin through supplement of yang.

2. *Invigorating yang*

This refers to the therapeutic principle of treating disorders of yang debilitation with yang-supplementing herbs. Yang debilitation is very common clinically, especially visceral deficiency of yang and general deficiency of yang. The former is mainly manifested as deficiency of kidney yang, heart yang, spleen-kidney yang and heart-kidney yang, etc. General debilitation of yang is a pathological manifestation of visceral insufficiency of yang. They can be treated by warming and nourishing the viscera such as warm-activation of heart yang and warm-nourishment of kidney yang, etc. The kidney is the root of yin and yang of the whole body, so kidney yang is closely related to general yang insufficiency. Since yang debilitation is marked by weakened functions, herbs warm in property and nourishing in action should be used instead of herbs pungent in flavor, warm in property and dispersing in action. The ancients once suggested nourishing kidney yang to restrict excessive yin. According to the inter-dependence and inter-promotion of yin and yang, when using yang-invigorating herbs, yin-nourishing herbs should be combined to supplement yang through replenishment of yin.

3. *Simultaneous nourishment of yin and yang*

This refers to the therapeutic principle of treating insufficiency of both yin and yang by supplementing yin and yang at the same time. Since yin and yang are both inter-promoted and inter-dependent, the relative debilitation of one side will inevitably lead to comparative deficiency of the other side, or simultaneous insufficiency of both sides. In this case, simultaneous nourishment of yin and yang can be applied. It should be noted that, in this situation, yin deficiency and yang deficiency are not at the same level, so nourishment of yin and nourishment of yang must be optimally sequenced in treatment after careful differentiation.

Regulation of Qi and Blood

Qi and blood are not only the basic substances constituting the human body, but also the material foundation for physiological activities of the viscera and meridians. Disorders of qi and blood may bring about a series of pathological changes, which can be treated by appropriate regulation.

1. Nourishing qi refers to the therapeutic principle of treating disorders of qi deficiency with qi-supplementing herbs. Qi originates from the congenital essence of parents, cereal nutrients of food, and fresh air in nature, so it is closely related to the physiological functions of the kidney, spleen, stomach and lung. During the application of nourishing qi, the above-mentioned viscera, particularly the spleen and stomach, should be regulated and reinforced.

2. Regulation of qi activities refers to the therapeutic principle of treating disorder of qi movements by using herbs or prescriptions with the function of regulating qi activities. The physiological characteristics of the related viscera in styles of qi movements should be paid attention to; for example, spleen qi is characterized by ascending, stomach qi is characterized by descending, liver qi is characterized by free moving, and lung qi is characterized by descending and purifying. If the liver fails to regulate qi, there will be qi stagnation, and if liver qi invades the stomach, there will be adverse rising of stomach qi. That is why we regulate qi activities according to the pathogenetic characteristics of different syndromes and symptoms.

3. Nourishing blood refers to the therapeutic principle of treating syndromes or disorders of blood deficiency by using herbs or prescriptions with the function of supplementing blood. Composed of nutrient qi and body fluid, blood is deprived from cereal nutrients. The production of

blood relies on the action of the lung and nutrient qi. Blood and essence are inter-promoted and inter-transformed, so blood is closely associated with the spleen, stomach, lung, kidney and liver. When the principle of nourishing blood is used, the abovementioned physiological functions of the viscera should be paid attention to.

4. Regulation of blood. This refers to the therapeutic principle of treating disorders of blood circulation by using herbs or prescriptions with the function of regulating blood movements. The disorders of blood circulation are mainly manifested as blood stasis, rampant flow of blood driven by heat, or even extravasation, etc. Blood stasis can be treated by activating blood and resolving stasis; rampancy of blood flow can be controlled by clearing away heat and cooling blood; and extravasation can be checked by nourishing qi, clearing away heat, or warming meridians after analyzing the etiology and pathogenesis.

Qi and blood, physiologically inter-dependent and pathologically inter-affected, often lead to the morbid state of qi disorder involving blood or blood disorder involving qi. When establishing the therapeutic principles, doctors should make full use of the relationship between qi and blood, giving consideration to both yet with emphasis on the primary aspect. The common methods are simultaneous nourishment of qi and blood, nourishing qi to produce blood, nourishing qi to control blood and regulating qi to activate blood, etc.

Daily Exercise

1. What are the basic principles of regulating yin and yang?
2. What are the basic principles of regulating qi and blood?

Regulation of the Viscera

The human body is an organic whole, and the balance among the viscera is a key link to the maintenance of the relative equilibrium of the internal environment and life activities. The normal performance of visceral functions is achieved through the concerted efforts of yin, yang, qi and blood; if they are in disorder, the visceral functions will be abnormal, too.

Besides, the pathogeneses of functional disorders of the viscera are various, so the regulative methods may be different.

Regulation of Qi, Blood, Yin and Yang of the Five Zang-organs

The disorders of heart yin and heart yang are mainly manifested as relative debilitation of heart yang, relative exuberance of heart yang, and insufficiency of heart yin. For deficiency of heart yang, it is advisable to warm and dredge heart yang; for hyperactivity of heart fire. It is advisable to clear the heart and purge the fire; for deficiency of heart yin, and it is advisable to nourish the heart yin. The imbalance of heart qi and heart blood is mainly manifested as relative debilitation of heart qi and heart blood, and obstruction of heart vessels. For deficiency of heart qi, it is advisable to nourish the heart qi; for deficiency of heart blood, it is advisable to nourish the heart blood; and for stagnation of heart vessels, it is advisable to activate blood and resolve stasis.

The disorders of yin, yang, qi and blood of the lung are manly manifested as the malfunction in lung qi and lung yin. For deficiency of lung qi, it is advisable to nourish the lung qi, for failure of the lung in dispersion and descent, it is advisable to disperse and descend the lung qi; for insufficiency of lung yin, it is advisable to nourish the lung yin; and for heat in the lung, it is advisable to disperse the lung and clear away heat.

The disorders of yin, yang, qi and blood of the spleen are mainly manifested as the debilitation of spleen yang, spleen qi and spleen yin. For deficiency of spleen yang, it is advisable to warm and nourish the spleen yang; for deficiency of spleen qi, it is advisable to nourish the spleen qi; for sinking of spleen qi, it is advisable to ascend spleen qi, for failure of spleen to control blood, it is advisable to nourish qi so as to stop bleeding; for insufficiency of spleen yin, it is advisable to nourish the spleen yin.

The disorders of qi, blood, yin and yang of the liver are mainly manifested as the relative hyperactivity of the liver qi and liver yang and the relative insufficiency of the liver yin and liver blood. For stagnation of liver qi, it is advisable to soothe the liver and regulate qi; for up-flaming of liver fire, it is advisable to subdue the liver and clear away fire; for hyperactivity of liver yang, it is advisable to subdue the liver and suppress yang; for internal stirring of liver wind, it is advisable to subdue the liver and extinguish wind; for deficiency of liver blood, it is advisable to nourish liver blood; for deficiency of liver yin, it is advisable to nourish liver yin.

The disorders of yin, yang, qi and blood of the kidney are mainly manifested as the insufficiency of the kidney essence, kidney yang, kidney yin, and kidney qi. For consumption of kidney essence, it is advisable to nourish the kidney essence; for deficiency of kidney yang, it is advisable to warm and nourish kidney yang; for insufficiency of kidney yin with deficiency-heat, it is advisable to nourish kidney yin so as to suppress yang; for weakness of kidney qi, it is advisable to nourish the kidney and secure the essence.

Regulation of Yin, Yang, Qi and Blood of the Six Fu-organs

The functional disorders of the gallbladder are mainly manifested as insufficiency of gallbladder qi, damp-heat in the gallbladder, and overflowing of bile, etc. For insufficiency of gallbladder qi, it is advisable to soothe the liver and warm the gallbladder; for damp-heat in the gallbladder, it is advisable to clear away heat and resolve dampness; for overflowing of bile, it is advisable to soothe the liver and relieve the gallbladder.

Functional disorders of stomach yin are mainly manifested as insufficiency of stomach qi and stomach yin, and relative exuberance of stomach yang, etc. For deficiency of stomach qi, it is advisable to nourish the spleen and stomach; for insufficiency of stomach yin, it is advisable to nourish stomach yin; for abundance of stomach heat, it is advisable to clear the stomach and purge fire; and for adverse rising of stomach qi, it is advisable to harmonize the stomach and descend qi.

The functional disorders of the urinary bladder are manifested as unsmooth qi-transformation and damp-heat in the urinary bladder, etc. For malfunction of qi-transformation of the urinary bladder, it is advisable to activate yang and drain water; for damp-heat invading the urinary bladder, it is advisable to clear away heat and resolve dampness.

The functional disorders of the triple energizer should be treated by focusing on the corresponding viscera. Clinically the methods of regulating qi activities of the triple energizer and dredging the waterways of the triple energizer are used to regulate the general qi movements and fluid metabolism.

The functional disorders of the large intestine and small intestine are often treated from the perspective of the spleen and stomach.

Regulation of the Inter-visceral Functions

According to the theory of inter-promotion and inter-restriction among the five elements, the internal organs are also inter-promoted and inter-restricted. This may shed light on the methods for regulating visceral functions. In *Nan Jing*, it was also pointed out, "reinforcing the mother organ to treat the deficiency syndrome and purging the child organ to treat the excess syndrome," which provides the principles for regulating the visceral functions.

1. *Reinforcing the mother organ to treat deficiency syndrome*

This is mainly applicable to the deficiency syndrome caused by the mother organ involving the child organ. The common methods are as follows:

(1) Tonifying water to nourish wood, or replenishing the kidney and liver, refers to the method of nourishing liver yin by tonifying the kidney yin. It is applicable to the treatment of insufficiency of liver yin and hyperactivity of liver yang due to deficiency of kidney yin. The kidney is the mother organ and the liver is the child organ, so physiologically the kidney-water will nourish the liver-wood and pathologically the deficiency of kidney yin may lead to insufficiency of liver yin. That is why this method is used to simultaneously treat the liver and kidney.

(2) Mutual promotion between metal and water, or mutual nourishment of the lung and kidney, refers to the tonification of the kidney yin by nourishing the lung qi and lung yin. It is applicable to the treatment of simultaneous deficiency of the lung yin and kidney yin due to insufficiency of the lung yin or kidney yin. The lung is the mother organ and the kidney is the child organ, so the lung-metal can generate kidney-water. By nourishing the lung qi and lung yin, the kidney yin is replenished and conversely, the nourishment of kidney yin is conducive to the supplement of lung yin. That is why it is called mutual promotion between metal and water.

(3) Consolidating earth to generate metal, or nourishing the spleen to supplement the lung, refers to the method for invigorating the lung qi by reinforcing the spleen qi and stomach qi. It is applicable to the treatment of simultaneous deficiency of the lung and spleen due to that the spleen and stomach are too weak to nourish the lung qi. The spleen is the mother organ and the lung is the child organ, so spleen earth can generate lung metal. By nourishing the spleen qi and stomach qi, the lung qi can be supplemented.

The principle of reinforcing the mother organ in case of deficiency can regulate some visceral actions and is used flexibly in the clinic. For example, deficiency of spleen yang can be treated by warming the kidney yang because the kidney yang is the foundation for all the viscera. In this sense, it can be treated by nourishing the kidney water to reinforce the spleen earth.

2. *Purging the child organ in case of excess*

This is applicable to the treatment of excess syndrome due to the child organ affecting or involving the mother organ. The common methods are as follows.

(1) Purging the spleen (stomach) to treat hyperactivity of heart fire is applicable to the treatment of syndromes or disorders marked by hyperactivity of heart fire due to stomach heat. The heart, pertaining to fire, is the mother organ; the spleen, pertaining to earth, is the child organ. Since fire produces earth, so the spleen and stomach heat disturbing the heart pericardium, called stomach heat subjugating the heart, can be treated by purging the heat of the spleen and stomach.

(2) Purging the heart fire to treat hyperactivity of the liver is applicable to the treatment of syndromes or disorders marked by hyperactivity of liver and heart fire. The liver, pertaining to wood, is the mother organ; the heart, pertaining to fire, is the child organ. Wood produces fire. Hyperactivity of heart fire generates liver fire, leading to simultaneous deficiency of both the liver fire and heart fire. So by purging the heart fire, the liver fire can be extinguished, too.

(3) Purging the liver fire to treat hyperactivity of the kidney is applicable to the treatment of syndromes or disorders marked by relative hyperactivity of liver and kidney fire. The kidney, pertaining to water, is the mother organ; the liver, pertaining to wood, is the child organ. Water produces wood, and the liver and kidney share the same origin. So when liver fire is abundant, the kidney will also be hyperactive. That is why purging liver fire is used to extinguish kidney fire.

3. *Restriction of the excessive and promotion of the inadequate*

This is a therapeutic principle established on the basis of the inter-restriction and inter-promotion of the five elements, is actually marked by suppressing the powerful and supporting the weak. The common methods are as follows.

(1) Purging the south to nourish the north, also called purging fire to nourish water, is a method to nourish the kidney by purging the heart. It is applicable to the treatment of imbalance between the heart and kidney due to insufficiency of kidney water and hyperactivity of heart fire. The heart controls fire, pertaining to the south; the kidney controls water, pertaining to the north. That is why it is called purging the south to nourish the north. Since the kidney yin is deficient and the heart fire is abundant, it is advisable to purge heart fire and nourish kidney water.

(2) Reinforcing earth to control water, also called invigorating the spleen to warm the kidney, is a method of treating retention of water and dampness by warming spleen yang or warming the kidney and invigorating the spleen. It is applicable to the treatment of edema due to deficiency of the spleen and overflowing of water and dampness. Since it is caused by spleen deficiency and malfunction of the spleen in transformation, the edema is treated by invigorating and warming the spleen.

(3) Suppressing wood to reinforce earth, also called subduing the liver to harmonize the stomach, is a method to treat deficiency of the spleen due to hyperactivity of the liver. It is performed by subduing the liver hyperactivity and nourishing the spleen deficiency, applicable to the disorder of liver qi invading the spleen.

(4) Supporting the lung to subdue the liver, also called clearing the lung by purging the liver, is a therapeutic method to restrict liver wood by clearing and purifying lung qi. It is applicable to the failure of the lung in purification due to hyperactivity of liver fire, also called wood fire scorching metal.

Besides, the visceral functions can be regulated through the exterior-interior relationship of the viscera. Commonly the fu-organs are purged to treat excess syndromes and the zang-organs are nourished to treat deficiency syndromes. For example, the small intestine fire is purged to clear away heart fire, the large intestine fire is purged to clear away lung heat and purify lung qi, the lung yin is nourished to moisten the bowels and promote defecation, the kidney qi is tonified to consolidate the urinary bladder, the spleen is invigorated to supplement the stomach, and the liver is enriched to treat gallbladder timidity. Clinically these methods should be used flexibly.

Daily Exercise

What are the basic principles for regulating the viscera?

Treatment in Accordance with the Triple Factors

Treatment in accordance with triple factors, namely climate, locality and individuality, refers to the establishment of appropriate therapies on the basis of analyzing seasonal climate, local environment, and individual conditions in terms of age, sex and constitution, etc. The concept of correspondence between man and nature holds that human beings are closely related to nature. The variations in nature will directly or indirectly influence the human body. Accordingly, the body will also respond to the changes, physiologically or pathologically. The occurrence and development are influenced by season and locality, and the difference in body constitution may also affect the onset and turnover of diseases. Hence, in the treatment of diseases, the above factors should be fully considered so as to properly and effectively treat diseases. This is a rule always stressed in TCM.

Treatment in Accordance with Climate

This refers to the establishment of principles for medication according to the climatic characteristics in different seasons. This may require the careful analysis of seasonal climatic characteristics during the diagnosis and treatment process.

The seasonal climatic variations in nature have a profound influence on both the physiology and pathology of the human body. In spring and summer when yang qi becomes predominant and the weather turns from warm to hot, everything flourishes, including the human body; the body's yang qi goes exuberant, and the skin and interstices also turn loose and open. At this stage, even if there is external contraction of wind-cold, herbs pungent in flavor and warm in property cannot be excessively used to disperse wind-cold lest profuse sweating should impair qi and yin. In autumn and winter when weather turns from cool to cold and everything hides inside, the body's yang qi astringes inwardly, making the skin and interstices compact and tight. At this stage, if external contraction of wind cold does not transform into high fever, herbs cool and cold in property cannot be excessively used so as to avoid impairment of yang qi. That is why it is said in *Su Wen*, "Administering cold-natured herbs with great caution in winter, cool in Autumn, warm in spring, and hot in summer; food taking is the same." When using herbs, the doctors should take full consideration of the seasonal and climatic factors.

1. The association between variation of seasons and occurrence of diseases is very close. For example, pathogenic summer-heat is predominant in hot summer and often accompanied by dampness, so it is often treated by removing summer-heat and resolving dampness. Pathogenic dryness is prevalent in autumn when weather is dry and solemn, so it is advisable to moisten dryness with herbs cool in property and pungent in flavor. These diseases, different from other exogenous febrile diseases such as wind-cold common cold and wind-warm ailments, should be properly differentiated and treated.

2. The development and changes of a disease is also related to the time variation within a day. In *Ling Shu* (*Miraculous Pivot*, 灵枢), it was pointed out that almost all diseases are marked by feeling comfortable in

the morning, being at ease in the daytime, worsening at dusk and deteriorating at night. In *Shang Han Lun*, it was recorded that shaoyin disorder is characterized by irascibility due to struggle with pathogens in the daytime, when yang qi is exuberant; it deteriorates at night due to decline of yang qi. A good understanding about the association between diseases and time is helpful for the doctor to diagnose and treat diseases on the basis of syndrome, e.g., selecting the optimal time for needling or taking medicine.

Treatment in Accordance with Locality

Treatment in accordance with locality refers to the principle for medication according to the different geographical or environmental characteristics. This requires the consideration of local geographical features during clinical diagnosis and treatment.

Owing to the differences in geographical environment, climatic conditions, lifestyles or habits, people from different locations have different physiological activities and pathological characteristics. Hence these factors should be taken into consideration when treating a disease. The ancient doctors have accumulated a rich collection of experience in this regard.

1. Pay attention to the influence of geographical environment and climate on diseases. For example, in northwest areas featured by cold and chilly weather, diseases are often marked by exterior cold and interior heat, so it should be treated by dispelling exterior cold and clearing away interior heat, taking into full consideration the geographical factors.

2. Refer to the lifestyles and habits in different localities: for example, in northwest plateau areas featured by chilly weather and lack of rain, common people live near the mountains or hills and consume fresh curds and whey or milk; so they are marked by strong constitution, powerful resistance against exogenous pathogenic factors, and yet susceptibility to internal damage. In southeast areas featured by low-lying swamps as well as warm, hot and rainy climate, common people have a preference for seafood and salty diet; so they are characterized by loose skin and muscle and susceptibility to exogenous diseases. The treatment should be adjusted to the specific conditions.

Treatment in Accordance with Individuality

This refers to the establishment of therapeutic principle according to age, gender, occupation, body constitution and lifestyle of the patients. That is to say, the individual characteristics of the patients should be fully considered during medication. This is the most important one in the triple factors for treatment. Any exogenous pathogen must manifest its symptoms through the body, which responds to different pathogenic factors with various manifestations; some pathogens may cause diseases and some may not. The difference in individuality plays a very significant role in the occurrence and development of diseases. That is why we emphasize the importance of treating diseases in accordance with individuality.

1. People of different ages vary in physiological function, disease-resistance ability and pathological characteristics. For example, senile people with debilitated organic functions, deficient blood and qi as well as weakened disease-resistance ability, is prone to deficiency syndromes or mixed deficiency-excess syndromes. This should be treated mainly by nourishing the deficiency so as to avoid impairment of healthy qi. Children are marked by exuberant vitality and yet are insufficient in qi, blood and delicate viscera. With infantile yin and infantile yang, children are apt to contract diseases cold or heaty in nature, or deficient or excess in essence. This should be treated mainly by expelling pathogenic factors or by other methods according to the specific conditions during clinical treatment.

2. Men and women are different in physiological functions and pathological characteristics because of their difference in gender. For example, physiologically and pathologically, women are closely related to menses, leucorrhea, pregnancy and delivery. These factors should be taken into consideration during treatment of either exogenous or endogenous diseases in females. While for males, it is not necessary to consider these factors.

3. Body constitution is an important factor in treatment according to individuality. In *Ling Shu* (*Miraculous Pivot*, 灵枢), the body constitution is classified into five types: taiyin, shaoyin, taiyang, shaoyang and moderate yin-yang. People with these five types of constitution are different in qi, blood, tendons and bones and so on, so the treatment also varies. It is

evident that TCM accords great importance to this aspect. Moreover, different body constitutions respond differently to the same pathogenic factor or the same medicine. The stronger one has a comparatively powerful resistance against medicine, while the weaker one is on the contrary. Some may be even allergic to medicine. This should be paid due attention to. Clinically the herbs should be used on the basis of syndrome differentiation and after analysis of the body constitution, making sure that whether it pertains to yin or yang, and deficiency or excess.

Besides, familiarity with the patients' occupation and lifestyle is also necessary for syndrome differentiation and medication, which is also required by the principle of treating diseases in accordance with individuality.

Treatment in accordance with tripe factors, embodying the concept of holism and the feature of syndrome differentiation and treatment in TCM, is very important in clinical treatment and must be mastered thoroughly.

Daily Exercise

What are the basic principles of treatment in accordance with triple factors?

Weekly Review

This weak, we discussed the therapeutic principles, and the rules for treating diseases. The commonly used basic therapeutic principles are treatment of disease before occurrence, treatment of disease in terms of root, regulation of yin and yang, regulation of qi and blood, regulation of the viscera, and treatment of disease in accordance with three factors (climate, individuality, and locality). Now we will make a review as follows.

Treating Diseases before Occurrence

This refers to the prevention of diseases or early treatment of diseases, preventing them from further development. Prevention before occurrence means the adoption of preventive measures to prevent diseases from occurring before their onset. Early treatment refers to the prompt diagnosis and treatment of a disease during its early stage so as to control the disease and prevent it from further developing. Early treatment requires a knee observation of the doctor who can discern the subtle signs of abnormality during the very beginning of a disease, and thus take timely measures to prevent it from deteriorating. The unaffected organs can be pre-treated so as to prevent the development of disease.

Treating Disease from the Root

This means that a disease must be treated by focusing on its root. In other words, the essence of the disease must be found and treated. It can be discussed from the following aspects: treatment of the primary aspect and treatment of the secondary aspect as well as routine treatment and contrary treatment. In the development of diseases, if some symptoms are extremely severe and life-threatening, or if some new acute disorders develop on the basis of old diseases, these symptoms and disorders should be addressed immediately even if they are the secondary aspects. In less severe or recovery period of a disease when healthy qi becomes deficient and pathogenic factors still remain, treatment of the primary aspect can be implemented if there are no acute symptoms or syndromes at this time. This is called treating the primary aspect in chronic diseases. Simultaneous treatment of the primary and secondary aspects refers to the treatment of the primary aspect and secondary aspect at the same time because both are severe, or closely related. Routine treatment refers to the therapeutic principle of treating diseases in contradiction to the manifestations. It is also called reverse treatment in which the actions of the herbs are contradictory to the manifestations of the disorder. Generally there are many principles of this kind such as treating cold syndrome with herbs hot in property, treating heat syndrome with herbs cold in property, treating deficiency syndrome with herbs tonifying in nature and treating excess syndrome with herbs purging in nature, etc. Contrary treatment, also called compliance treatment, refers to the therapeutic principle of treating disease in compliance with false manifestations. There are many types of this principle, such as treating heat syndromes with herbs hot in nature, treating cold syndromes with herbs hot in nature, treating obstructive disorders with herbs nourishing in nature and treating diarrhea with herbs dredging in nature, etc.

Reinforcing Healthy Qi and Eliminating Pathogenic Factors

Reinforcing the healthy qi refers to the supplement of healthy qi, the strengthening of body constitution, and the improvement of body's resistance against diseases. The types of deficiency should be firstly clarified before applying this principle so as to effectively reinforce the healthy qi. Expelling of pathogenic factors refers to the therapeutic principle of elimination of pathogens to ensure health with herbs purging in action. The nature of pathogenic factors should be firstly clarified so as to adopt the corresponding methods.

Regulation of Yin and Yang

This principle is widely used clinically, but we will only introduce two aspects: subduing relative exuberance and supplementing relative debilitation. The common practices of subduing relative exuberance are subduing exuberance of yin and subduing exuberance of yang. Subduing exuberance of yang refers to the treatment of disorders with relative exuberance of yang and non-debilitation of yin by purging heat or descending fire. Subduing exuberance of yin refers to the treatment of disorders with relative exuberance of yin and non-debilitation of yang by warming yang and dissipating cold. Supplementing relative debilitation refers to the adoption of nourishing yin, nourishing yang or simultaneous nourishment of yin and yang to treat diseases according to the conditions of yin deficiency or yang deficiency.

Regulation of Qi and Blood

It refers to the treatment of disorders of qi and blood by nourishing qi, regulating qi activities, nourishing blood and regulating blood circulation.

Nourishing qi refers to the therapeutic principle of treating disorders of qi deficiency with qi-supplementing herbs. Regulation of qi activities refers to the therapeutic principle of treating disorder of qi movements by using herbs or prescriptions with the function of regulating qi activities. Nourishing blood refers to the therapeutic principle of treating syndromes or disorders of blood deficiency by using herbs or prescriptions with the function of supplementing blood. Regulation of blood refers to the therapeutic principle of treating disorders of blood circulation by using herbs or prescriptions with the function of regulating blood movements. The commonly used ones are activating blood to resolve stasis, and clearing away heat to cool blood and stop bleeding, etc.

Regulating the Viscera

It is mainly classified as regulation of qi, blood, yin and yang of the five zang-organs, regulation of qi, blood, yin and yang of the six fu-organs, and regulation of the physiological functions among different viscera.

1. Regulation of qi, blood, yin and yang of the five zang-organs

For deficiency of heart yang, it is advisable to warm and dredge heart yang; for hyperactivity of heart fire, it is advisable to clear the heart and purge fire; for deficiency of heart yin, and it is advisable to nourish heart yin. For deficiency of heart qi, it is advisable to nourish heart qi; for deficiency of heart blood, it is advisable to nourish heart blood; and for stagnation of heart vessels, it is advisable to activate blood and resolve stasis.

For deficiency of lung qi, it is advisable to nourish lung qi, for failure of the lung in dispersion and descent, it is advisable to disperse and descend lung qi; for insufficiency of lung yin, it is advisable to nourish lung yin; and for heat in the lung, it is advisable to disperse the lung and clear away heat.

For deficiency of spleen yang, it is advisable to warm and nourish the spleen yang; for deficiency of spleen qi, it is advisable to nourish the spleen qi; for sinking of spleen qi, it is advisable to ascend spleen qi; for failure of spleen to control blood, it is advisable to nourish qi so as to stop bleeding; for consumption of kidney essence, it is advisable to nourish the kidney essence; for deficiency of kidney yang, it is advisable to warm and nourish kidney yang; for insufficiency of kidney yin, it is advisable to nourish kidney yin; for weakness of kidney qi, it is advisable to nourish the kidney and secure the essence.

2. Regulation of yin, yang, qi and blood of the six fu-organs

For insufficiency of gallbladder qi, it is advisable to soothe the liver and warm the gallbladder; for damp-heat in the gallbladder, it is advisable to clear away heat and resolve dampness; for overflowing of bile, it is advisable to soothe the liver and relieve the gallbladder.

For deficiency of stomach qi, it is advisable to nourish the spleen and stomach; for insufficiency of stomach yin, it is advisable to nourish stomach yin; for abundance of stomach heat, it is advisable to clear the stomach and purge fire; and for adverse rising of stomach qi, it is advisable to harmonize the stomach and descend qi.

For malfunction of qi-transformation of the urinary bladder, it is advisable to activate yang and drain water; for damp-heat invading the urinary bladder, it is advisable to clear away heat and resolve dampness.

For functional disorders of the triple energizer, it is advisable to regulate its qi activities.

3. *Regulation of the inter-visceral functions*

According to the theory of inter-promotion and inter-restriction among the five elements, the internal organs are also inter-promoted and inter-restricted. This may shed light on the methods for regulating visceral functions.

(1) Reinforcing the mother organ in case of deficiency

Tonifying water to nourish wood, or replenishment of the kidney and liver, refers to the method of nourishing liver yin by tonifying the kidney yin. The kidney is the mother organ and the liver is the child organ, so pathologically the deficiency of kidney yin may lead to insufficiency of liver yin. That is why this method is used to simultaneously treat the liver and kidney.

Mutual promotion between metal and water, or mutual nourishment of the lung and kidney, refers to the tonification of the kidney yin by nourishing the lung qi and lung yin. The lung is the mother organ and the kidney is the child organ, so by nourishing the lung qi and lung yin, the kidney yin is replenished.

Consolidating earth to generate metal, or nourishing the spleen to supplement the lung, refers to the method for supplement of lung qi by reinforcing the spleen qi and stomach qi. The spleen is the mother organ and the lung is the child organ, so by nourishing the spleen qi and stomach qi, the lung qi is supplemented.

(2) Purging the child organ in case of excess

Purging the spleen (stomach) to treat hyperactivity of heart fire is applicable to the treatment of syndromes or disorders marked by hyperactivity of heart fire due to stomach heat. The heart, pertaining to fire, is the mother organ; the spleen, pertaining to earth, is the child organ. So heart fire can be treated by purging the heat of the spleen and stomach.

Purging the heart fire to treat hyperactivity of the liver is applicable to the treatment of syndromes or disorders marked by hyperactivity of liver and heart fire. The liver, pertaining to wood, is the mother organ; the heart, pertaining to fire, is the child organ. So by purging the heart fire, the liver fire can be extinguished, too.

Purging the liver fire to treat hyperactivity of the kidney is a method applicable to the treatment of syndromes or disorders marked by relative hyperactivity of kidney fire. The kidney, pertaining to water, is the mother organ; the liver, pertaining to wood, is the child organ. That is why purging liver fire is used to extinguish kidney fire.

(3) Restriction of the excessive and promotion of the inadequate

Purging the south to nourish the north, also called purging fire to nourish water, is a method to nourish the kidney by purging the heart. The heart controls fire, pertaining to the south; the kidney controls water, pertaining to the north. Since the kidney yin is deficient and the heart fire is abundant, it is advisable to purge heart fire and nourish kidney water.

Reinforcing earth to control water, also called invigorating the spleen to warm the kidney, is a method to treat retention of water and dampness by warming spleen yang or warming the kidney and invigorating the spleen. The spleen pertains to earth and the kidney controls water. Since it is caused by spleen deficiency the edema is treated by invigorating the earth to control water.

Suppressing wood to reinforce earth is a method to treat deficiency of the spleen due to hyperactivity of the liver. This method is applicable to the disorder of liver qi invading the spleen.

Supporting the lung to subdue the liver is a therapeutic method to restrict liver wood by clearing and purifying lung qi. It is applicable to liver fire scorching lung metal.

Treatment in Accordance with Triple Factors

Treatment in accordance with climate refers to the establishment of principles for medication according to the climatic characteristics in different seasons.

Treatment in accordance with locality refers to the principle for medication according to the different geographical or environmental characteristics and lifestyles.

Treatment in accordance with individuality refers to the establishment of therapeutic principle according to age, gender, occupation, body constitution and lifestyle of the patients.

Daily Exercises

1. Master the therapeutic principles of treating diseases before occurrence, treating diseases in terms of root, reinforcing the healthy qi and expelling pathogens, regulating qi and blood, and regulating the viscera, etc.
2. Understand the principle of treatment in accordance with triple factors.

THE FOURTEENTH WEEK

SECTION 3　THERAPEUTIC METHODS

Therapeutic methods, a constituent part of syndrome differentiation, refer to the ways to cure diseases. They are established to treat certain diseases on the basis of clarifying the causes and pathogenesis as well as the nature of the diseases. Therapeutic principles are general laws for treating diseases whereas therapeutic methods are the specific ways to treat diseases under the guidance of the principles. There are many theories and practices about therapeutic methods in *Nei Jing*, such as sweating and purging in treatment of febrile diseases. Zhang Zhongjing, a great physician in the Eastern Han dynasty, wrote *Shang Han Za Bing Lun* in which the system of syndrome differentiation and treatment is established, thus further developing the therapeutic methods in *Nei Jing*. As early as the period when *Shang Han Lun* and *Jin Gui Yao Lue* were complied, the eight therapeutic methods we use today have already existed. The eight methods were further developed by later generations. For example, Cheng Zhongling has clearly put forth the eight therapeutic methods in his *Yi Xue Xin Wu* (*Understandings on Medicine*) that the causative factors are either endogenous or exogenous; the disease conditions can be generalized into cold and heat, deficiency and excess, interior and exterior, or yin and yang; while the therapeutic methods are represented by sweating, harmonizing, purging, resolving, vomiting, clearing, warming and nourishing. These eight methods are a generalization of the main content of therapeutic methods.

The Eight Therapeutic Methods

Sweating Method

This is a method of opening sweat pores, regulating the defensive qi and nutrient qi, and promoting perspiration so as to expel exterior pathogenic factors. Sweating is applicable to exterior syndromes. It is used to expel pathogenic factors out of the body through the sweat pores when there is struggle between the pathogens and healthy qi, marked by fever, aversion to cold and floating pulse, etc. Because sweating can expel the pathogenic factors out of the body through the skin and muscles, this method is not only used for exterior syndromes, but also applicable to some types of edema marked mainly by swelling over the waist, to ulcers and sores at the initial stage marked by aversion to cold and fever, or to newly erupted measles marked by inconspicuous rashes without pus discharge. Because the characteristics of pathogens and body constitutions are different, sweating can be divided into pungent-warm sweating and pungent-cool sweating, and is often combined with other methods such as nourishing and purging. For patients with deficiency syndromes, such as profuse bleeding, deficiency of qi and blood due to chronic diseases, or massive loss of body fluid due to drastic vomiting or purging, this method should be used with caution or combined with nourishing method even if there are exterior syndromes. In hot summer, the interstices of the skin tend to be loose and people are liable to sweat; in this case, try not to use herbs warm in property and pungent in flavor because they may promote sweating excessively and damage the body fluid; instead, moderate sweating is applicable if it is necessary.

Vomiting Method

Vomiting refers to the therapeutic method of removing phlegm, food or toxic substances retained in the throat, chest, diaphragm, and stomach. It is a method conducted in light of the general tendency by lifting the retained substances in relatively high positions up out of the body through the mouth. It is applicable to situations such as accumulation of phlegm in the throat or chest, obstruction of food in the gastric region, or retention of toxic substances in the stomach. Since it is drastic and fierce in action, clinically this method is used exclusively to remove pathogenic excess in the upper energizer. Besides some specified medicinal substances, other objects such as fingers, goose feather, rooster feather, chopsticks or tongue depressor, can be used alone or together with medicines to induce vomiting. It is normally used only once and should be discontinued promptly as soon as there is improvement. After vomiting, the patient may take a small amount of porridge to protect the stomach qi, in addition to a good rest. Vomiting is a method for emergency and will produce immediate effect if used appropriately; however, if used improperly, it may damage the healthy qi and even cause accidents. For this reason, it should be used only when necessary. It is not advisable for old patients or those with weak constitutions.

Purging Method

This is a therapeutic method of promoting defecation and removing stagnation or retention of water and fluid with purgative herbs. This method is applicable to the removal of dry stools, food, phlegm, fluid and water retained in the body. So it is often used to eliminate pathogens in the intestine and stomach, internal accumulation of dry stools, retention of phlegm and fluid, blood stasis, edema, and heat-obstructed diarrhea, etc. Since diseases may be marked by either cold or heat, and healthy is either strong or weak, this method can be subdivided into cold purgation, warm purgation, moistening purgation, purgation of water, and simultaneous application of purgation and nourishment. It can also be used together with other therapeutic methods. Purging is marked by drastic and fierce action, so it is used exclusively to treat syndromes of interior excess. It is inapplicable to patients with unrelieved exterior syndromes; patients of advanced age or with weak constitution, insufficient body fluid, and constipation; patients with postpartum insufficiency of nutrient blood and unsmooth defection, etc. Besides, it cannot be used in pregnant women unless it is necessary.

Harmonizing Method

This refers to the therapeutic method of expelling pathogenic factors by regulation or harmonization. The method was initially introduced to treat shaoyang disorder in the half-interior and half-exterior region. Later on it was developed to expel pathogens in moyuan (space between the exterior and interior where the pathogens of epidemic febrile disease tend to settle), to regulate the liver and spleen, to soothe the liver and stomach, to harmonize the intestine and stomach, and to eliminate pathogens from the upper and lower separately, etc. It is evident that the scope of harmonization has been expanded. And this method can be used to treat syndromes or disorders due to pathogenic factors in shaoyang or moyuan, imbalance of liver and spleen, intestinal cold with stomach heat, disorder of qi and blood and disharmony of nutrient qi and defensive qi. However, it is inadvisable to treat such cases as existence of pathogenic factors in the exterior rather than in the shaoyang region, or cold syndromes of the triple yin.

Warming Method

This is a therapeutic method of treating cold syndrome with herbs warm and hot in property. This is called "heating the cold" or "warming the over-strained." Cold syndromes are caused by either external invasion or internal damage, such as direct attack into the interior by pathogenic cold, impairment of healthy qi due to improper treatment, or endogenous production of cold due to innate deficiency of yang qi. Cold syndromes are located in either zang-organs or fu-organs or meridians, so the corresponding warming therapies can be divided into three categories: warming the interior to dispel cold, restoring yang for resuscitation, and warming meridians to dissipate cold. Clinically warming is often combined with nourishing. Exterior cold syndrome is treated by sweating instead of warming, so it does not belong to this category. Warming is used exclusively for cold syndromes, so it is inapplicable to yang syndrome of excess heat. Besides, it is also inapplicable to syndrome of genuine heat and false cold due to heat hidden in the interior. For hyperactivity of fire due to yin deficiency complicated by cold manifestations, this method should be used with caution, or used in combination with other methods.

Clearing Methods

This is a therapeutic method of treating interior heat syndrome by using herbs with the function of clearing away heat and purging fire. This is called "expelling heat pathogens with cold herbs" or "clearing away warm pathogens with cold herbs." Clinically this method is used widely for all heat syndromes, especially the syndromes marked by abundance of interior heat with relieved exterior syndrome. Syndrome of interior heat covers a wide range, from heat in the qi phase, nutrient phase and blood phase, to heat in the yangming meridian. Hence, clearing method can be subdivided into the following types: clearing heat in qi phase, clearing heat in nutrient and blood phase, simultaneous clearing of qi and blood, clearing heat and removing toxin, and clearing heat in the viscera and meridians, etc. Because interior abundance of heat tends to impair the body fluid and healthy qi, clearing method is often combined with herbs working to produce body fluid and replenish qi. At the late stage of febrile diseases when yin fluid is damaged, yin-nourishing method is often used in addition to clearing away heat. Exterior heat syndrome relived with herbs pungent in flavor and cool in property, however, does not belong to this category. Owing to the cool or cold nature of herbs used to clear away heat, this method is unsuitable for constitution of yang deficiency, interior coldness of the viscera with loose stool, or syndrome of genuine cold and false heat due to exuberance of yin rejecting yang. For syndrome of deficiency heat due to insufficiency of yin fluid, it should be used in combination with nourishing.

Nourishing Method

This is a therapeutic method of nourishing qi, blood, yin and yang of the body to treat various deficiency syndromes. This is called "supplementing the impaired" in *Su Wen*. Nourishing method can regulate and balance the visceral qi, blood, yin and yang, reinforce healthy qi and improve disease-resistance ability through the action of herbs nourishing in nature. Syndrome of deficiency covers a wide range, from insufficiency of qi, blood, yin and yang to impairment of the viscera. For this reason, nourishing methods are subdivided into the following types such as nourishing qi, nourishing blood, nourishing yin and nourishing yang as well as nourishing the viscera. According to the severity or degree of deficiency, different approaches such as drastic purgation, gradual purgation and mild purgation are adopted. Nourishing method is used exclusively for deficiency syndromes. So before implementing this method, the digestive function of the spleen and stomach must be examined. If the spleen fails to transport and transform normally, there will hardly be any satisfactory effects. If the pathogens still linger on, simultaneous nourishment and purgation should be applied to avoid leaving the pathogens behind. Moreover, medicines that are too oily or greasy cannot be used for fear of impairing the stomach.

Resolving Method

This is a therapeutic method of treating stagnation of food, qi and blood, or painful abdominal masses by using herbs with the functions of promoting digestion, removing obstruction and dissipating stasis, etc. This is referred to as "softening the hard" or "dispersing the stagnated" in *Su Wen*. It is applicable to many syndromes or disorders, so this method is subdivided into different types such as promoting digestion and removing stagnation, dispersing mass and dissipating accumulation, resolving phlegm and expelling water, relieving accumulation due to malnutrition and killing parasites, healing ulcer and subduing carbuncle, etc. These methods are often used to treat different syndromes with their own specific causes. However, if improperly used, they may cause damages. For example, it is inapplicable to drum belly due to qi deficiency and abdominal obstruction, edema due to deficient spleen failing to control water, diarrhea due to deficient spleen failing to transform, and suppressed menstruation due to blood deficiency, etc.

The above-mentioned are the main content of the eight principles. For complicated syndromes and disorders, a single method may not be effective, so two or three methods are often used in combination. From the above, we can see that it is important to deeply comprehend and flexibly implement the eight principles.

Daily Exercises

Describe the main content of the eight principles.

Chinese Medicinals

Chinese medicinals are the main material for disease treatment in TCM, including plants, animal parts, minerals or chemicals, etc. Its actions are recognized and accumulated in the living and working of the ancient people and their struggle against diseases. It is a major part of TCM. The related knowledge on this area is indispensable to a qualified doctor in the treatment of diseases. In this section, we will only discuss the general knowledge about the nature, seven relationships, incompatibility and dosage of Chinese materia medica. For further study on this aspect, you can learn the book titled *Studying Chinese Materia Medica in 100 Days*.

The Nature of Chinese Herbs

The basic functions of Chinese herbs are to expel pathogenic factors, remove the root of disease, supplement the insufficiency of qi, blood, yin and yang, and restore the coordination among different viscera, thus recovering the normal state of the human body so as to perform the physiological activities properly. These actions are attributable to the herbs' property, flavor, meridian attribution, and functional tendency of ascending, descending, floating and sinking, etc.

1. *Four properties and five flavors*

Every herb has its own property and flavor. The property is concluded from numerous tests on the therapeutic efficacy and serves as a generalization of the remedial functions of the herbs according to their nature; whereas the flavor is summarized through tasting. In this way the connection between the tastes of the herbs and their therapeutic effects is revealed. In other words, the flavors of herbs are indicative of their practical functions.

(1) Four properties refer to the characteristics of cold, heat, warm and cool, of which warm and heat pertain to yang and cold and cool pertain to yin. Cool and cold, as well as warm and heat, vary only in degree, and therefore warm may be divided into super warm and slight warm while cold may be classified into great cold and mild cold. The four properties of herbs can be reflected by the reactions of the body after administration, e.g., herbs with the action of treating cold syndromes can be deemed as cold or cool in property and herbs with the action of treating heat syndromes can be regarded as warm or hot in property. Besides, some herbs are mild in nature, yet they are still considered to be slightly cool or warm, so they also pertain to the general classification of four properties. A mastery of the four properties of Chinese medicinal herbs can be very helpful for us to treat diseases.

(2) Five flavors refer to the five tastes of pungency, sourness, sweetness, bitterness, and saltiness; besides, there are also uncommon ones such as bland flavor and astringent flavor. Because the five flavors are the basic ones, commonly we only discuss these five tastes, which are associated with the five viscera. For example, in *Su Wen*, it was recorded, "sourness enters the liver, pungency enters the lung, bitterness enters the heart, saltiness enters the kidney and sweetness enters the spleen." This can be used to direct clinical medication and to address the relative exuberance and debilitation of the viscera. Generally the remedial actions of different flavors are concluded as follows.

Herbs pungent in flavor can disperse stagnation, move qi and circulate blood. They are used to treat exterior syndromes or obstruction of qi and blood.

Herbs sour in flavor, with the action of astringing and consolidating, can treat sweating with deficiency, or diarrhea, etc.

Herbs sweet in flavor, with the functions of nourishing the insufficient, harmonizing the middle and reliving the urgent, can be used to treat deficiency syndromes and regulate the actions of herbs.

Herbs bitter in flavor, with the function of purging and drying, can be used to treat syndromes of excess-heat in the interior or disorders with cold-damp or damp-heat.

Herbs salty in flavor, with the actions of softening hardness, dispersing nodules and purging stagnation, can be used to treat scrofula, phlegmatic nodules, abdominal masses, and constipation with heat accumulation, etc.

The flavors can be divided into two major categories: yin and yang. That is, pungency, sweetness and blandness pertain to yang, while sourness, bitterness and saltiness pertain to yin. The nature of herbs is composed of four properties and five flavors, which are inseparable. Herbs with the same flavor may differ in property, and herbs with the same property may vary in flavor, which is an embodiment of the multiple functions of the herbs. Therefore, only after fully recognizing and mastering the entire properties of every herb and the difference between herbs with the same property or flavor, can we completely understand the actions of herbs and use them accurately.

2. *Ascending, descending, floating and sinking*

This refers to the functional tendency of herbs. Ascending means moving upward while descending refers to moving downward; floating is marked by dispersing and sinking is characterized by infiltrating or draining. Herbs floating in tendency are marked by moving upward and outward; pertaining to yang, they have the functions of lifting, dispersing, wind-expelling, dredging, and interior-warming. Herbs sinking in tendency are marked by moving downward and inward; pertaining to yin, they have the functions of yang-subduing, descending, astringing, draining and purging, etc. A few herbs, however, have no apparent tendency of ascending, descending, floating or sinking, and there are still others have dual tendencies, but only in small numbers.

The tendency of ascending, descending, floating and sinking is closely related to the property and flavor of herbs. For example, herbs pungent and sweet in flavor and warm and hot in property are marked by ascending and floating; herbs bitter, sour and salty in flavor and cold in property are characterized by sinking and descending; medicinal flowers or leaves as well as herbs light in weight and loose in texture are marked by ascending and floating; and medicinal seeds or fruits as well as herbs heavy in weight and turbid in nature are characterized by descending and sinking. These functional tendencies are also influenced by the preparing process. For example, some herbs fired with salty water can have the tendency of moving downward whereas herbs fired with wine can have the tendency of going upward. In compound formulas, the functional tendency of one herb may be affected by that of another. Hence, the ascending, descending, floating and sinking of herbs can be modified, controlled and transformed purposefully under certain circumstances.

3. *Meridian attribution*

This refers to the connection between actions of herbs and the five zang-organs, six fu-organs and twelve meridians. It is intended to indicate that some herbs act mainly on certain viscera and meridians. The four properties, five flavors and the theories of yin-yang and five elements play an important role in meridian attribution, especially the attribution of five flavors to the five viscera. Many herbs are attributed to a certain meridian according to the five colors, five flavors and five elements. Taking the following for example:

Herbs green in color, sour in flavor and pertaining to wood enter the liver meridian of foot jueyin and the gallbladder meridian of foot shaoyang.

Herbs red in color, bitter in flavor and pertaining to fire enter the heart meridian of hand shaoyin and the small intestine meridian of hand taiyang.

Herbs yellow in color, sweet in flavor and pertaining to earth enter the spleen meridian of foot taiyin and the stomach meridian of foot yangming.

426 Fundamentals of Traditional Chinese Medicine

Herbs white in color, pungent in flavor and pertaining to metal enter the lung meridian of hand taiyin and the large intestine meridian of hand yangming.

Herbs black in color, salty in flavor and pertaining to water enter the kidney meridian of foot shaoyin and the urinary bladder meridian of foot taiyang.

The aforementioned meridian attributions are not invariably the same, and clinically they should be used flexibly according to the functions of herbs. On the basis of meridian attribution, the ancients have also summarized some messenger herbs, which can be used according to the specific conditions.

4. *The seven relationships*

The ancients have generalized the application of a single herb and the compatibility between two or more herbs into seven aspects: Single application, mutual reinforcement, mutual assistance, mutual restraint, mutual suppression, mutual inhibition, and antagonism.

Single application refers to the treatment of disease with a single herb.

Mutual reinforcement refers to the synthetic application of herbs with similar actions so as to strengthen their therapeutic effects.

Mutual assistance refers to the application of a main herb added by another herb with similar effects or actions. In this case the auxiliary herb may strengthen the effect of the main herb.

Mutual restraint means that the toxic and side-effect of one herb may be relieved or inhibited by another herb.

Mutual suppression refers to that one herb may relieve or eliminate the toxic and side-effect of another herb.

Mutual inhibition refers to the reducing of the curative effects of one herb by the other herb if the two are used in combination.

Antagonism means that when two herbs are used together, there may be severe toxic or side-effects.

The above-mentioned seven relationships, except for the first one, indicate that the compatibility of herbs should be conducted with caution. Mutual reinforcement and mutual assistance can be applied as often as possible to better exert their effects. Mutual restraint and mutual suppression should be paid attention to when using herbs with toxic or side-effects. Mutual inhibition and antagonism are taboos in herbal combination.

Contraindications

The contraindications of herbs can be discussed as follows.

1. *Prohibited combination*

In compound prescriptions, some herbs should not be used together to avoid certain side-effects, commonly known as mutual inhibition and antagonism, which are generalized as "the 19 incompatibilities" and "18 antagonisms."

The 19 incompatibilities. Liuhuang (sublimed sulfur) is incompatible with Puxiao (Mirabilitum Depuratum), Shuiyin (Mercury) with Pishuang (Arsenolite), Langdu (Wolf's Bane) with Mituosheng (Litharge), Badou (Croton Fruit) with Qianniu (Pharbitis), Dingxiang (Clore) with Yujin (Turmeric Root Tuber), Chuanwu (Common Monkshood Mother Root) and Caowu (Kusnezoff Monkshood Root) with Xijiao (Rhino Horn), Yaxiao (Mirabilite) with Sanleng (Common Burreed Tuber), Guangui (Cortex Cinnamomi) with Shizhi (Red Halloysite), and Renshen (Ginseng) with Wulingzhi (Excrementum Pteropi).

The 18 antagonisms. Gancao (Radix Glycyrrhizae) contradicts with Gansui (Gansui Root), Daji (Radix), Haizao (Seaweed), and Yuanhua (Lilac Daphne Flower Bud); Wutou (Aconite Root) contradicts with Beimu (Fritillaria), Gualou (Snakegourd Fruit), Banxia (Pinellia Tuber), Bailian (Japanese Ampelopsis Root) and Baiji (Common Bletilla Tuber); Lilu (Eranthis hyemalis) contradicts with Renshen (Ginseng), Shashen (Root of Straight Ladybell), Danshen (Danshen Root), Xuanshen (Figwort Root), Xixin (Manchurian Wildginger) and Shaoyao (Paeonia).

The above-mentioned rules are not absolute, and some herbs can be used together in certain occasions such as the combination of Gancao (Radix Glycyrrhizae) and Haizao (Seaweed) in Haizao Yuhu Decoction, and the combination of Wutou (Aconite Root) and Xijiao (Rhino Horn) in Dahuoluo Dan. These combinations are of no apparent toxicity and side-effects. But some combinations do cause severe toxicity such as the simultaneous application of Xixin (Manchurian Wildginger) and Lilu (Eranthis hyemalis), which may lead to the intoxication or even death of animals in the lab. That is why we should pay special attention to these conditions.

2. *Contraindication in pregnancy*

Certain herbs taken during pregnancy may impair the fetus or even cause abortion. These herbs are prohibited for pregnant women, such as Badou (Croton Fruit), Daji (Radix), Qinniu (Pharbitis), Shanglu (Pokeberry Root), Shexiang (Musk), Sanleng (Common Burreed Tuber), Erzhu (Zedoray Rhizome), Shuizhi (Leech), and Mangchong (Gadfly). Some are used only when necessary, such as Taoren (Peach Seed), Honghua (Safflower), Dahuang (Rhubarb), Fuzi (Prepared Common Monkshood Daughter Root), and Rougui (Cassia Bark), etc.

3. *Diet taboo*

Also called dietetic restraint, it refers to the prohibition of certain food during the medication period. For instance, in *Shang Han Lun*, raw and cold food, greasy food, meat or wheaten food, pungent food, wine and cream, or foul substances are prohibited when taking Gui Zhi Decoction.

Therefore, during the period of medication, irritant food or food impeding the absorption of medicine are inadvisable.

Dosage

Dosage should be adopted according to certain principles, such as the nature, compatibility and form of the medicinals, as well as the severity of the diseases and the body constitution of the patients.

Medicines with drastic action should be used in and started from small doses; medicinal flowers and leaves, or aromatic herbs, can be used in small doses; medicinal minerals and shells, or greasy substances, can be used in large doses. In mild cases, or for the old, the young and the weak, it is advisable to take the medicine in small dosages; while in severe cases, or for the strong and the middle-aged, it is advisable to take the medicine in large dosages. For more specific information, please refer to the book entitled *Science of Chinese Materia Medica* or the *Pharmacopeia*.

Daily Exercises

1. What is the main content of the nature of Chinese herbs?
2. What is the main content of the seven relationships?
3. To which aspects should we pay attention in terms of the contraindication and dosage of Chinese herbs?

Prescriptions

Prescription is a further improvement of the application of a single herb. It is a major part of the complete system of principle, method, prescription and herb. The different herbs, combined in a particular fashion, can form a prescription so as to perform their functions synthetically in the treatment of diseases. Prescriptions are the accumulation of medical experience of the ancient physicians, so the conscientious study of prescriptions is of great significance to clinical syndrome differentiation and treatment.

Principles of Formulation

The principles of formulating a prescription are based on the hierarchy of the monarch, minister, assistant, and envoy.

1. Monarch herb

This refers to the herb which plays the leading role in treating the main disorder or syndrome. It is indispensable to a prescription.

2. Minister herb

In one aspect, this refers to the herb which helps the monarch herb to reinforce the effect in treating the main disorder or syndrome; for another, this refers to the herbs that treat the accompanying disorder or syndrome.

3. *Assistant herb*

This has three actions. The first is to assist the monarch or minister herb to reinforce therapeutic effects, or to treat the secondary symptoms; the second is to inhibit or attenuate the toxic effect of the monarch or minister herb, or to suppress the drastic and strong actions of the monarch or minister herb; the third is to serve as a corrigent when the body resists the monarch herb, thus facilitating the treatment with counteractive actions.

4. *Messenger herb*

This refers to the herb with the action of regulating other herbs in a prescription or the herb with the function of directing other herbs in the prescription to target at the location of diseases.

From the above, we can learn that apart from the monarch herb, the minister herb, assistant herb and messenger herb all have more than two actions, and there is no fixed pattern of formulation. The number of ingredients, or the combination of the monarch herb, the minister herb, assistant herb and messenger herb, depends on the severity of the disease or syndrome and the therapeutic requirements. Generally the monarch herb is indispensable to a prescription, and has a larger dosage than the minister herb, assistant herb and messenger herb. During the preparation of a prescription, it should be taken into consideration that the herbs should be kept in accordance with the nature of the syndrome or disorder as well as the therapeutic method so as to better address the disease.

Classification

There are many classifications of prescription such as the "seven prescriptions" and "ten formulas."

The seven prescriptions refer to the large, small, mild, acute, odd-numbered, even-numbered and multi-numbered prescriptions. In *Shang Han Ming Li Lu*, Cheng Wuji modified the multi-numbered prescription into compound prescription.

The ten formulas was created by Xu Zicai in the North Qi dynasty, namely dispersing, dredging, nourishing, purging, dispelling, subduing, astringing, lubricating, drying and dampening formulas. They are capable of dispersing accumulation, dredging stagnation, nourishing deficiency, purging obstruction, dispelling excess, subduing timidity, astringing slippage, lubricating stickiness, drying dampness and dampening dryness. The clinical medication is not only confined to the ten formulas. So the classification is further developed by later generations according to syndromes, therapeutics, major prescription and etiology, etc.

Dosage Forms

To improve the clinical efficacy, prescriptions should be made into proper forms to fit different syndromes or disorders. The ancients have accumulated a rich collection of experience in this regard, and created many different forms such as decoction, pill, powder, plaster, pellet, distillate, lozenge, and medical cake, etc. Later, the form of medication was further developed and many more forms began to appear. Now we may introduce them as follows:

1. *Decoction*

This is made by decocting the herbs with water or wine and then abandoning the gruffs. It can be quickly absorbed and thus may take effect rapidly. As the form of medication used most widely in the clinic, it is suitable for many acute or chronic diseases.

2. *Pills*

These are made by grinding medicinal materials into fine powders, and then mixing them with honey, water, rice paste, flour paste, wine, or medicated juice, etc. Honeyed pills are made by mixing medicinal powders with prepared honey; watered pills are made by mixing medicinal powders with cold boiled water, wine, vinegar, or medicated juice; and paste pills are made by mixing medicinal powders with rice paste or flour paste. Condensed pills are made by mixing certain ointment condensed from some medicinal decoctions with other medicinal powders and, after drying and pulverizing the mixture, blending it with water, wine or other medicated juice.

3. *Medicated powders*

These are made by grinding herbs into dry powders. They are used for either internal or external application. For the former, they can be directly taken with water, or taken after decocted in water. For the latter, they can be applied on the local area after mixing with water, or directly applied on the surface of the ulcers, or directly added into the slurry for external application.

4. *Slurry*

This is made by condensing medicinal substances with water or vegetable oil into paste, or ointment. It is applied either internally or externally. Liquid extract, common extract, and decocted extract are used internally; soft plaster and hard plaster are used externally. Liquid extract is made by leaching out the effective substances with solvent, evaporating a part of the solvent in low temperature, and adjusting the concentration and alcohol content to the required standard. Common extract refers to the semi-solid or solid solvent extract containing dissoluble and effective medicinal substances. Decocted extract is made by repeatedly decocting medicinal water into condensed juice to which honey, candy sugar or brown sugar are added, shaping into a paste in the end. Soft plaster is also called ointment, which is made by evenly mixing proper base materials with medicinal materials into semi-solid preparation convenient for external application on the skin or membrane. Hard plaster is made by decocting medicinal materials to a certain extent, and then abandoning the gruffs and adding yellow lead or white wax to the condensed juice. Also called back plaster, it is a dark black preparation pasted to cloth or paper for external application on the skin.

5. *Dan or pellet*

This is used either externally or internally with no fixed forms. Some are made by grinding medicinal materials into fine powders, while others are added with sticky medicinal fluid so as to shape them into different forms. Pellets are in essence not different from common pills, but they are mostly made of expensive or refined medicinal materials. That is why they are referred to as Dan or pellet instead of pill.

6. *Medicinal alcohol, or medicinal wine*

This is made by dissolving the effective substance of the medicinal materials into alcohols (distillate spirit or yellow wine), or decocting them together in high temperature. After the removal of gruffs, the medicinal fluid can be used either internally or externally.

7. *Medicinal tea*

It is a solid preparation made by mixing the coarse powders of the medicinal materials with adhesives. After infusing the preparation into hot water, it can be served as tea for oral administration.

8. *Distillate*

This is made by distilling fresh and volatile medicinal substances in hot water. The collected distillate is used for oral administration.

9. *Lozenges and medicinal cakes*

These are made by grinding medicinal materials into fine powders. These can be used in this preliminary form or be made into different forms if added with proper amount of aleurone, honey or adhesives. It can be used either internally or externally.

Besides, there are other forms of medicated roll, medicated thread, medicated moxa, syrup, tablet, granule, or injection, etc.

Daily Exercises

1. What are the principles for formulating a prescription?
2. What are the common dosage forms of prescription?

Acupuncture and Moxibustion

Acupuncture and moxibustion are characteristic to TCM in treating diseases. It stimulates certain acupoints on the body by various needling manipulations to reinforce, reduce, or regulate the yin, yang, qi and blood of the body so as to produce reaction in varying degrees and thus cure diseases.

Acupuncture and moxibustion are two different therapeutic methods. The former refers to the production of the sensations of sourness, distension, numbness and heaviness by inserting metallic needles into related acupoints and performing manipulations of reinforcement or reduction. The latter refers to the production of warm or scorching sensation of the local area by applying ignited moxa wool. They are both conducted on certain acupoints, and have different indications and contraindications. Clinically acupuncture and moxibustion, simple in performance and significant in efficacy, are indispensable to TCM. Here we will only brief some basics of acupuncture and moxibustion.

Meridians and Collaterals

Meridians and collaterals can connect the interior with exterior or upper with lower, associate different internal organs, promote circulation of qi and blood, nourish the viscera and tissues, receive messages and regulate different functions of the body. Meridian theory is the foundation for this therapy, and is also indispensable to its theory and practice. In this sense, we must have a good command of meridian theory.

Acupoints

Shu Xue, also called "acupoints," "needling points" or "energy points," have specific meanings. "Shu" refers to the transportation and infusion of meridian qi; "Xue" means apertures or interstices where meridian qi occupies. Acupoints are the regions where qi and blood from the viscera and meridians effuse and infuse beneath the body. They are closely related to the viscera through the meridians, and can reflect the physiological or pathological reactions of the viscera and, more importantly, receive various stimuli (by acupuncture, moxibustion, massage, or medicinal injection, etc.) so as to regulate the viscera and treat diseases.

1. Generally acupoints can be classified into three categories: meridian acupoints, extraordinary acupoints and ashi acupoints.

(1) Meridian acupoints, also known as acupoints of the 14 meridians, refer to the acupoints located on the 12 meridians as well as the

governor vessel and conception vessel. *Huang Di Nei Jing* (*The Yellow Emperor's Canon of Medicine*, 黄帝内经) recorded 365 acupoints, called acupoints of 14 meridians.

(2) Extraordinary acupoints were discovered gradually by generations of doctors and are also located at the regions where meridian qi infuses and effuses. They are also of therapeutic effects, but are excluded out of the 14-meridian system. Commonly there are about 200 of them.

(3) Ashi acupoints refer to the tenderness points during the development of diseases. They have no fixed location and can only be discovered by palpation of the affected area. So they are also called "unfixed acupoints," "heaven-correspondent acupoints" and "pain-reactive acupoints."

There are still some special acupoints, classified according to the difference in region and action, such as the Back-Shu acupoints, Front-Mu acupoints, Jing-Well acupoints, Ying-Spring acupoints, Shu-Stream acupoints, Yuan-Source acupoints, Jing-River acupoints, He-Sea acupoints, Luo-Connective acupoints, Xi-Cleft acupoints, and eight Convergence acupoints, etc.

2. The correct location of acupoints is very important to the therapeutic methods and necessitates some special methods. Now they are introduced as follows:

Location of points according to proportional bone measurement. Also called bone-length measurement, this refers to the method of locating acupoints by dividing the human body into different equations, and each equation is called one cun, which varies from individual to individual. So clinically they are often used as a reliable method to locate the acupoints.

Location of points according to finger-cun measurement. Also called body-cun measurement, this refers to the method of acupoint selection by using the width of the finger as the criterion to measure the distance between points. If the doctor has the same body size with the patient, the doctor can use his own finger for measurement. This method is simple in performance, but poor in accuracy compared with the above-mentioned one.

Location of points according to anatomic landmarks. This refers to the method of acupoint selection by using different anatomic landmarks on the body surface. Some of them are fixed while others can only appear when the body takes a particular position.

Acupuncture Methods

Acupuncture method, or needling method, refers to the way to regulate qi and blood, dredge meridians and cure diseases by inserting specific needling tools into the appropriate acupoints selected based on the nature of diseases.

In *Ling Shu (Miraculous Pivot,* 灵枢), nine classical needling tools were recorded such as sharp needle, round-shaped needle, long needle and large needle, etc. The commonly used ones at present are filiform needle, triple-edged needle, and dermal needle.

Filiform needle. This varies from 3 to 3.5 cun in length, and also different in diameter. Round and smooth in appearance, it is made of metal wire, and is widely used clinically.

Triple-edged needle. This is a triple-edged needle with a sharp point, varying in length and diameter. Commonly it is used for blood pricking.

Dermal needle. This is also called seven-star needle, because its head of the handle resembling the seedpod of a lotus, with five or seven tiny needles fixed to it. It is mostly used for these who are fearful of pain. Before the performance, the patient must take a proper position.

Moxibustion

Moxibustion is a method for prevention and treatment of diseases by warming and dredging meridians with ignited moxa products fumigating around the acupoints or affected regions.

The raw materials for moxibustion are argy wormwood leaves; they are made into moxa cone or moxa stick for clinical treatment.

Moxibustion methods refer to direct moxibustion, indirect moxibustion, and other methods for moxibustion.

1. Indirect moxibustion includes Moxibustion with moxa cone and moxibustion with moxa stick.

(1) Moxibustion with moxa cone. This is conducted by putting the ignited moxa cone on acupoints. After it is burned out or when the patient feels pain, the cone is replaced with another one. Generally three to five moxa cones are used.

(2) Moxibustion with moxa stick. This is performed by fumigating the selected acupoints with ignited moxa stick till the affected area turns red and moist or till the patient feels hot, and yet the pain is tolerable. Generally this is conducted for 3–5 minutes.

2. Indirect moxibustion is conducted by first putting medicinal materials on the selected acupoints and then placing ignited moxa cones. Generally there are ginger moxibustion, salt moxibustion, and garlic moxibustion, etc.

(1) Ginger moxibustion. First cut fresh ginger into thin slices 0.5 fen in thickness and 0.5 cun in diameter, and then pierce several holes with needle into the slices. Later, put the pierced slices on the acupoints, and then place ignited moxa cone on the ginger slice and replace it with another one when the patient feels hot and intolerable. If the ginger slice is dried out, replace it with another one.

(2) Salt moxibustion. This is mostly applied on Shenque (RN 8), or the umbilicus. First fill the umbilicus with salt and then put the ignited moxa cone on it. Replace the moxa cone with another one when the patient feels hot and intolerable.

(3) Garlic moxibustion. Cut garlic into slices and practice the moxibustion in the same way as the aforementioned one.

Ginger moxibustion is the most frequently used one. Besides, there are also needle-warming moxibustion by burning the end of the needle, natural moxibustion by blistering the local skin with chemicals, tube-warming moxibustion with a cylinder, and mulberry moxibustion in surgeries, etc.

When conducting moxibustion, try to avoid burning the skin, make the moxa cone placed in the right position, and prevent it from rolling; try not to deflagrate the bedclothes during the moxibustion with moxa stick.

The local skin generally turns slightly red after moxibustion and needs no treatment. If the skin turns dark red with apparent burning sensation, apply factice onto the local area and prevent it from infection.

Daily Exercises

1. What is the main content of acupuncture?
2. What are the main methods of moxibustion?

Tuina

Tuina, or Chinese massage, is a therapeutic method unique to TCM. It employs certain manipulations of the hands, combined with some specific body movements, to stimulate the meridians, acupoints, or the affected areas of the body so that the qi, yang, qi and blood of the body are regulated, thus preventing and treating diseases.

Chinese massage has a long history. It was recorded even in *Nei Jing*. As the precious legacy from our ancestors and an important part of TCM, this therapy is easy to learn and significant in efficacy. In this section, we will introduce some basic knowledge about it.

Meridians and Acupoints

Chinese massage is developed on the basis of the meridian theory. It promotes circulation of qi and blood and balance of yin and yang by stimulating the meridians and acupoints. For example, article swelling and pain with stagnation of qi and blood due to sudden sprain and contusion can be treated by massaging the related meridians so as to disperse the depressed qi, unblock the obstruction, dissipate the stagnation, promote circulation of qi and blood, smooth the joints and stop pain. For sudden abdominal pain, it can be treated by pressing forcefully the corresponding acupoints of the urinary bladder meridian. For gastric and intestinal disorders, they can be treated by pushing Zhongwan (RN 12) and pressing Zusanli (ST 36) so as to regulate the stomach qi and promote digestion; besides, pressing or pushing Daheng (SP 15), Pishu (BL 20) or Jiashu can also be helpful. So the theory of meridian and the knowledge about acupoints are indispensable to the mastery of tuina therapy.

The Classification of Tuina

According to the aims and manipulations of tuina, it can be classified into the following types: medical massage, healthcare massage, passive massage, self-massage, etc.

Medical massage refers to the selection of massage manipulations by professional doctors to treat diseases according to the nature of diseases and the principle of syndrome differentiation.

Healthcare massage refers to the tuina therapies for strengthening the body, improving health, as well as preventing and treating diseases. It is often combined with some exercises of the body or limbs.

Passive massage is conducted by professional doctors, as is seen in most cases in the clinic.

Self-massage is conducted by the patients themselves so as to expel pathogenic factors and strength the body. Healthcare massage mentioned above is also a kind of self-massage.

Tuina techniques are methods for manipulation with hands, limbs or the body and, occasionally, some instruments. As one of the essentials of tuina, the techniques should be durable, forceful, rhythmic and gentle so as to act on the location of disease deep inside. Syndrome differentiation and treatment should be put into effect when carrying out the tuina therapy in the clinic in order to better perform its therapeutic effects. Tuina techniques are various, and here we shall introduce a few common ones.

Pushing manipulation. First, place the tip, pad or sideway of the thumb onto certain region or acupoint, then lower the shoulder and elbow, suspend and sway the wrist, and bend and stretch the thumb joint, constantly exerting force on the acupoint.

Grasping manipulation. Squeeze and relax certain region or acupoint alternately with the thumb, the index finger, and the middle finger, or with the thumb and the remaining four fingers.

Palpating manipulation. Press certain region and acupoint with the thumb or the end of the palm, exert force gradually, and retain it for a while.

Rubbing manipulation. First, press the palm or the pad of the forefinger, middle finger and ring finger on certain region or acupoint, then stroke the area rhythmically in a rotary movement. The force is exerted by the movements of the wrist joint and the forearm.

Scrubbing manipulation. First place the palm, thenar eminence, or hypothenar eminence partially on certain regions or acupoints, then scrub the related area to and fro in a straight line.

Rotating manipulation. Fix the hand dorsum adjacent to the little finger, or the metacarpophalangeal joints of the little finger, ring finger and middle finger to certain regions, then bend and stretch the wrist joint as well as rotate the joint outwardly and continuously.

Kneading manipulation. Fix the thenar eminence, the end of the palm, or the pad of the fingers to certain regions or acupoints, and then knead the related area circularly, gently and slowly.

Swaying manipulation. Hold the proximal end of the joint with one hand, and grasp the distal end of the joint with the other, then rotate the joint slowly and gently.

Pulling manipulation. Pull or turn the body with both hands and exert force in the opposite or same direction.

Patting-percussing manipulation. Patting is conducted by tapping the body surface with the palm, whereas percussing is applied by knocking the body surface with the back of the fist, the end of the palm and the palmar hypothenar eminence, or the mulberry twig specially prepared.

Twisting manipulation. First, hold certain parts of the body with both palms, then twist it rapidly to and fro or up and down.

Shaking manipulation. First, hold the distal extremity of the upper limb or lower limb, and then shake it up and down in small amplitude with continuous and gentle force so as to loosen and relax the joints.

Twirling manipulation. Pinch certain parts of the body with the pads of the thumb and forefinger and twist it with relative forces.

Brushing manipulation. Brush the skin with the thumb pad of one or both hands up and down, or to and fro.

Back-carrying manipulation. Standing back to back, the doctor carries the patient onto his back by holding the elbows of the patient with both his arms, and then the doctor bends his waist, flexes his knees, raises his buttocks, lifts up the patient, shakes the patient with his buttocks, and stretches the spine of the patient.

Stepping manipulation. The doctor steps on the affected part of the patient with one foot or both feet and move his heel up and down.

Stretching manipulation. Stretching is used for bone-setting to relocate dislocation of joint or displacement due to fracture.

Daily Exercises

What are the commonly used tuina manipulations?

Weekly Review

This week we have studied therapeutic methods (the eight curative methods), Chinese materia medica, Chinese prescriptions, acupuncture, moxibustion, and tuina. Now we will make a review as follows.

Therapeutic methods, a major part of syndrome differentiation, refer to the ways to cure diseases. They are established to treat certain diseases on the basis of clarifying the cause, pathogenesis, and nature of the diseases. Therapeutic methods are the specific ways to treat diseases under the guidance of the principles. The commonly used ones are the eight curative methods.

Sweating method is a method of opening striae of the skin, regulating ying and wei, and promoting sweating so as to expel exterior pathogenic factors.

Vomiting method refers to the therapeutic method of removing the phlegm, food or toxic substances retained in the throat, chest, diaphragm, and stomach out of the body through the mouth.

Purging method is a therapeutic method of promoting defecation and removing stagnation or retention of water and fluid with purgative herbs.

Harmonizing method refers to the therapeutic method of expelling pathogenic factors by regulation or harmonization.

Warming method is a therapeutic method of treating cold syndrome with herbs warm and hot in property.

Clearing method is a therapeutic method of treating interior heat syndromes by using herbs with the functions of clearing away heat and purging fire.

Nourishing method is a therapeutic method of nourishing qi, blood, yin and yang of the body to treat various deficiency syndromes.

Resolving method is a therapeutic method of treating stagnation of food, qi and blood, or painful abdominal masses by using herbs with the functions of promoting digestion, removing obstruction and dissipating stasis, etc.

Chinese materia medica is the main material for disease treatment in TCM, including plants, animal parts, minerals or chemicals, etc.

Chinese herbs have four properties, five flavors, meridian attribution, and functional tendency of ascending, descending, floating and sinking, etc.

Four properties refer to the characteristics of cold, heat, warmth and cool, of which warmth and heat pertain to yang and cold and cool pertain to yin. Herbs cool and cold in property can be used to treat heat diseases, whereas herbs warm and hot in property can be used to treat cold syndromes. Besides, some herbs are mild in nature, yet still slightly cool or warm, so they also pertain to the general classification of the four properties.

Five flavors refer to the five tastes of pungency, sourness, sweetness, bitterness, and saltiness; besides, there are also uncommon flavors such as blandness and astringency. However, the five flavors are the basic ones, so commonly we only discuss these five tastes, which are associated with the five viscera. A good command of the four properties and five flavors of the herbs can be very helpful in the treatment of diseases.

Ascending, descending, floating and sinking refer to the functional tendency of herbs. Ascending refers to moving upward while descending to moving downward; floating is marked by dispersing and sinking by infiltrating or draining. Herbs floating in tendency are marked by moving upward and outward; pertaining to yang, they have the functions of lifting, dispersing, wind-expelling, dredging, and interior-warming. Herbs sinking in tendency are marked by moving downward and inward; pertaining to yin, they have the functions of yang-subduing, descending, astringing, draining and purging, etc. The tendency of ascending, descending, floating and sinking is closely related to the property, flavor, preparation and combination of herbs.

Meridian attribution refers to the connection between the action of herbs and the five zang-organs, six fu-organs and 12 meridians; in other words, some herbs act mainly on certain viscera and meridians. The four properties, five flavors and the theories of yin-yang and five elements play an important role in meridian attribution.

The ancients have generalized the application of a single herb and the compatibility between two or more herbs into seven aspects, namely single application, mutual reinforcement, mutual assistance, mutual restraint, mutual suppression, mutual inhibition, and antagonism. Mutual reinforcement and mutual assistance can be applied as often as possible to better exert their effects. Mutual restraint and mutual suppression should be paid attention to when using herbs with toxin and side-effects. Mutual inhibition and antagonism are taboos in herbal combination.

The 19 incompatibilities and the 18 antagonisms are not absolute, but they should be paid due attention to. Pregnancy prohibitions and diet taboos should also be taken note of. Dosage should be adopted according to certain principles, such as the nature, compatibility and form of the medicines, as well as the severity of the diseases and the body constitution of the patients. For more specific information, please refer to *Science of Chinese Materia Medica* or *Pharmacopeia*.

Prescription is a further improvement of the application of a single herb. It is an important part of the complete system of principle, method, prescription and herb. The principles of formulating a prescription are based on the hierarchy of the monarch, minister, assistant, and envoy.

Monarch herb refers to the herb which plays the leading role in treating the main disorder or syndrome. It is indispensable to a prescription.

Minister herb refers to the herb which helps the monarch herb to reinforce the effect in treating the main disorder or syndrome; besides, it refers to the herbs that treat the accompanying disorder or syndrome.

Assistant herb has three actions. The first is to assist the monarch or minister herb to reinforce therapeutic effects, or to treat the secondary symptoms; the second is to inhibit or attenuate the toxic effect of the monarch or minister herb, or to suppress the drastic and strong actions of the monarch or minister herb; the third is to serve as a corrigent when the body resists the monarch herb, thus facilitating the treatment with counteractive actions.

Messenger herb refers to the herb with the action of regulating other herbs in a prescription or the herb with the function of directing other herbs in the prescription to target at the location of diseases.

There are many classifications of prescription, such as the "seven prescriptions" and "ten formulas."

To improve the clinical efficacy, the prescriptions should be made into proper forms to fit different syndromes or disorders. The ancients have accumulated a rich collection of experience in this aspect, and created many different forms such as decoction, pill, powder, plaster, pellet, distillate, lozenge, and medical cake, etc. The preparing methods and characteristics of the common dosage forms should be mastered.

Acupuncture and moxibustion are external therapies unique to TCM. It stimulates certain acupoints on the body through various needling manipulations to reinforce, reduce, or regulate the yin, yang, qi and blood of the body so as to produce reactions in varying degrees and cure diseases.

Acupuncture refers to the production of the sensations of sourness, distension, numbness and heaviness by inserting metallic needles into related acupoints and performing manipulations of reinforcement or reduction. Meridian theory is the foundation for this therapy, and is also indispensable to its theory and practice. Therefore, we must have a good command of the meridian theory.

Generally acupoints can be classified into three categories: meridian acupoints, extraordinary acupoints and ashi acupoints. Besides, there are still some special acupoints, classified according to the difference in location and action, such as the Back-Shu acupoints, Front-Mu acupoints, Jing-Well acupoints, Ying-Spring acupoints, Shu-Stream acupoints, Yuan-Source acupoints, Jing-River acupoints, He-Sea acupoints, Luo-Connective acupoints, Xi-Cleft acupoints, and eight Convergence acupoints, etc.

The methods for locating the acupoints are proportional bone measurement, finger-cun measurement and anatomic landmark measurement.

Acupuncture method, or needling method, are commonly conducted with filiform needle, triple-edged needle, and dermal needle.

Moxibustion refers to the production of warm or scorching sensation of the local area by applying ignited moxa wool or heat or light source to warm and dredge the meridians as well as prevent and treat diseases.

Moxibustion methods refer to the direct moxibustion, indirect moxibustion as well as other ways. Direction moxibustion includes moxibustion with moxa cone and moxibustion with moxa stick, whereas indirect moxibustion includes ginger moxibustion, salt moxibustion and garlic moxibustion, etc.

Tuina, or Chinese massage, is an external therapeutic method unique to TCM. It employs certain manipulations of the hands, combined with some specific body movements, to stimulate the meridians, acupoints, or the affected areas of the body so that yin, yang, qi and blood of the body are regulated and the diseases are prevented and cured.

Chinese massage is developed on the basis of the meridian theory.

According to the aims and manipulations of tuina, it can be classified into the following types: medical massage, healthcare massage, passive massage and self-massage, etc.

Tuina techniques are various, and commonly there are pushing manipulation, grasping manipulation, palpating manipulation, rubbing manipulation, scrubbing manipulation, rotating manipulation, kneading manipulation, swaying manipulation, pulling manipulation, patting-percussing manipulation, twisting manipulation, shaking manipulation, twirling manipulation, brushing manipulation, back-carrying manipulation, stepping manipulation, and stretching manipulation, etc.

Daily Exercises

1. Get a command of the definitions of the eight therapeutic methods.
2. Get a command of the main content of Chinese materia medica and prescriptions.
3. Get a command of the main content of acupuncture and moxibustion.
4. Understand the common tuina manipulations.

Index